THE SUPPLEMENT HANDBOOK

A Trusted Expert's Guide to **What Works** & **What's Worthless** for More Than **100** Conditions

MARK MOYAD, MD, MPH

Jenkins/Pokempner Director of Complementary and Alternative Medicine
at the University of Michigan Medical Center

with Janet Lee, LAc

RODALE

This book is dedicated to my wife Mia (the consummate social worker), who has been my best friend since the day we met. To say I won the lottery when I met her and raised our two wonderful kids Holly & Nicholas is actually an understatement (and, of course, our dog Chauncey, too).

It is also dedicated to my dad—and doctor—Robert Moyad, my mother Eva Moyad, my two brothers Andy and Tom Moyad, and my current boss and long-time mentor Dr. David Bloom.

And finally, this book is dedicated to the individuals—Epstein, Jenkins, Pokempner, and Thompson— who invested in the dream, which allow Mia and I to still make a difference, one starfish at a time.

Rodale books may be purchased for business or promotional use or for special sales.
For information, please write to:
Special Markets Department, Rodale Inc., 733 Third Avenue, New York, NY 10017

Printed in the United States of America
Rodale Inc. makes every effort to use acid-free ⊗ recycled paper ♻

Book design by Elizabeth Neal

Library of Congress Cataloging-in-Publication Data is on file with the publisher.
ISBN 978-1-62336-035-1

Distributed to the trade by Macmillan
2   4   6   8   10   9   7   5   3   1   paperback

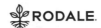

We inspire and enable people to improve their lives and the world around them.
rodalebooks.com

CONTENTS

INTRODUCTION

> *"The master in the art of living makes little distinction between his work and his play, his labor and his leisure, his mind and his body, his education and his recreation, his love and his religion. He hardly knows which is which. He simply pursues his vision of excellence at whatever he does, leaving others to decide whether he is working or playing. To him he is always doing both."*
>
> **—L.P. JACKS**

HOW I BECAME "THE SUPPLEMENT DOCTOR"

I never intended to specialize in diet, lifestyle, and dietary supplements. I was supposed to be a urologist and join my father's practice in Ann Arbor, Michigan, so we could do surgery side by side. But I realized very early in my medical career that I had about as much talent for surgery as my dog Chauncey did. I greatly appreciate the sheer beauty of what some surgeons, like my brother (Tom) and father (Robert), can do, but I simply didn't like it.

Instead, when I was just 22 years old, I researched, wrote, and published my first medical paper, with the help of Dr. Michael Kern from the College of Wooster in Ohio, on the effects of cottonseed oil on health. Shortly thereafter, I was one of the primary investigators of the L-tryptophan dietary supplement debacle in Florida; a huge tainted batch of supplements caused at least 37 deaths and 1,500 permanent disabilities. I interviewed patients to try to piece together what happened (it turned out it was a problem with the manufacturer; impurities produced at the plant got into the supplements). In the process of working on the medical paper and investigating what went wrong with L-tryptophan, I spent years doing extensive research on supplements. The seed was planted and this work became the foundation for what I do now.

Several years after the L-tryptophan incident, my cousin Firouzeh Moayyed died of breast cancer at the age of 38. Her death seemed so senseless, and I was so distraught that I made the emotional decision to tell her story wherever I could. I went on a speaking tour of the 50 states and encouraged people to contact their representatives in Washington, DC, to increase funding for cancer research. I thought this was the sole purpose of my tour, but something odd—or perhaps spiritual—happened during that time. Wherever I lectured, cancer patients came up to me to ask about their diets and especially dietary supplements.

Back then, there was no Internet (hard to fathom, I know) and there really wasn't any education in medical school in the area of dietary supplements, so patients were desperate for answers. Does selenium fight prostate cancer? Does fish oil protect against breast cancer? What supplements will reduce the side effects of chemotherapy? Does a vegan diet improve the chances of surviving lymphoma? Does vitamin C reduce side effects from surgery? I was inundated everywhere I spoke and would spend 3 to 4 hours answering questions, almost all of which were about supplements. I think the audience was shocked that I could answer all their questions, so they just kept 'em coming!

I ended my trip by delivering the signatures I had gathered along the way to senators in Washington, DC, which eventually helped to increase funding for cancer research. After DC, I started thinking that maybe I could make a career out of special-izing in dietary supplements, so I set up a consulting practice at the University of Michigan Medical Center in the department of urology. It had always been a dream of mine to work for this university, and I really wanted to do cancer-related research. At that time, the urology department was unusually open to conducting diet- and supplement-related research on many types of cancers. (Thanks go out to my current wonderful mentor and boss, Dr. David Bloom, and my former boss and mentor, Dr. Jim Montie, both world-renowned urologic surgeons, as well as Dr. Ken Pienta, a world-famous oncologist who's running an entire cancer research department at Johns Hopkins and whom I still miss very much.) When our research began, I was flooded with all kinds of patients (suffering from breast, colon, prostate cancer—you name it) asking for dietary and supplement advice. Soon, people started coming to see me from all over the world. I was shocked, pleased, and spiritually moved; I felt like this was a way to honor my cousin's memory.

During my first year at the University of Michigan, I met a patient with cancer named Phil Jenkins. Though I thought he came into my life so that I could help and heal him, it was he who helped me—and changed my life. I had been giving him diet and supplement advice for his condition, and he asked me why no doctors were working full-time in this area. I told him the system was simply not set up to educate or train doctors in this category and that financially it was a dead end. (After they have accumulated more than $100,000 in debt during school, doctors want a job that can help pay the bills!)

One day I joked (and it was a joke) that if he contributed $1.5 million to a supplement endowment (which would be the first of its kind in the world), I could devote my life to studying dietary supplements and wouldn't have to charge people for my advice if they were indigent. A few days later, Mr. Jenkins wrote a check for $1.5 million (I still shake my head in disbelief over this). Now, more than 20 years later, I have the same position, but the endowment has grown substantially thanks to other notable donors, including Josh Pokempner and his wife Gretchen (who were not patients but simply wanted to fund a position for a full-time doctor who focused solely on nutrition and supplements), Robert and Ellen Thompson, Daniel and Phyllis Epstein, and many more.

Thanks to Mr. Jenkins and these other very generous people, I've been able to have a remarkable impact on people's lives. I'm able to spend real time with patients and groups and help "one starfish at a time," as I like to say to them (in reference to the Loren Eiseley essay about a man saving otherwise doomed starfish that had washed up on a beach). This endowment has allowed me to do things differently. I get to spend an hour or two with each patient, often in the comfort of their own homes, in addition to teaching, conducting research, lecturing to various groups, and consulting with supplement and pharmaceutical companies to help them do a better job. I've written 10 books, given more than 5,000 lectures around the world to

health care professionals and consumers, published more than 130 articles, and served as the editor-in-chief of a complementary and alternative medicine journal. I have been fortunate to consult with people from all walks of life—from CEOs and celebrities to coal miners. What a life!

Some have said that I may be the top expert in the world right now in this area, but I would argue that I am just a trailblazer, clearing the way for other doctors and health care professionals to specialize in this growing field. Part of that "blazing," if you will, was creating a book—this book—on supplements that would be the gold standard, a resource for health care professionals and consumers alike.

CREATING SYNERGY IN HEALTH CARE

I realize there aren't many people out there who specialize in supplements the way I do, so the chances that your doctor is up to date on the most recent research on CoQ10, vitamin E, and SAM-e are slim. Throughout this book, however, I advise you to ask your doctor before beginning to take a supplement, especially when it comes to drug interactions, which may seem contradictory. My hope is that you arm yourself with this book and open a dialogue with the physician you trust the most with your health so you can work together to land on the best treatment—be it a drug, a supplement, or a combination—for you. I'm passionate about supplements, but that doesn't mean I think everyone should get a battery of nutritional tests and an assortment of supplements as a solution for everything that ails them. A good physician (naturopath, MD, or DO) should be willing to take the time to discuss with you what drugs or supplements work, which ones are worthless, and whether using them (or even combining them) offers any advantages or disadvantages. In addition, the physician should be willing to refer you to health care experts in the field who can provide more insight into this unique discipline. This is a synergistic, multidisciplinary approach to health care—utilizing a variety of resources to find the best answer—and it's how medicine is practiced throughout the world except when it comes to dietary supplementation. I think the time has arrived for supplements to be included in these everyday health decisions, and it's up to you as a patient to advocate for this.

BE YOUR OWN JUDGE

This book is not about Chinese herbal medicines, tinctures, drops, potions, homeopathy, and other esoteric products that can be hard to come by and even harder to understand. It's not about listing every possible drug interaction and side effect: This is overwhelming and rarely helpful (or necessary). The science I reference in each section is ever-evolving and very individualized— what works for one person may be ineffective or even harmful for another. I want people who are reading this book to be able to have a conversation with their doctor or pharmacist about their options and also use it to navigate the supplement aisles at their local grocery, pharmacy, or health food store.

One of the key concepts I'd like every reader to take away from this book is that drugs and supplements are very similar. To that end, some are worthless and some are effective. Deciding whether one works or not comes down to looking at a preponderance of the evidence, just like in a courtroom. It also always depends on a benefit-versus-risk scenario for the individual.

It's time to treat dietary supplements as a full-time discipline or specialty that needs constant objective review and surveillance: One that teases out the evolving pros and cons of each and every pill out there for most medical conditions, and one that truly reviews the benefit-versus-risk scenario for different pills so health care professionals and consumers can make the right decision in each situation. In this book, I have compiled the sum of my life's work to help inform your supplement decisions, and I hope that you find it a valuable resource in your journey toward health.

Love and bear hugs,
Mark A. Moyad, MD, MPH,
Jenkins / Pokempner Director of
Complementary and Alternative Medicine at
the University of Michigan Medical Center

P.S. Go Blue Baby! (Sorry, but I had to throw that in. We are all happily and voluntarily brainwashed here in Ann Arbor, and there is no dietary supplement that can cure this wonderful lifelong "disease." Winning just makes it a heckuva lot worse, thank goodness!)

PART
1

[1]

NAVIGATING THE
SUPPLEMENT WORLD

MAYBE YOU CAME TO THIS BOOK because you'd like a better understanding of the supplements you're already taking. More likely, though, you're probably baffled and confused as to where to begin. The supplement world can be overwhelming, to say the least, but I am here to help.

Too often, in an attempt to navigate and make sense of the excess of choices, barrage of information, and varying opinions in the supplement market, consumers take the crowd-sourcing approach: polling their friends to see what pills they're popping, doing an exhaustive Internet search, then heading to the store to stock up on a host of supplements.

I believe the days of dabbling in dietary supplements are over. Thousands of products debut every year and hundreds (sometimes thousands) of research studies come out every month, just in the areas of diet and supplements! If an "expert" is only dabbling part-time in this area but dishing out information to you, he is being reckless, especially since so many supplements are the equivalent of drugs.

I've been in the dietary supplement world for more than 30 years, and it is truly my passion. I don't just look at the bottom line in an abstract or at the conclusion or focus of one study. I go through a detailed, 70-point checklist (see page 461) of criteria to truly decipher whether anything can be gleaned from a study or a summary of studies. I draw on my own experience of working with patients on a daily basis. I take a hard look at specific conditions and ailments and deduce when a drug might work better than a supplement. When I have a question about the latest cancer treatment, I call an oncologist. When some of the world's top doctors have supplement questions, they call me.

I know the world of supplements can be complicated and convoluted. That's why I wrote this book as a guide to help you steer through it. Each year, just when I think I've heard every

THE MIDDLE WAY

I use the excerpt below from *The Teaching of Buddha* to describe my approach to diet and lifestyle as well as supplements: Be educated but not extreme.

"To those who choose the path that leads to Enlightenment, there are two extremes that should be carefully avoided. First, there is the extreme of indulgence in the desires of the body. Second, there is the opposite extreme of ascetic discipline, torturing one's body and mind unreasonably."

question, comment, or conspiracy theory about dietary supplements and nutrition recommendations, someone surprises me with a new one! So I'm giving you a small sampling of my responses to some common questions and declarations from the 5,000 lectures I've given in every corner of the world. I have also sprinkled some myth-busting information throughout, labeled as "FACT" or "FALSE," as well as some of my favorite factoids, labeled as "Moyad Fact" (which you'll find throughout the book). My hope is that this chapter will help you navigate and understand more clearly the massive world of supplements.

BEFORE YOU BEGIN

"Why should I be taking supplements?"

You don't necessarily need to take a supplement if you're perfectly healthy, just like you wouldn't take a drug if you didn't have any health issues. If you do have a health condition, though, or you're at higher risk of a disease, such as heart disease or diabe-

tes due to lifestyle or family history, you may want to consider taking a supplement just like you would consider taking a drug. What I've found over the last 30 years is that virtually all people have their own unique story that involves some health concern, large or small. In other words, almost everyone could potentially benefit from some type of supplement, even if it's something as simple as a multivitamin to reduce cancer or cataract risk.

"How are supplements different from drugs?"

To me, there is no difference between an effective supplement and a drug for a specific medical condition. Some of the most interesting supplements mimic the actions of pharmaceuticals, or vice versa (for example, red yeast rice extract versus statins for lowering cholesterol or capsaicin in low concentration versus the higher concentration prescription-only form for neuropathic pain). When a supplement works like an available drug, you should have more confidence in its ability to have a tangible effect (and, like drugs, not necessarily without side effects). In fact, many supplements sold in the United States are only available as drugs in other countries. (The over-the-counter supplement alpha-lipoic acid, to give you just one example, is sold as a prescription drug in parts of Europe and Asia.)

On the flip side, many drugs are derived from natural sources, including some of the biggest-selling drugs of all time: Cholesterol-lowering statins originally came from a fungus/yeast; metformin, used to treat diabetes, originates from the French lilac; and aspirin, a pain reliever and over-the-counter anti–heart attack pill, was created from willow bark. Bottom line: The difference between a drug and an effective supplement is only perception, not reality. I'm hoping this book will spur a change. Throughout, for each ailment and condition, I will give you the full answer: If a drug is more effective than a supplement in a specific situation, I have no problem saying so.

"Do I need an annual checkup to determine my supplement needs?"

Not necessarily, but you should have an annual discussion with a trusted doctor.

A research review of nine clinical trials, published in the *Cochrane Database of Systematic Reviews*, looked at 182,000 participants and found annual checkups did not improve health and often led to harmful or unnecessary tests. In fact, having an annual checkup did not appear to reduce

the risk of hospitalization or disability, referrals to a specialist, or time missed from work. Sometimes when you're looking for a tractor in a haystack, you find a needle. In other words, even though you're typically being screened for "big" issues at a checkup, sometimes your doctor will find a small issue that you might then feel compelled to treat. Often, the benefits do not outweigh the negative side effects of treatment. This is why some cancer screening tests (prostate, breast, and thyroid, for example) are more controversial now. Let me give you an example: You go to the doctor for some complaint or maybe for an annual checkup. She notices that your PSA (prostate-specific antigen) levels are elevated, so she orders a biopsy. Then, she finds a small tumor in your prostate and now you're completely stressed out and anxious. You opt for treatment and endure significant side effects, including incontinence and erectile dysfunction. But it's very possible that the tumor, although malignant, would never have been fatal in the first place because they don't always grow to be life-threatening, and you would have been perfectly fine without treatment. In cases like these, the treatment is worse than the problem.

Of course, this doesn't mean you should never be tested for these cancers; screening saves lives. It just means many Americans are being overtested, which can lead to unnecessary procedures, prescriptions, and supplements. However, I am a fan of personalized risk assessment for anyone who's concerned about cardiovascular disease (see Chapter 2), so talk with your doctor about that.

"How do I know if a supplement will help or hurt me?"

People come up to me at lectures or in the clinic all the time to tell me that they read something negative about a supplement they're taking and are concerned but don't want to stop using it. One of the best ways to get to the bottom of any potential issue is to stop taking the supplement and see what happens. I call this the guinea pig effect. Likewise, one of the best ways to figure out if a supplement could help a condition is to start taking it at a low dosage.

"Should a ton of studies be done before a supplement is considered safe?"

I frequently recommend supplements that don't have large, randomized, double-blind placebo studies to back them up as long as they are inexpensive and safe; they have preliminary research for the condition in question and minimal side effects; and there are few other options (or those options are costly). For example, the research on vitamin B_2 for migraine prevention is still preliminary, but it's impressive. The vitamin is dirt cheap and the side effects are negligible, so it's worth a try. The prescription options for migraines are expensive, have side effects, and don't always work. Plus, up to 50 percent of users have trouble functioning after taking them, so better alternatives are needed.

This is the essence of benefit versus risk.

I would love to live in a world where every supplement fulfills all my research criteria (see the Appendix), but even conventional drugs don't work this way; it's part of the art of medicine. Few things in medicine come with a 100 percent assurance of effectiveness, so it comes down to probability and your willingness to accept a certain amount of risk to gain certain benefits.

"Are quality-control testing organizations useful?"

They can be. Both *Consumer Reports* and ConsumerLab.com tend to watch the supplement industry. ConsumerLab.com gets criticized for not being a "real" lab—they send out samples to reputable testing facilities—but I think they're providing a decent service.

The only problem I have with some of the quality-control testing labs in the United States, which will remain nameless, is that they are discriminatory. For example, these labs will not test sexual enhancement products, either because they have to do with sex (gasp!) or because of the sordid, negative associations they anticipate for getting in bed (pun intended) with these products. This is one of the largest categories within supplements! And they should all be allowed equal testing. Erectile dysfunction and female sexual dysfunction are *real* medical conditions that should be handled like any other, but instead the testing labs see them as stereotypes. I look forward to these labs being exposed for their at times discriminatory behavior.

"What's the difference between a dietary study and a dietary supplement study?"

I'll often see a dietary study referenced as support for a supplement or, more rarely, vice versa. A dietary study looks at the nutrients in certain foods, while a dietary supplement study looks at taking a specific supplement. You can't apply the conclusions about nutrients in the diet, say omega-3s or vitamin D, to the individual supplements. It's like comparing apples and tennis balls. For example, based on *dietary* studies, researchers believed beta-carotene was the active component in many plant foods that was reducing the risk of heart disease and cancer. But in several *supplement* studies of beta-carotene, people who took the pill ended up with an increased risk of lung cancer if they were current or possibly even former smokers, and in all the other trials, it showed no health benefit. (And there went hundreds of millions of dollars on clinical trial research!) Similarly, eating foods with selenium might reduce the risk of cancer, but taking selenium to prevent cancer has shown no benefit (and, again, it cost hundreds of millions of taxpayer dollars to show this).

The take-home message here is, if someone is selling you a supplement and referring to dietary studies with that ingredient, it proves nothing and it's likely a waste of your money. Always look at how the supplement itself has performed in clinical trials. As I was writing this section, I came across an "expert" on the Internet using studies of magnesium rich–food that showed a reduced risk of bone fractures and high blood pressure as a reason to buy a special magnesium supplement. And the beat goes on!

"The supplement business is a racket! There are huge quality control and safety issues!"

I hear this all the time. Those who bash dietary supplements across the board, claiming that drug-supplement interactions have reached epidemic proportions and quality control is nonexistent, just spread misinformation and panic. The biggest pill problem in the United States, by far, is death from an unintentional prescription drug overdose. And about 70 people die each day as a result of this, according to the latest report from the Centers for Disease Control and Prevention; that's more than 27,000 deaths per year and one every 19 minutes! Pain, antianxiety, and insomnia medications are most often to blame.

I have worked on supplement investigations where people have died, and it's always a tragedy, but those cases don't compare to the 70 people dying each day—or the thousands of others who become seriously and dangerously addicted to these medicines. Yes, we need to drastically improve quality control in the supplement world, but let's put it in perspective, folks.

"Do I need blood testing to check for multiple nutrient deficiencies?"

There are clearly some cases in which you need a blood test if your doctor suspects a nutrient deficiency—say, with potassium, magnesium, iron, or vitamin B_{12}—especially when a drug increases the risk of one. (For example, the cancer drug Zytiga reduces blood potassium in many patients.) Iron blood testing for anemia is a gold standard for women with fatigue from excessive blood loss from menstruation, and B_{12} and magnesium testing may be warranted if you're on acid reflux medication long term.

Nutritional deficiency testing should always be handled on a case-by-case basis. Most people do not need a massive nutritional panel that looks at amino acids, vitamins, and minerals, where inevitably something shows up low and you're told you need a supplement to correct it. If your panel does reveal some deficiencies, always ask if correcting them (taking more of whatever nutrient is low) will produce a tangible, beneficial result. Let me explain: Hundreds of millions of dollars have been spent on studies looking at how high doses of vitamins B_6 and B_{12} and folic acid affect a compound in the blood called homocysteine, which experts believe is a marker for cardiovascular disease in most individuals. The Bs did, in fact, lower blood homocyste-

ine levels, and supplement companies jumped on that. But after several decades, experts are realizing that lowering homocysteine doesn't really have much impact on heart health for most people. In other words, just because a blood test improves does not mean *you* will improve—with the exception of the obvious ones, such as cholesterol and glucose.

Again, some individual tests are worthwhile, but the majority are absolute nonsense. Be leery about extensive blood panel tests for the following:

Amino acids

Antioxidants

B-complex vitamins

Fatty acids

Metabolites

Minerals

Vitamins

I often hear from people who have been dealing with celiac disease or Crohn's disease for years, both of which can impact nutrient absorption, or from those who've been on long-term extreme diets and are curious about possible nutrient deficiencies. If you're in a similar situation, please read the Bariatric Surgery section (see page 90), which lists a comprehensive panel of proven nutrient deficiency tests that can help you determine your own nutritional issues.

Researchers are starting to better understand that high doses of drugs (such as cholesterol-, acid-, and glucose-lowering medications) can lead to deficiencies because of the way they impact the production and absorption of some nutrients. Yet in medical school, students are still being taught about deficiencies that result from not getting enough nutrients in our diets (like scurvy from vitamin C deficiency) despite the fact that today's nutritional shortcomings are often due to excess medications and extreme diets.

"My doctor is the best person to ask about supplements, right?"

When it comes to dietary supplements, companies have to say "check with your doctor." But it's often a hollow statement because there's a general lack of education and knowledge about dietary supplements in health care, and the manufacturers know that! This is slowly changing though, maybe thanks to the $30 billion that's now being plowed into the supplement industry annually. Whether you're seeing a conventional or alternative practitioner, investigate the supplements you're interested in, and when you go to consult with them, take this book with you. Supplement research is moving as fast as any research now, and it's up to you to help your practitioner arrive at the right decision.

"Should I trust the supplements my doctor sells?"

This used to appall me since there is usually such a large markup and an overall lack of scientific knowledge about the products, but over time I've relaxed my take on this a little bit. If a patient benefits

from a doctor selling supplements at his office—often called nutraceuticals—then I think it's okay, as long as the patient knows this is a moneymaking venture. Ideally, the health care professional should let patients know that they can look for whatever the active ingredient is in another product. Unless there is outstanding quality control and the product has been well tested, I would look for a cheaper alternative.

"I'm on the _____ diet. Should I take supplements to counteract deficiencies?"

Every fad diet has the potential to cause nutrient deficiencies because it usually involves eliminating a particular aspect of a normal diet. It's your job to thoroughly investigate the plan to see what might be lacking. Juicing diets can lack sufficient fiber. Vegans might get less iron, zinc, B_{12}, or vitamin D and may need to take a multivitamin or two daily and religiously. Ketogenic dieters (those whose diets consist of 70 to 90 percent fat, low protein, and virtually no carbs) might need extra calcium, vitamin D, and fiber.

The problem with making blanket statements about what supplements are needed with certain diets is that most dieters only follow some version of the diet or they're not 100 percent compliant every day. I always recommend keeping a food diary for a week and then analyzing what you might be missing (and first trying to fill that gap with food when possible). Another related but much more

9

FACT: DIET AND EXERCISE CAN REPLACE PILLS OR IMPROVE THEIR EFFECT.

The question you should always ask before you pop any pill (apart from benefit versus risk) is "Can I make lifestyle changes instead of taking this?" If the answer is "yes," then do it! If not, lifestyle changes can make almost any pill work better. Recent research has shown that diet and exercise work as well as many prescription medications, and I believe they work as well as supplements, too. Naturally, it's also true that the worse your lifestyle is, the less you can expect from your pills. Recently, cholesterol-lowering medications and Viagra were found to work much better in people who exercised compared to more sedentary individuals.

Along these same lines, lifestyle can also affect blood tests (for example, a big breakfast the day of your blood draw can reduce your testosterone temporarily, and weight gain can cause reductions in vitamin D levels), so always check the latest information on how to take a blood test, especially if your doctor is using it to prescribe a supplement or drug.

involved solution is to compare the nutrients in your diet with the contents of a children's multivitamin (or you can have a dietitian do it for you). This gives you a baseline of what you should be getting through food. Just don't let a magazine or book tell you what you *have* to supplement; investigate it for yourself.

"Can't I just get my 'rainbow' of fruit and veggies in a pill?"

Some supplement companies claim that swallowing pills with fruit and vegetable extracts is the same as eating whole fruits and veggies. What about the thousands of published research articles showing the health benefits of eating whole fruits and veggies compared to just a handful of preliminary studies of these capsules? And what

about fiber? These capsules are fabulous for those who can't tolerate fruits or vegetables for various reasons, but the vast majority of folks should just eat the real thing.

"Can genetic tests tell me which supplements I need?"

I get so depressed when people tell me about their high-priced genetic tests (try an online search for the "23andMe" genetic test, which I discouraged, but many people were desperate to believe). They think the results can somehow predict a clinical event—like a heart attack, stroke, or something else—and it's just not true! Obviously, there are rare exceptions—breast and ovarian cancer screening for harmful genes, for example—where genetic testing may be beneficial, but most of these tests

FALSE: LEVELS OF _____ DROP AS YOU GET OLDER.

Estrogen, progesterone, testosterone, vitamins, minerals—they all tend to decrease with age, but that doesn't mean taking them in the form of a supplement will cure your aging problem or improve your health. Bodies don't really do things by accident; they're pretty smart machines. In some cases, these declines are a physiological advantage and may even protect us from certain diseases, such as cancer. When the hormone DHEA (dehydroepiandrosterone) hit the market, it was a big seller because advertisers showed graphs depicting declining DHEA levels and increasing disease incidence with age. Please! DHEA has failed to show benefits against various medical conditions in almost every trial. "My age made me do it" is not a good reason to buy a supplement. Don't fall for it!

are bogus. Genetic testing to determine the dietary supplements you need should be treated with the same skepticism. Don't get me wrong, genetics research is fascinating, and it may change the way we practice medicine someday. But so far, it's not a great diagnostic or preventive tool. These tests only amp up your anxiety and make you buy a lot of pills!

The truth is, while you do inherit your genes, you *can* still change them. Genes are like light switches that can be turned on and off, or made easier to turn off and on. And your lifestyle and environment have an impact on determining whether some bad genes get expressed. For example, exercise has been shown to impact thousands of genes, even in fat cells! As a result, it's been linked to a reduced risk of conditions, such as breast and prostate cancers, to name just a couple. In fact, if you reduce your risk of cardiovascular disease to as

close to zero as possible, you can reduce your genetic risk for most conditions.

Think about it this way: Some people come into the world like expensive, finely tuned cars that never feel any bumps in the road. Others are more like a cheap, used car that could break down at any moment. But if you give that old car enough TLC, you can get 100,000 or 200,000 miles or more out of it. This is how our genes work! Although you may have inherited a bad set of genes (like me), you can improve them.

"Big Pharma is evil, right?"

I get tired of all the "us" versus "them" talk about pharmaceutical and supplement companies. "They just want to make money!" people scream. And supplement companies don't?

At least once a month I get a call at home from someone somewhere in the world who's dying. They don't really want my advice; they just want to know if I have any connections to the latest, greatest drugs going through clinical trials at some big pharma company. From AIDS to breast cancer to hepatitis C, big pharma has made the difference between life and death for millions of people. We should never forget this. But at the same time, of course, there are pharmaceutical companies that gouge consumers and others that serve very little purpose but to spin similar versions of the same drug in order to keep the patent and high prices going as long as possible.

I think it's a myth that big pharma does not want to cure, control, or prevent anything. Let's consider a few real-world examples: The hepatitis B vaccine and countless others are dramatically reducing the damage these infectious agents can do (from liver damage to pneumonia to early death). Some point to statin drugs and claim that they're overprescribed. In reality, statins have done more good in terms of reducing health care costs and dramatically reducing the need for expensive procedures (and big pharma profits from the materials used in these procedures). And the drug companies are doing such a great job at preventing heart disease—for pennies a day—that soon cardiovascular disease will no longer be the number one cause of death in men and women.

Of course, there's always a profit motive, but are you not going to take a drug that can make your life better and longer in hopes of cutting into a company's bottom line? Of course statins are overprescribed,

but I would rather have a nation overprescribed on these pills than a nation waiting in line to get their chests cracked open or a nation of fatherless (like my wife) or motherless sons and daughters because their parents died too early of a preventable cause. *That* is a tragedy.

Many big pharmaceutical companies, from Bayer to Pfizer, now make their own supplements. In general, the price is pretty low and the quality control is usually very good. I'm grateful they have entered the market to keep prices down and research interest up.

I have been the co-chair of a volunteer committee that worked with pharmaceutical companies to secure free drugs for more than 1,000 cancer patients. These were people who had run out of treatment options and were waiting for a drug to be FDA approved, so it was an early/expanded access program. We put pressure on companies to do this, and it worked. So maybe big pharma isn't the enemy we'd like to believe it is.

"Are supplements safe for women who are pregnant or breastfeeding?"

Never use any herbal product or dietary supplement while pregnant or breastfeeding until you have reviewed the latest research with your doctor. Most dietary supplements suffer from a lack of safety research in the area of pregnancy and breastfeeding. It is just that simple, folks. Some doctors allow ginger supplements for nausea or cranberry supplements to prevent urinary tract infections during pregnancy. But, overall, the fewer herbal products you take while you're pregnant the better; the risk can outweigh the benefit.

"What do you mean when you say 'do you qualify for a supplement'?"

A supplement, just like a drug, can make your life better if you need it and worse if you don't. In other words, don't take it if you don't need it. A doctor would never give a cholesterol-lowering drug to improve hair growth or vitamin E supplements to reduce prostate cancer risk in men. Before you go on a pill, first see if you can solve the problem through lifestyle changes (weight loss; exercise; alcohol, sodium, and stress reduction; following a healthy diet—whatever it takes). If those don't work, then it may be time for a drug. And before recommending any supplement, I employ the same qualification process. This means having the patient undergo relevant medical questioning and potentially testing as well as looking at the research (see the Appendix). Was the supplement tested in people with the same or similar conditions (or lack of conditions) and of the same age, gender, race, and so on? If the supplement was tested on people with diabetes and you don't have this disease, then it may not be right for you.

"Can I take supplements if I'm having surgery?"

I don't recommend it. There are so many herbals or supplements (feverfew, garlic, ginger, ginkgo, goldenseal, licorice, St.

John's wort, valerian) that can mess with you during surgery, maybe by increasing the risk of bleeding, increasing or decreasing blood pressure, or impacting the sedative effects of anesthetics. It's just not worth the risk. For almost 30 years I have told health care professionals to have patients stop all dietary supplements ideally 2 to 3 weeks before a procedure. (After you recover, you can consider starting again.) There will indeed be exceptions to this rule as more and better research becomes available. For example, vitamin C supplementation before and after some cardiac procedures may reduce the risk of postoperative atrial fibrillation.

"Don't supplements come with side effects?"

Do you ever watch those comical pharmaceutical commercials where at the end the voice-over artist rattles off a long list of potential side effects and contraindications? "Taking _____ can cause acid reflux, anemia, certain types of cancer, diabetes, death, depression, dizziness, heart attacks, headaches, hearing problems, hot flashes, insomnia, itching, mood swings, nausea and vomiting, rash, sexual dysfunction, stroke, or visual disturbances. Talk to your doctor before taking _____." This is the CYA or "cover your gluteus maximus" info. In many cases, these side effects are rare or do not exist, but the company has to mention them for legal reasons. People just tune this part out. I feel the same way about drug-supplement

13

interactions. You should tune these out for three reasons.

1. Many conventional "experts" like to list anything bad that was ever reported with a supplement ingredient, even if it was in combination with other products, the result of contamination, or a one in a million occurrence from a case study. This is a ridiculous way to handle the situation and only leads to fear mongering or desensitization and a lack of supplement education.

2. We don't even really know about 99.9 percent of the potential drug-supplement interactions. This is because companies are not required to test their specific supplement against other drugs, which is probably a good thing because many would go broke. Most clinical trials also don't test these interactions either. Even when a company does report drug-supplement interactions, it's probably inaccurate because the final product includes a whole list of other ingredients—its "unique blend."

3. Science progresses so fast when it comes to drug and supplement research that interactions are a moving target. It can take a year for a study to get published, so by the time you read about it, it could be old news. In a perfect world, we'd see drug-supplement interactions updated weekly or monthly.

If you really want to know about drug-supplement interactions, you have to be willing to do your research (talk with a pharmacist or another health care professional or search online, such as at pubmed.gov) and accept some risk. It's hard to keep up with the research on benefits, much less side effects and drug interactions, so the primary onus is on you, as it should be with prescription drugs as well.

"Can supplements help me detox?"

No! The liver is great at eliminating toxins, and fiber (in foods or powder form) is good for getting rid of some intestinal toxins. Pills don't help. Let me repeat: PILLS DON'T HELP! Now, there are cases when someone is exposed to toxic amounts of a substance, and a supplement or drug can help prevent damage from this overdose (acetaminophen overdose is treated in the emergency room with N-acetylcysteine, or NAC, which is a drug and a supplement), but that's rare. If you really want to reduce toxin exposure, take fewer pills, exercise more, maintain a healthy weight, and avoid drinking too much and smoking. These healthy habits allow your body to work at its maximum capacity.

BUYING SUPPLEMENTS

"Are higher-priced supplements absorbed better?"

No! Some supplement companies will tell you their product is absorbed better than another product that has fewer bells and whistles. But I always have to ask, apart from a much higher price, what does this

FALSE: CELEBRITIES ARE DIETARY SUPPLEMENT EXPERTS.

Actresses, athletes, and models love to talk about their diets and exercise regimens, but I have never met one who could teach a dietary supplement course at a major university or even accurately refer to the science. Sure, celebs help boost sales and awareness, but when stars endorse or formulate a product, I don't get excited about it. I just want more proof of how it's better or different, and I always expect to pay more. (Full disclosure: Sometimes the actual person who creates the product behind the scenes is someone like me. And yes, I have been guilty of this in the past.) I can handle the celebrity endorsement part; that's how the game is played. But creating the product? That's like me playing in the NBA or starring in an episode of *The Big Bang Theory* (a.k.a. my favorite show—"Bazinga!").

This leads me to something else: Don't be fooled by some of these daytime doctor talk show guests. They can be helpful, but often viewers think the "expert" is only mentioning products that she knows work best. They don't realize that sometimes these guests get rewarded or paid for mentioning a product. I agree with the Federal Trade Commission's stance that if someone is getting paid to endorse a product, that person should have to disclose it so the audience is aware of the potential conflict of interest. I've tried to do this throughout the book where it's applicable. I consult for AbbVie Pharmaceuticals—formerly part of Abbott Laboratories—and speak for the company about lifestyle changes and supplements. I also occasionally consult for Max International and Farr Labs (and receive no royalties from sales). I own stock in the Park City Group, which produces and implements a quality-control software product for food and supplements known as ReposiTrak.

expensive supplement do better *clinically* (in the real world) than the plain, old cheap stuff? If it has not been proven to do anything better (like reduce pain, bone loss, or cholesterol or improve mood), then I don't recommend it.

"Should I pay more for an enteric or special coating?"

Most of the time, no. For example, aspirin comes in all sorts of forms—immediate release and enteric coated—and, in the end, these forms don't appear to have an impact on effectiveness or side effects. Sometimes they can even make things worse: Slow-release niacin has a higher rate of liver toxicity compared to immediate or extended release. Rarely is a pill worth more money because of its coating, but there are exceptions. Enteric-coated fish oil pills could be easier to take because the coating reduces the fishy aftertaste; specially coated peppermint oil can keep the pill from breaking down before it gets to the intestines; and some probiotics also need a coating to resist stomach acid. But these are rare cases. Most studies don't use supplements with an expensive added coating either. If an enteric or special coating is preferable, I note that in the individual supplement entries in this book.

"Is there an ideal dietary supplement?"

There is no ideal dietary supplement, but below is a partial list of some of the characteristics many people look for in the "perfect" product (these would be reported either on the packaging or the supplement's Web site).

Heart healthy

Safe for mental health

Safe during pregnancy and for children

Respected quality-control testing and monitoring methods employed

Supplement fact panel on the label is in a readable size and font (People misread things all the time because the type is just too small)

Vegetarian or even vegan friendly (contains no animal products)

BPA-free container

Biodegradable container (or otherwise environmentally friendly)

Phthalates free

No artificial coloring

No artificial flavoring

No sugar or artificial sweeteners

No fragrances

No gluten

Non-GMO

No hormones

No lactose

No pesticides or herbicides

No preservatives

No or low sodium

No starch

No yeast

No allergens (including soy, peanuts, tree nuts, etc.)

Halal friendly

Kosher friendly

Tested for heavy metals (such as arsenic, cadmium, lead, mercury)

Tested for total bacteria count, yeast and mold, salmonella, *E. coli*, *Staphylococcus aureus*, and bile-tolerant gram-negative bacteria

Quality assurance report available online

This long list incorporates some of the issues that people have asked me about over the years. Personally, I just want to make sure that the company producing the dietary supplement uses incredible quality-control testing and monitoring methods and that the supplement contains few to no contaminants that are hurting

(continued on page 18)

FALSE: WHAT YOU BUY IS WHAT YOU GET.

First, the good news: The quality control of supplements is getting better overall, and part of this is due to the FDA slightly stepping up quality-control standards. Now, the bad news: The journey of most supplement products—from when they came out of the dirt (the way most herbals do) all the way to the store shelf—can't be traced. So you don't know if your valerian came from Brazil, China, or India since the supplier isn't required to tell you.

There should be a mandate in place to force these suppliers to reveal their sources all the way back to the place the herb originated. Why is this so critical? If a product or ingredient cannot be traced back to the dirt that it was grown in and there is a contaminated batch or lot number, how fast and how confidently can a company recall the product? While some programs and policies are in the works (such as the Park City Group's Reposi-Trak, a software program that would enable all manufacturers and suppliers to provide certification and transparency), there is still much to be done. Until more progress is made with regulation and transparency, NSF (nsf.org), NPA (npainfo.org), and USP (usp.org) labels are helpful.

Here's an example that will drive home my point: Recently, researchers at the University of Guelph in Ontario, Canada, purchased 44 single-ingredient herbal products manufactured by 12 different companies from stores in the Toronto area and via mail from the United States. They used DNA barcoding, a groovy gene-testing method, to identify the plant species in each product, and they found that 33 percent of the dietary supplements did *not* contain the botanical listed on the label! Incredibly, 59 percent contained material from plants not listed on the label, and 9 percent contained only rice or wheat. One St. John's wort product contained only senna, a well-known laxative. Not surprisingly, the researchers suggested that herbal supplement providers "embrace DNA barcoding for authenticating herbal products."

It's not as hard as it may sound to investigate this kind of thing. Look for quality-control statements on manufacturers' and suppliers' Web sites, and don't hesitate to call their customer service numbers and ask them directly. Keep an eye out for those NSF, NPA, and USP labels as well. You have to think of this process as part of being a smart, educated supplement consumer.

the environment or my body. Bottom line: Learn about supplements and decide what you're willing to spend, what kind of quality control you want, and what factors are most important to you (you may not care about whether the pill contains gluten or sodium, for instance).

"Are naturally derived supplements better than synthetics?"

There's no way to know if there's a difference between natural and synthetic products and their ability to prevent and treat diseases until they're actually tested on people. Take the case of one of the best and largest vitamin E supplement trials in the world, called SELECT. In it, researchers found that 400 IU of synthetic vitamin E significantly increased the risk of prostate cancer in healthy men. Another group, in the Physicians' Health Study II trial, tested 400 IU of synthetic vitamin E in healthy men and found no impact on reducing the risk of cancer or cardiovascular disease but a significantly increased risk of hemorrhagic stroke.

Some critics suggested that it was the synthetic source that caused the negative and/or neutral findings. But another major study—called HOPE-TOO—used the same dosage of natural vitamin E (400 IU) and found it did not prevent cancer or major cardiovascular disease and appeared to significantly increase the risk of heart failure and hospitalizations for heart failure (these were patients with vascular disease or diabetes). So, yes, there could be a difference between natural and synthetic vitamin E; one might increase your risk of prostate cancer and the other might increase your risk of heart failure in different populations of people. People want to believe that "natural" is always better, but our cells may not see it that way. It all comes down to the research.

Now, I've heard some critics say that the real problem is not one form of natural or synthetic vitamin E but more expensive and, at times, complex forms (gamma-tocopherol or the mixed tocotrienols). And I wonder, *How many more hundreds of millions of dollars should we waste on this issue?* The truth is, we know enough: The cheapest high-dose (2,000 IU/day) form of synthetic vitamin E can help some Alzheimer's patients and the cheapest high-dose form of natural vitamin E (800 IU/day) can help some NASH (nonalcoholic steatohepatitis) patients, so just try to copy what worked in the clinical research.

When people in the supplement industry continue to fight for a product that has been adequately tested with consistently negative results, they're no different than someone in the pharmaceutical industry who fights for a drug that has failed many times or who illegally promotes an off-label use that does not have proof. The line between natural and synthetic can be a fuzzy one. In reality, drugs are derived from natural sources in at least one-third of cases, and most supplements are really a hodgepodge of natural and synthetic ingredients.

Finally, the argument about natural versus synthetic is rarely an objective one;

it's more about getting you to spend your money. I think it's ridiculous to tell people that bioidentical hormones—like estrogen, progesterone, and testosterone—are better than synthetic or FDA-approved drugs. They have not been tested head-to-head, and almost all of the research is on the FDA-approved versions. If you want to use bioidenticals, then you should educate yourself on the benefit versus the risk. Bioidentical hormones have no proven long-term safety and efficacy and no FDA oversight; the dosage may not be accurate (I have seen so many cases of overexposure); and the purity is not monitored. I think people should use synthetic drugs or bioidenticals based on personal choice and an objective overview; if you use bioidenticals, it should be at your own risk.

"Should I care about ORAC scores?"

ORAC, or oxygen radical absorbance capacity, was originally a scientific scoring method used by the USDA to estimate the overall antioxidant potential of certain foods and beverages (mainly fruits and veggies). In theory, the higher the ORAC score, the higher the antioxidant potential. Some supplement companies jumped on this idea and started providing their own ORAC scores or other antioxidant measurements in an effort to impress consumers. But the USDA recently abandoned this system when it couldn't find a correlation between ORAC scores and efficacy (remember what I said earlier about being impressed not by a test result but rather by whether the supplement makes a difference?).

In addition, there are absolutely no credible guidelines for how many ORAC units you need daily. A food or beverage with a high ORAC or antioxidant value is not necessarily healthier because in studies these superfoods have not been found to be clinically healthier than the boring "non-super" foods. Spinach and alfalfa sprouts have lower ORAC values than blueberries and strawberries. Who cares? All of this stuff is healthy. Do not allow yourself to make purchasing decisions based on an ORAC or antioxidant score, or based on any of the many scoring systems that will no doubt replace these in the future. Human research and quality control should be your guide.

"Is it better to get a prescription dietary supplement? Is there a difference?"

There are a variety of supplements that are only available through your doctor with a prescription, such as NicAzel, higher dosages of vitamin B_6 for nausea, Niaspan (niacin), Rozerem (which acts somewhat similar to melatonin), and some omega-3s. Supplements can turn into prescription drugs when higher doses are needed or an alternative form is created that may work the same as or better than the over-the-counter (OTC) version.

My advice: Pick the cheapest one (usually OTC) and see if it works first. If not, then you might want to try the more expensive product. For example, OTC melatonin and fish oil work just fine and generally have good quality control. But

FACT: YOU DO *NOT* ALWAYS GET WHAT YOU PAY FOR.

In the supplement world, as in life, some of the least expensive products work almost as well as, and sometimes better than, the most expensive ones. Calcium, vitamin D, CoQ10, and omega-3s are just a few examples. Since the supplement business is so lucrative, everyone wants a piece, which has caused a massive shift in competition and more consumer choices than we had even 5 years ago. Of course, there are exceptions, and you need to make sure that the supplement contains the active ingredient(s) that make it effective and that it's low in contaminants. But don't just assume that the pricier product is better.

prescription Niaspan is much easier to take than OTC niacin pills and has fewer side effects (although the latest research suggests niacin might not be as great for heart disease as was once thought, so I wouldn't bother). In some cases, like with B_6, you can just take a few more OTC pills to match the prescription dosage. In other cases, such as with NicAzel, it is tough to find OTC products with the same combination of ingredients that are proven to be beneficial in studies. Again, this book will help guide you in regard to dosage and effective and noneffective products. And remember: Just because a doctor is offering a product does not mean you should get it or that it has good quality control.

"Medical food" is a special category where some supplements become pseudo prescriptions, meaning they're recommended by a doctor (although you may not need an actual prescription) and supposed to be used under a doctor's supervision. But many of these items aren't much better than less expensive nonmedical food supplements, plus they don't undergo any FDA evaluation. For the most part, these "medical foods" are really just a way to overcharge patients (of course, there are exceptions, which I mention in some parts of this book).

TAKING SUPPLEMENTS

"What's the best time to take a supplement?"

The best time to take a supplement is when you can remember to do it! Take this example, for instance: Some doctors recommend taking cholesterol-lowering pills at night because that's when the liver makes the most cholesterol. However, in clinical trials where the pills actually saved lives, people downed them at all hours of the day.

If you take a pill regularly, you will

eventually reach what is called a steady state, which is a stable concentration of the supplement or drug in your body. Half-life is the time it takes for a supplement or drug to reach half its concentration in the blood; the longer the half-life, the longer it stays in your body. When you take your pills consistently (daily) and the drug has a decent half-life, it usually won't make a difference if you happen to miss a dose.

Finally, always try to take your supplement with or right after a meal, unless the directions or your doctor tells you to take it on an empty stomach. Taking it with a meal maximizes your stomach acid, which aids absorption, and minimizes the chances of getting gastrointestinal upset—research lingo for an upset stomach, a common side effect of supplements.

"Is it okay to start with a lower dose?"

Absolutely! "Start low and go slow and you'll save side effects and dough" is usually my mantra with supplements. Children's supplements, which are usually cheaper, are great options for adults, especially considering that many companies are making larger and larger pills that are based on marketing tactics, not science. Some people simply cannot take large doses of certain supplements due to side effects, and in many cases, a large dose isn't needed anyway. Look at antiallergy drugs like Claritin and Benadryl. Adults who take the children's version of these drugs often have an excellent response. The children's version, as with a multivitamin, is often easier to take and

safer. Remember, you don't have to start with the recommended dosage—that's just a guideline. (See page 24 for the benefits of taking a multivitamin and for more on children's supplements.)

"How long do I have to take my _____ supplement?"

My mantra throughout this book and my career with any drug or supplement is to take the lowest effective dose at the lowest price for the shortest time (based on the research). Following this simple rule will keep you from developing a tolerance or resistance or becoming addicted (if this is a possibility), and it will help you maintain your focus on making healthy lifestyle changes. If your health care professional does not subscribe to this mantra, I would find another doctor.

Every year, a handful of my wealthiest clients become enamored with some doctor pushing the latest, greatest drugs, supplements, or injections. Usually it's an "anti-aging" doctor who starts selling pills or potions for aging, then it's growth hormone injections, then it's painkillers. This doctor is selling unnecessary products, but the client gets sucked in, like with a gateway drug. And every time the patient goes in, he walks out with 15 more pills and starts to feel like he *needs* them. I've watched this happen hundreds of times! The goal of any doctor-patient relationship should be to create independence and educational empowerment, not dependence and a self-medication philosophy.

FACT: YOU *CAN* GET TOO MUCH OF A GOOD THING!

Some people like to talk about all the supplements they take every day as if it's a healthy thing. But all those pills make the liver work extra hard to metabolize and detoxify the ingredients (virtually every supplement contains contaminants—such as heavy metals or silicon dioxide, which is sand—even if it's just small amounts). When I hear about a celebrity taking more than 100 supplements a day, it just seems like a form of self-medication (and in my experience with some of these celebrities, that is exactly what it was).

They may not be treated like prescription drugs, but supplements can still hurt you. A few well-done studies have shown that too much selenium (200 micrograms a day) has been associated with an increased risk of type 2 diabetes, aggressive prostate cancer, and skin cancer recurrence, and with no benefit for heart health. Selenium is a wonderful and probably disease-preventing nutrient where both too little and too much can be harmful. Here are some other ways you can OD on supplements.

Too much vitamin A = liver toxicity

Too much calcium, vitamin D, vitamin C, or inosine = kidney stones

Too much red yeast rice extract = muscle pain, liver toxicity

Too much 5-HTP or St. John's wort = nausea

Too much vitamin B_6 = sensory peripheral neuropathy

Too much fish oil = gastrointestinal upset and an increase in bad cholesterol (LDL)

Too much zinc = loss of taste and smell

Too much iron = constipation

Too much magnesium = diarrhea

Too much iodine = thyroid problems

Too much L-arginine = unsafe drop in blood pressure

I could go on with every supplement ever invented, but I think you get the point. I always recommend taking the lowest dosage possible in every case.

SUPPLEMENT-SPECIFIC QUESTIONS

"Is taking antioxidants the best way to ward off disease?"

Antioxidants help fight the ravages of time (normal wear and tear on the body) and the effects of toxins (tobacco, pollution) on the cells. They can be very beneficial, but in the wrong situation, every antioxidant can become a pro-oxidant, *creating* free radicals and causing damage. In some cases, they can keep the body from activating its own natural response system and even feed the enemy. For example, ROS (reactive oxygen species) kill cancer cells; certain antioxidants can block them and even keep medications from working.

Antioxidants are a complex subject, and (as with any supplement) you should consider the benefit-to-risk factor. Throughout this book, I will give information on antioxidants that are commonly recommended for certain conditions. This information, as well as personal research on the benefits of taking an antioxidant and an honest discussion with your doctor, should be taken into account before popping any pill.

"Do supplements that claim to boost the immune system really work?"

Have you ever heard of autoimmune diseases? Or allergies? These occur when your immune system is "boosted" or in overdrive. Not a good thing, folks. I'm always surprised by how often people get impressed by this claim. Your goal should be to have a normal immune system with normal immune surveillance—not too high or too low (suppressed).

The best supplements for immune health—vitamin C, zinc, and yeast-based supplements—improve immune function and surveillance; they don't turbocharge the immune system. I find it interesting that our newest cancer drugs, which are designed to help boost the immune system, have some autoimmune side effects where the immune system actually attacks various organs! The tips in Chapter 2 will help your immune system almost as much as any pill.

"Do you recommend B vitamins, especially B_{12} shots, for energy?"

Sorry, unless you're anemic, there is no good research showing that B vitamins increase energy or fight fatigue. B vitamins help convert food into energy, but not the "hit the gym, run a million errands, chase your kids, and dance all night" kind of energy. It's the kind needed to fuel natural body processes, like digestion.

There are a few cases where a blood test for B_{12} may be warranted, however, such as if you are 65 or older, are a heavy drinker, or take acid reflux or diabetes medication. Also, some people swear by B vitamin shots over pills, but unless you have absorption problems, research continues to show they're both absorbed equally well. Taking a multivitamin can help you avoid mild nutrient deficiencies like this.

"Is it true that calcium and vitamin D are overhyped as supplements?"

Absolutely! I agree, for the most part, with the Institute of Medicine, which recently updated the calcium and vitamin D guidelines. For people up to the age of 70, the Institute of Medicine recommends getting 600 IU per day of D; above age 70, it's 800 IU per day. (I would recommend 800 to 1,000 IU per day, but it's close enough.) I believe in getting one vitamin D blood test every 3 to 5 years to make sure you're not terribly low (below 10 ng/mL). The recommendation for calcium is 1,000 to 1,200 milligrams per day for most adults, and the majority of this should—and usually does—come from diet (versus a pill). Because so many foods now have calcium and vitamin D added to them, most people don't need to take more than one calcium pill, if they need one at all.

"Is there anything super about superfood supplements?"

Whenever I read the latest, greatest news report about some exotic berry, fruit, or herb that increases longevity and boosts health, I have to laugh (and yawn). The only thing proven to increase life expectancy and quality of life consistently, apart from genetics, is a heart-healthy lifestyle (see Chapter 2). Everything else is just theory or a gimmick. I have seen acai, goji, mangosteen, maqui berry, raspberry ketones, resveratrol, and more come and go. Unless a product improves weight, blood pressure, blood glucose, or blood cholesterol, supplement manufacturers are just trying to make people believe they can outwit the body's innate system.

"Are multivitamins really worth the money? Do they even work?"

While multivitamins are arguably the number one selling dietary supplement in the world, they've drawn controversial headlines for the last 5 or so years. The largest and only randomized multivitamin trial ever conducted on healthy individuals—the Physicians' Health Study II (PHS II) trial—followed 14,600 incredibly healthy physicians over 11 years and came to some strong conclusions about multivitamins (specifically, Centrum Silver) and their benefits.

1. A multivitamin modestly (but still statistically significantly) reduces the risk of cancer in men, including those with a personal history of cancer and those with an outstanding diet and lifestyle.

2. It modestly (but still statistically, clinically, and significantly) reduces the risk of nuclear cataracts (the most common type) in men and women.

3. It corrects some nutritional insufficiencies or deficiencies.

4. It is heart safe (even heart healthy).

5. It has similar side effects to a placebo.

6. The cheapest multivitamins in the lowest dosages have the most research.

No pill—except this particular multivitamin—has ever been found to reduce the risk of cancer and cataracts in healthy individuals *and* with the same overall side effects as a placebo. Some critics argue that these benefits weren't impressive enough to warrant telling most people to take a daily multivitamin, and they cite lower-quality studies to make their point. I say: Cancer will soon be overtaking cardiovascular disease as the leading global killer and cataracts are the most common cause of blindness around the world. So if spending a few pennies a day has the ability to reduce the risk of cancer and cataracts even modestly and can help prevent any nutritional deficiencies, then I'm going to take one daily and recommend it to other adults.

The Centrum Silver used in the study (in the 1990s) was similar to many children's multivitamins that are sold in the United States today. Over the years, multivitamin dosages have increased faster than McDonald's french fry servings or American waist sizes, for no good reason (it's not based on science). If you want to take a multivitamin that has all the evidence today, take a Centrum Silver or a children's multivitamin. In fact, compare the dosages used in the PHS II study (below) with your multi.

The final line of the PHS II report states, "Although the main reason to take

VITAMIN AND MINERAL CONTENT IN CENTRUM SILVER IN THE PHS II STUDY

Vitamin A = 5,000 IU (50% as beta-carotene)	Vitamin B_{12} = 25 mcg	Copper = 2 mg
Vitamin C = 60 mg	Biotin = 30 mcg	Manganese = 3.5 mg
Vitamin D = 400 IU	Pantothenic acid = 10 mg	Chromium = 130 mcg
Vitamin E = 45 IU	Calcium = 200 mg	Molybdenum = 160 mcg
Vitamin K = 10 mcg	Iron = 4 mg	Chloride = 72.6 mg
Vitamin B_1 = 1.5 mg	Phosphorus = 48 mg	Potassium = 80 mg
Vitamin B_2 = 1.7 mg	Iodine = 150 mcg	Boron = 150 mcg
Niacin = 20 mg	Magnesium = 100 mg	Nickel = 5 mcg
Vitamin B_6 = 3 mg	Zinc = 15 mg	Vanadium = 10 mcg
Folic acid = 400 mcg	Selenium = 20 mcg	Silicon = 2 mg

Note: IU = international units, mg = milligrams, mcg = micrograms (also symbolized by "µg" on some supplement containers)

multivitamins is to prevent nutritional deficiency, these data provide support for the potential use of multivitamin supplements in the prevention of cancer in middle-aged and older men." It would have been nice to do a similar clinical trial with women, but for now I can only hypothesize that they would benefit in a similar fashion to men. A large Italian study done in 2008 and published in the journal *Opthalmology* tested Centrum in women and men for cataract reduction and showed a potential overall benefit, which is also why I assume similar results for women.

"What should children take in terms of a multivitamin?"

Just like we didn't know for more than 50 years if adults really needed a multivitamin, we don't know if children need multis now. There is just no research on this, not even strong preliminary clinical research. That said, I let my kid have one children's multivitamin a day. There's no evidence it can help him, but the dosages don't worry me. He's vegan (for now) and it covers his iron, vitamin D, and B_{12} needs, which are all difficult to get in many vegan diets. I am a "nagev"—the opposite of a vegan—but he is getting me to eat more plant-based foods (good boy!).

"How do you feel about protein supplements?"

I talk about these in several chapters of this book. Many so-called experts will tell you that we get too much protein, but I would argue that we're not getting enough of it in healthy forms. We're eating it surrounded by fat and especially carbs. Most healthy people should eat a maximum of half their weight in grams of protein per day (so, a 200-pound person should eat no more than 100 grams of protein daily). This much is necessary because as we age, protein is needed to help build muscle and prevent muscle wasting.

The older generation of protein powders—egg white, whey, soy, and casein—generally taste better than the newer products that are made with hemp, rice, pea, and potato, but the choice is yours. Look for an "isolate," which means the powder is just protein, no (or very little) sugars or added ingredients. My favorite whey protein isolate has 25 grams of protein and less than 1 gram of sugar in 120 calories.

Most protein bars are a waste; they have too much sugar and fancy extras and too little protein for the calories (the only thing you should get from a bar is a beer, in my book; and this *is* my book). Protein pills are a pain to take, and I rarely recommend them because you end up needing a ton of them. Just get the powder and save yourself some money.

"Is it true that certain supplements increase telomere length?"

No! Over the last several years, scientists have been investigating the tiny segments at the tips of each chromosome (DNA) called telomeres (think of them as the plastic tips at the end of your shoelaces that keep your laces from unraveling). They protect your chromosomes, or genetic information, from damage. The latest thinking is that the longer they are, the greater your chances of living longer—maybe. Exercise has been shown to reduce stress-related telomere shortening and so might losing weight, but whether these people actually live longer or are healthier down the road is still unknown. I will be long gone by the time this one is figured out, so it's not worth using it as a reason to take supplements.

The heart-healthy tips in Chapter 2 will arguably be more predictive of your life expectancy than any telomere study. The bottom line: If a company reports that its supplement improves telomere length, do not buy it. The company is just riding the coattails of the latest scientific theory. The societies around the world that have the greatest longevity tend to not take many pills, and my guess is these people are not worrying about their telomeres.

[2]

SEVEN WAYS TO LIVE LONGER, BETTER, AND STRONGER

ULTIMATELY, I THINK ANY PHYSICIAN has to first want to maximize health without creating a dependency on pills. This is the essence of the statement in the Hippocratic oath that says, "First do no harm." Otherwise, health care workers continue to add to the epidemic of what I call the self-medication generation. Making some basic changes to your lifestyle can help reduce or eliminate the need for most pills, increase longevity, and improve your life. I am not a pill-pusher, despite my passion for supplements. Above all, I'm a healthy-lifestyle advocate.

I believe the foundation of good health starts with your heart. If you make sure this vital organ is taken care of, all of the other major systems of the body are better able to do what they do best. You'll see this concept repeatedly throughout the book. Whether it's your eyes, your liver, or your genitals, your body functions best when your heart is healthy (see "The Heart's Connected to the . . . " on page 34).

Cardiovascular disease (CVD) has been the number one cause of death in women and men for 114 of the last 115 years! It was surpassed only once, in 1918, by the great influenza epidemic (and even then it was number two). CVD claims more lives each year than cancer, chronic lower respiratory disease, and accidents combined. While some people are very aware of how serious CVD is, many others aren't, or they've become desensitized to it—or are just plain tired of hearing about it—since every week seems to bring new research about what causes it, what makes it worse, and which interventions can reduce the risk of dying from it. I think the last reason may give people a false sense of complacency: *Medicine will fix it! All I need is a statin for my cholesterol and a stent to prop open the artery and I'm good to go! How bad could it be?*

However, even with all of our medical advances (and the fact that the vast majority of health research dollars are spent on CVD and cancer research), we have only taken a massive

28

epidemic and turned it into a normal-size epidemic. Did you know that of the more than 800,000 men and women who died from CVD in the past year, approximately 150,000 were younger than 65? This is an epidemic of the young and old: In fact, recent research has found that the first hints of CVD begin to show up in our teens!

So, the more you do to lower your risk of CVD, the better your chances of enjoying a longer and healthier life and the lower your chances of having to rely on drugs, including supplements. Here's what's key: I would like to see people making these changes *before* they start taking supplements. Naturally, in some cases you'll want to alleviate your symptoms as soon as possible, but at the very least you should be making these changes concurrently with taking supplements. If you're truly committed to getting better— *feeling* better—you need to commit to adopting the following heart-healthy habits.

THE SEVEN HEART-HEALTHY HABITS

These seven habits for heart health (and therefore *overall* health) are synergistic, which means the more of them you do, the greater your reduction in risk of major diseases and the longer your life span. In fact, each one you carry out accounts for a 10 to 15 percent improvement in health; accomplishing all seven would mean you've reduced your risk of major diseases as much as 90 to 95 percent and increased your odds of living to age 85 or longer (with no or little physical or mental disability) by 80 to

90 percent. There are no other antiaging strategies that can match these effects. If a pill did all this, it would receive a Nobel Prize in medicine. These habits are also cheaper than taking a pill daily, and they're doable!

While these recommendations may seem pretty basic and easy to accomplish, most people can't seem to follow them. They'd rather take a drug—or die early. I'm hoping this book will help change that mind-set. These strategies take a lifetime of commitment (once you get into the habit, it's not that hard), but every time you conquer just *one*, you change your life dramatically.

1. **Exercise regularly.** Aim for a minimum of 30 minutes 5 or 6 days a week; if you're working out at a vigorous level—where you're really huffing and puffing—you can get away with less time. Cardiovascular exercise and resistance training are both important. Also, make sure to choose activities that you'll actually do (if you don't like running, don't run!).

2. **Eat a moderately healthy diet.** This means emphasizing vegetables, fruits, lean proteins, complex carbohydrates (like fiber), and healthy fats and limiting unhealthy fats, processed carbohydrates (think cookies, crackers, white-flour pasta), and sugar (not just cakes and candy but also sugary drinks). You're not aiming for perfection or deprivation here; you're just trying to eat in a way that helps you feel better and helps get your CVD risk numbers to a normal level. For the most part, I believe that if a diet is reasonable, lowers your CVD risk, and

keeps you happy, it is the right one—whether it is low carb, moderate carb, high protein, high good fat, low fat, vegan, Paleo, etc.—and this is what I encounter working with patients and in the research, too.

3. **Eliminate all tobacco exposure** (cigarettes, secondhand smoke, and smokeless sources). Smoking is a leading risk factor for CVD and most other diseases as well.

4. **Maintain a normal blood pressure** (120/80 or less).

5. **Maintain a normal blood sugar level** (less than 100 mg/dL after fasting).

6. **Maintain healthy cholesterol levels** (an LDL of less than 100 mg/dL, an HDL of 50 mg/dL or higher, and triglycerides of less than 100 mg/dL after fasting).

7. **Maintain a healthy weight or waist size.** Ideally, you want a body mass index of 18.5 to 24.9 or a waist circumference of less than 32.5 inches for women and 35 inches for men.

THE MEDITERRANEAN WAY

Andorra is a tiny principality—roughly the size of New Orleans—squeezed between the borders of France and Spain. It is also the region of the world with the longest life expectancy—an average of 83.5 years (although it's common for Andorrans to live to 90 or even 100). Why? The locals there seem to follow many of the heart-healthy habits just listed. Located in the Pyrenees (a mountain range), Andorra is crisscrossed by hiking and biking trails, so there are lots of opportunities for exercise. In addition, there are many public (and pristine) swimming pools and gyms that are free or low cost. And the local diet is healthy, consisting of classic Mediterranean fare—lean meat, red wine (even served in the hospitals—I kid you not), fish (trout is local and popular), vegetables, and olive oil. Andorra also enjoys generous health care for its population; it's not unusual for people to have surgery in their 80s and even 90s.

Socialization is also an integral part of life in this country. Every parish has free "leisure centers" where people gather to talk, play games, read, and discuss current events. Strong family and other social connections are the rule, not the exception. Other longevity factors include a safe water supply and sanitation, 100 percent employment and literacy, and minimal to no crime. It should come as no surprise, then, that stress appears to be very low in this country.

Now, here's something that will completely surprise you and doesn't often get reported in stories about Andorra. Many Andorrans smoke! This just goes to show that increasing your longevity and health is really about the sum of what you do. They smoke, but they also do pretty much everything else right. Don't get me wrong, this is not an endorsement for smoking; I think life expectancy there could be even higher if they quit smoking.

(continued on page 32)

THE OBESITY EPIDEMIC

Obesity has just overtaken smoking as the primary *preventable* cause of illness and premature death. Like with smoking, the health impact of obesity is absolutely staggering. You cannot be obese and healthy. Having a body mass index of 30 or higher (the official definition of obesity) increases the risk of so many conditions, including:

Acid reflux (GERD)

Atrial fibrillation

Blood clots

Breathlessness

Cancers (such as breast, cervix, colon and rectum, endometrial, esophageal, gallbladder, kidney, liver, multiple myeloma, non-Hodgkin's lymphoma, ovarian, pancreas, and prostate; obesity may also increase the risk of getting a more aggressive form of cancer)

Complications from surgical procedures

Diabetes

Eye disease that can lead to blindness

Fetal defects from maternal obesity

Gallbladder disease

Gout (high uric acid levels)

Heart disease

Heart failure

Hiatal hernia

High blood pressure

High cholesterol

Hot flashes

Immobility

Incontinence

Infertility (men and women)

Low back pain (chronic)

Low testosterone

NASH (a.k.a. fatty liver disease)

Osteoarthritis

Pregnancy complications (such as preeclampsia)

Sexual dysfunction (erectile dysfunction and female sexual dysfunction)

Sleep apnea

Stroke

Urinary tract infection

MOYAD FACT: Chronic diseases (CVD, cancer, arthritis, Alzheimer's) do not exist in a vacuum. If an area or country has high levels of CVD, it also likely has high rates of other chronic problems. That's why having a low rate of CVD can increase average life expectancy so much; rates of other chronic diseases tend to be low, too.

THE PENDULUM OF GOOD HEALTH

You might notice that the seven heart-healthy habits discussed earlier don't explicitly mention other well-known causes of accelerated aging and disease, such as lack of sleep, stress, high sodium intake, and depression. These are, indeed, critical factors that can impact the quality and length of your life. However, it turns out that when you follow the tips on page 29, depression, stress, and insomnia are more likely to go away or be dramatically reduced. This is because in medicine there is something called a pendulum effect: When you make a healthy change, it triggers other healthy transformations. For instance, you improve your diet, which lowers your cholesterol, blood sugar, and blood pressure and boosts your sex life. Or you start exercising, which alleviates stress, reduces depression, and helps you sleep better. And these positive changes then spark other healthy habits, such as wearing sunscreen, limiting alcohol, and so on.

Unfortunately, the pendulum of health swings in both directions. So if you take up smoking, you are less likely to improve your diet and exercise and more likely to see your blood pressure increase. Or if you don't exercise regularly, you are more likely to have an unhealthy diet, gain weight, and see an increase in cholesterol, blood pressure, and blood sugar levels—all of which can cause you to fall into a depression.

Which way is your pendulum swinging?

ISN'T THERE AN APP FOR THAT?

Now you may be thinking, *In this day and age, isn't there just a pill I can take that will do all of this?* Of course, some people are taking pills to achieve healthy blood pressure or cholesterol levels, and that's better than living with unhealthy levels. The magic of the seven habits in this chapter is that they can make the pills you take work better so you may be able to get by with a lower dosage. Let me give you two classic examples.

1. Sexual dysfunction drugs are an embarrassment in terms of price—running $5, $10, even $20 dollars per pill—but they can help. Yet, no prescription pill for sexual dysfunction in the United States has ever been FDA-approved to improve sex drive or libido. In a beautifully done European clinical trial, however, individuals who exercised several times a week and took these pills reported improved libido. Plus, there was a greater chance of the pills working effectively in the exercise group compared to the nonexercise bunch.

2. In a 10-year US study, participants with high cholesterol who were fit and taking a cholesterol-lowering drug reduced their risk of dying of all causes by 70 percent (yes, that's right, *70 percent*!) compared to those taking cholesterol medicine who weren't as fit and couldn't exercise as intensely.

So, your pills will work far better when you follow the seven heart-healthy habits outlined earlier. If you go to Andorra or Singapore (I have many times for research), there are plenty of healthy folks taking prescription drugs and supplements. They're getting the most from their pills and taking less or relying less on them because they follow the seven heart-healthy strategies. In the United States, where more than two-thirds of Americans are overweight or obese, it is safe to say we are getting the *minimum* benefit from the more than $300 billion we're spending on prescriptions each year!

KEEP YOUR EYES ON THE BIG PICTURE

I know my strategies aren't sexy or scandalous or fear-inducing (although they should be!). They'll never get the attention they deserve, especially compared to these (mostly) health-related topics that vie for your attention every day.

- Acai vs. goji berry
- Alkaline water
- Amalgam fillings
- Antibiotics in meat
- Arsenic in rice
- Artificial sweeteners
- Bird flu
- Bottled vs. tap water
- Cell phones and brain tumors
- Colon cleanses
- Farmed vs. wild salmon
- Flesh-eating bacteria (!)
- Genetic testing
- Gluten-free for people without a gluten sensitivity
- GMOs
- Heterocyclic amines
- High-fructose corn syrup
- Mad cow disease
- Mercury in fish
- Mercury in vaccines
- Natural vs. synthetic hormones
- Nitrites in cured meats
- Organic vs. conventional fruits and veggies
- Pink slime in meat (!!)
- Power lines and cancer
- Probiotics vs. prebiotics
- Radiation from the microwave
- Raw milk vs. regular milk

33

THE HEART'S CONNECTED TO THE . . .

It can be confusing to try to remember which study said what about which disease, so just remember: Heart healthy =

BLADDER healthy (reduces risk of bladder cancer)

BONE healthy (reduces risk of osteoporosis and life-threatening bone fractures)

BRAIN healthy (reduces risk of Alzheimer's/dementia/Parkinson's)

BREAST healthy (reduces risk of dying from breast cancer)

COLON healthy (reduces risk of dying from colon cancer)

EAR healthy (reduces risk of hearing loss)

EYE healthy (reduces risk of most major eye diseases)

HORMONE healthy (reduces risk of hormonal changes that increase some cancers)

IMMUNE SYSTEM healthy (reduces risk of being hospitalized for and dying from infectious diseases like the flu or pneumonia)

JOINT healthy (reduces risk of crippling pain from osteoarthritis and the need for invasive procedures)

KIDNEY healthy (reduces risk of kidney cancer and kidney failure)

LIMB healthy (reduces risk of blood clots and circulation problems)

LIVER healthy (reduces risk of fatty liver and liver damage and the need for liver transplants)

LUNG healthy (reduces risk of lung cancer)

PANCREAS healthy (reduces risk of pancreatic damage, diabetes, and pancreatic cancer)

PROSTATE healthy (reduces risk of dying from prostate cancer)

SEXUALLY healthy (reduces risk of erectile and female sexual dysfunction)

SKIN healthy (reduces risk of skin damage and signs of aging)

- Shopping carts and bacteria

- Soy and thyroid problems

- Sugar and cancer

- Trans fats

- Vaccines and autism

- Insert your favorite health controversy here _____

Don't get me wrong: Most of these issues are important and need answers, but for some people they can serve as distractions from achieving an all-around healthy lifestyle. I can't tell you how many people I talk to every year who are anxious about GMOs or meat by-products or flesh-eating bacteria yet have no idea what their LDL or blood glucose levels are. It's like being fixated on getting hit by an asteroid while you're driving 100 miles an hour toward the edge of the Grand Canyon!

You have only so much time to dedicate to your health, and when the latest headline-news health controversy grabs your attention, it shifts your focus away from the things that matter most for a long, healthy life. These distractions are part of the reason so few people can master the seven heart-healthy habits! They are also part of the reason that physical education and proper nutrition aren't a priority in schools—these things are just not a priority for most Americans. If the United States really committed to the steps for better health given in this chapter, it would completely transform policy and public opinion.

So the next time you get worked up about whether to use a water filter or rinse your rice, please ask yourself how you are doing with maintaining the heart-healthy habits; 99 percent of us, including myself, need to keep working on them.

[PART 2]

CONDITIONS

HOW TO USE THIS BOOK

The following sections cover common diseases/conditions as well as popular health goals (such as performance enhancement, weight loss, healthy travel, and antiaging). All told, there are more than 100 conditions and goals here. If you've got it (or aspire to achieve it), it's probably in here! For those conditions and goals with a significant amount of supplement research, either good or bad, you'll see the following information.

DR. MOYAD SECRET. I'll start each section with a quick insight on the "state of the condition," so to speak. It's my take on current controversies or trends surrounding a disease or health aspiration, treatment issues related to the drugs or supplements used to address it, or frightening statistics.

WHAT IS IT? This section provides a brief explanation of the condition or health goal. It's not meant to be a comprehensive account of all the potential problems or symptoms that can arise, since that's not what this book is focused on.

WHAT WORKS. Here, I give you my top three picks for supplements based on the science and my 30 years of experience. Usually, these are in order based on the strength of the evidence; in other cases, there may be ties for first, second, or third place. While I usually try to give you at least my top three options, occasionally only one or two have earned my stamp of approval.

HONORABLE MENTION(S). These are supplements that have promising research, but it's just not enough yet to bump them into one of the top three slots. You should definitely keep your eye on them, though.

WHAT'S WORTHLESS. This is where I go over the supplements that have no impact on the condition or health goal—again, based on the research as well as my experience—or that could potentially make the condition worse, render the goal harder to achieve, or cause other issues. Usually these are supplements that are being hyped for a condition. I'm not afraid to call foul on any of these, as you'll quickly see.

LIFESTYLE CHANGES. This could very well be the most important advice in each section because, as you've figured out by now, lifestyle is the foundation of health. I might give you diet and exercise tips or just simple things you can do at home to help, such as meditating. You'll almost always see "heart healthy = _____ healthy" here as well since your cardiovascular health impacts every other part of your body.

WHAT ARE THE OPTIONS FOR KIDS? In most cases, the recommendations in these sections are for adults. I include options for children only when there's evidence that a supplement may be able to help and is safe.

WHAT ELSE DO I NEED TO KNOW? I've saved any other nuggets I've gleaned about the condition or health goal over the years for this component, which shows up only in select sections. It may be regarding a new drug that's worth discussing with your doctor or some other treatment option.

MOYAD FACTS and MOYAD TIPS. I've sprinkled these in many of the following sections to highlight interesting statistics or tidbits about certain supplements or the conditions and health goals themselves.

Interspersed throughout the book, you'll also see smaller sections on various conditions and goals for which **"The Jury's Still Out."** Put simply, these are topics that just don't have a ton of research or options, but I still wanted to arm you with what I know. I might give you only one supplement, inform you about an option with limited but promising evidence, or tell you about only one product that's worthless (so you can avoid it). I wanted to at least give you something to research more and discuss with your doctor.

Acid Reflux/Heartburn/Indigestion

Dr. Moyad Secret Have you seen those commercials with the funny, slightly corpulent (more on this later) guy with an engaging Southern accent who takes the acid reflux pill daily for "zero heartburn" and wants you to do the same while you ignore the small print at the bottom of the screen? He seems so endearing that you want to give him a hug and invite him over for dinner, beers, football, and arm wrestling. Don't be charmed, though. Acid reflux drugs might as well be crack cocaine or heroin. They work so well and so quickly that you can become addicted to them, but you shouldn't take them long term.

Acid reflux drugs increase the risk of vitamin B_{12} and magnesium deficiencies, which can (in rare cases) cause muscle spasms and irregular heartbeats. They can also reduce the absorption of iron and increase the risk of pneumonia, bone loss, fractures, and a nasty bacterial infection (*Clostridium difficile*) that can cause terrible diarrhea and lead to hospitalization or worse. Some people who quit these drugs after becoming dependent on them develop higher levels of gastric acid, which then requires another prescription and leads to further dependency! I have also personally seen several cases of people taking acid reflux medications long term who have had false positive tests for a rare cancer marker for neuroendocrine/pancreatic tumors.

Do you get my not-so-subtle drift here? Prescription and over-the-counter acid reducers work very well and are very necessary in some cases, but too many people are becoming reliant on them. In most cases, you should take the lowest dose for the shortest period of time. In fact, based on multiple studies, 75 percent of users could reduce their dosage or stop taking these pills altogether if they made some heart-healthy lifestyle changes (like losing weight, increasing fiber intake, and reducing stress).

WHAT IS IT?

Acid reflux occurs when some of the stomach's acidic contents move up into the esophagus (some people refer to this as heartburn, but that's only one symptom). It can be caused by weight gain, lifestyle changes, genetics, and medications (antibiotics, antidepressants, cancer treatments, steroid or immune-suppressing drugs, OTC and prescription pain drugs, and long-term antacid use). Regardless, the acid irritates, inflames, and erodes the esophageal lining over time, which can increase your risk of esophageal cancer.

Chronic acid reflux, where it occurs

several times weekly or starts to interfere with everyday life, is known as gastro-esophageal reflux disease or GERD. In the United States, approximately 20 percent of the adult population experiences GERD weekly. In addition to a burning sensation in your chest (heartburn), symptoms also include a sour taste, regurgitated food in the back of your mouth, indigestion, and trouble swallowing. Some people don't realize they're experiencing acid reflux because their symptoms seem unrelated, but a chronic cough, wheezing, and even mild chest pain (especially while lying down at night) can be signs of GERD.

One thing to keep in mind is that stomach acid is part of your immune system; it kills foreign microorganisms on contact. It's also critical for breaking down food so your intestines can absorb all the nutrients. Now you can see why shutting down acid production for a long period of time increases the risk of several problems.

WHAT WORKS

Note: The side effects of prescription acid reflux drugs that I mentioned earlier (nutrient deficiencies, intestinal infection, pneumonia) can also happen with supplements for acid reflux (until proven otherwise) because they primarily work by reducing acid levels in the stomach.

1. Calcium carbonate 500 milligrams once or twice a day

Products that contain calcium carbonate—like Tums, Rolaids, and even Os-Cal—can relieve heartburn within 30 minutes and can work for several hours. This mineral neutralizes esophageal acid and can prevent reflux. More recent research suggests that it can also improve esophageal movements (peristalsis), clearing more acid. Nevertheless, even something as benign as this supplement increases your risk for rebound reflux when you quit, so taper your dosage gradually or over several weeks. As long as you're taking this product, you don't need another calcium supplement for bone loss. If you have to be on acid reflux drugs indefinitely, however, and want to take a calcium supplement for bone loss, then opt for calcium citrate because it's absorbed just as well with or without stomach acid and should not increase your risk of kidney stones.

2. (tie) Artichoke leaf extract (*Cynara scolymus*) 640 milligrams (two pills) three times a day for 6 weeks maximum, primarily for indigestion

Functional dyspepsia, or indigestion, is slightly different from acid reflux or GERD. Symptoms include upper abdominal pain and discomfort with bloating, nausea, and a feeling of uncomfortable fullness. Artichoke leaf extract (ALE) contains a bitter compound called cynaropicrin, which has antispasmodic and other gastrointestinal benefits. In studies, ALE (two 320-milligram pills three times a day for 6 weeks) reduced bloating and fullness and improved overall quality of life, but it didn't reduce pain and nausea much better than a placebo. However, six pills a day is a little tough to stomach for a lot of people, especially if you're taking other pills as well. I get nervous when a supplement only works at high doses because the more you take of anything, the greater the odds that you'll experience side effects. Also note, ALE comes from the daisy family; an allergic reaction or rash is a common side effect.

2. (tie) Alpha-galactosidase
(Beano) follow package directions and use as needed

Bloating, gas, and flatulence (the GI triple threat) are common with functional dyspepsia. And enzyme-based dietary supplements like alpha-galactosidase can help reduce gas in the digestive tract that's caused by the carbohydrates (sugars) in soybeans and other legumes as well as some veggies. (Soy products—like tofu, tempeh, miso, and soy protein—have been processed and the sugars have been removed, so they're easier to digest than soybeans.) If you have diabetes, check with your doctor before taking alpha-galactosidase supplements because they might impact your blood sugar. Similar OTC products contain simethicone (like Gas-X), which is an antifoaming agent and a pseudo natural product mixture of silica gel and polydimethylsiloxane.

3. Melatonin 1 to 3 milligrams once a day before bed for acid reflux and heartburn symptoms

Say what? Though melatonin is best known as a sleep aid, it also reduces acid secretion. There isn't a plethora of clinical research on this yet, but the benefit far outweighs the risk, so it receives my bronze medal. I've had people from all over the country tell me they notice a difference with their GERD symptoms while taking melatonin. This hormone is produced not only by the tiny pineal gland in your brain but also by cells within the gastrointestinal tract that affect movement. In fact, recent research suggests that the GI tract secretes several hundred times more melatonin than the pineal gland, and it appears that melatonin's role in the GI tract is to protect the esophageal, stomach, and intestinal tissue.

In small studies where researchers used either melatonin alone, conventional proton pump inhibitor (PPI) medication, or a combination of the two, it was found that the combo worked better for pain and heartburn than the drug by itself. Melatonin has a similar chemical structure to some PPIs, such as omeprazole, and in one study it actually beat this acid reflux drug. Some of these trials used 3 milligrams of melatonin at bedtime by itself or with a PPI or other acid reflux medication, but I recommend starting with a lower dose, such as 1 milligram. The most exciting ongoing research with melatonin is whether it can prevent ulcers or accelerate their healing when it's combined with conventional medicine. Man, I dig this stuff!

WHAT'S WORTHLESS

Note: There are more supplements that can make acid reflux worse than can help it.

Ginger. Ginger supplements reduce nausea, but they can make acid reflux worse by relaxing the opening between the esophagus and stomach, making it easier for acid to move upstream.

Peppermint oil. This herb can settle the stomach, but it can also open up the esophageal sphincter and make acid reflux worse. If you're taking peppermint oil supplements for conditions such as irritable bowel syndrome, make sure they're enteric coated, which means they won't dissolve until they reach the small intestine.

Deglycyrrhizinated licorice (DGL). This dietary supplement has been promoted in alternative medicine books for ulcers, heartburn, acid reflux, and all kinds of gastrointestinal disorders, but some of the best studies failed to show any clinical benefit. In the very best case scenario, it may be as effective as some older generic drugs for acid reflux (e.g., cimetidine), but even then you have to take it several times a day and it doesn't go down easy (it tastes bad). Still, it doesn't come close to working as well as newer medications or supplements. Licorice dietary supplements, which are closely related, are much more of a problem in terms of side effects—including blood pressure swings and hormonal changes—and should not be used at all for reflux. (I can feel the heat coming off the heads of some alternative medicine experts after reading that DGL is not recommended for acid reflux. Boy am I going to get some hate mail from them, which I'll add to the letters from the acid reflux drug manufacturers.)

Capsaicin. In capsule form, this fiery active ingredient in hot peppers has been shown to—surprise!—increase the risk of heartburn. I love capsaicin topically for neuropathy or arthritis pain, but it's too *caliente* for acid reflux.

Ascorbic acid (vitamin C). The name is a dead giveaway. It's known as an acid for a reason, my friends. It can make reflux and indigestion worse and only increases levels of acidity. In fact, any supplement that contains the word *acid* should be put on the "be leery" list. If you have to take C, look for nonacidic alternatives, such as calcium ascorbate or buffered vitamin C (pH neutral), which aren't as harsh on the stomach.

Fish oil. It's prone to causing reflux partly because of the size and number of pills needed and partly because fish oil can reduce lower esophageal sphincter pressure, allowing backflow. It's also known for causing regurgitation or "fish burps," which you can avoid by taking an

MOYAD TIP: A drug or supplement that has shown a benefit for ulcers is not necessarily good for someone who only has acid reflux or GERD. Ulcers can kill, and there is no supplement yet that I'm willing to risk a person's life with based on minimal data. This book makes no claim to treat an ulcer with supplements.

enteric-coated product. (Some experts recommend storing them in the freezer to prevent this problem, but I say, "no thanks"; I don't recommend taking pills that are too cold or too hot because they can cause esophageal irritation and damage.)

Fiber. These dietary supplements and powders can cause regurgitation and esophageal irritation, making GERD and even bloating worse. However, fiber from foods could be really helpful (see the following section on lifestyle).

LIFESTYLE CHANGES

Heart healthy = less acid reflux and GERD. Losing weight, eating more fiber-rich foods, and kicking the tobacco habit can help reduce acid reflux *and* your risk of cardiovascular disease. The more you can avoid or reduce your reliance on reflux medications through lifestyle changes, the better off you'll be.

Limit caffeine and alcohol. They both increase acid reflux from the stomach into the esophagus when used in excess.

Pare off pounds. Losing just a little bit of weight (especially in the waist) takes some pressure off the stomach and can immediately reduce reflux. If the obesity epidemic were cut in half overnight, companies making acid reflux drugs and supplements would see their profits halved as well!

Loosen your belt. Avoid tight-fitting clothing unless you're headed to a disco or Speedo bathing suit convention. Seriously,

tight-fitting clothes increase abdominal pressure and can make acid reflux worse (just like weight gain).

Sleep with your head slightly elevated or on your left side. This is just gravity. The slope keeps stomach acid where it belongs. And besides losing weight, this is the second best thing you can do lifestyle-wise to relieve GERD. Snoozing on your right side relaxes the esophageal sphincter, allowing acid to creep up into the esophagus; lying on your left keeps the area between the esophagus and stomach above the level of gastric acid in the stomach (so remember: left is right!).

Eat smaller meals. This is especially important at dinner and before bedtime. Lower-carbohydrate diets with increased protein can have a calming effect on digestion, too.

Eliminate trigger foods. Fried, fatty, and greasy foods; fruit beverages; and acidic pills (like vitamin C) can make your condition worse.

Eat more fiber. It's your best friend. Flaxseed, chia seed, oatmeal, and bran cereals work like a sponge to mop up acid. It's one of the only things in your diet that clinical research has found can consistently reduce acid reflux and possibly even the risk of esophageal cancer that can result from chronic GERD. Try to get 25 to 30 grams total (a combination of both soluble and insoluble fiber) per day through diet, not pills. The problem with taking fiber pills and powders is that they can expand in the throat or irritate an already inflamed esophagus. Stick with high-fiber cereals, like Fiber One or All-Bran Buds, or look for a fiber bar that has insoluble and soluble fiber.

Breathe deeply. New research suggests that performing abdominal breathing exercises before meals or at least 1 hour afterward can strengthen the lower esophageal sphincter and train it to tighten or open appropriately, reducing symptoms of reflux and reliance on medication. This is still preliminary, but I think it's interesting and exciting! You can search online for proper abdominal breathing exercise techniques, but they basically involve standing, sitting, or lying on your back while breathing through your nose as deeply as possible, making sure your stomach rises when you inhale and falls when you exhale. Even if the research ends up debunking this, rhythmic breathing exercises are known to improve several conditions, such as hot flashes and stress or anxiety, so it won't do you harm.

Get needled. Preliminary studies have shown that acupuncture may help reduce regurgitation and heartburn.

WHAT ELSE DO I NEED TO KNOW?

Many patients have asked me about a drug found in Canada and Europe called domperidone (no, not the champagne), which they claim helped to alleviate the symptoms of acid reflux better than any drug or supplement they have ever tried. The FDA, however, has concerns about cardiovascular toxicity with this drug, so it's not one to take lightly. If you run out of options for your GERD, talk to your doctor about it.

Acne

Dr. Moyad Secret I get tired of hearing so-called experts say things like, "A poor diet and stress are the primary reasons for most acne problems, and only antibiotics can really treat acne." To this I say, "Whatever!" While diet and stress do have some impact on acne, for many individuals these are only a small part of the cause. And most people should not take antibiotics to prevent or treat acne because the harm outweighs the benefit. One of my favorite recommendations is to make your own topical treatment to fight acne. Simply crush four to six noncoated, plain, full-size aspirin, mix them in a cup with several tablespoons of water to form a paste (if too pasty, add more water; if not pasty enough, add another aspirin), and then apply it to the pimples with an applicator (like a cotton swab). Leave the mixture on for 10 to 15 minutes, and do this two or three times a week (make a new batch each time). Otherwise, many over-the-counter products work well.

WHAT IS IT?

The most common skin condition in the United States, acne is caused by hair follicles that become plugged with oil, dead skin cells, and, ultimately, bacteria (such as *Propionibacterium acnes*). It can range from a small, noninflammatory blackhead (called an open comedone, in doctor circles) to angry, red pimples (known as inflammatory acne), and it can appear on the face, neck, chest, back, and shoulders. As I said earlier, stress and diet can be contributing causes, but so can hormonal fluctuations, genetics, and hygiene. Here's a surprise: Although we usually associate acne with teenagers, one-third or more of acne sufferers are in their thirties, forties, and fifties.

WHAT WORKS

1. Zinc 15 milligrams of elemental zinc gluconate twice a day

Zinc's infection-fighting abilities and its antibacterial and healing properties make it a natural for treating inflammatory acne. (I've noticed that when some individuals use topical sunscreen with zinc oxide, their skin improves!) In some men and women, zinc also blocks the conversion of testosterone into a more potent form of testosterone, which can encourage acne growth. Be careful not to exceed 15 milligrams of elemental zinc per dose (that's why I have recommended taking it in two doses) or you may experience nausea and even vomiting, and always take it with food. In general, most of the good clinical studies that have been done have not exceeded 3 months. You can take it longer, but there is no evidence of how effective and safe it is beyond that point. There are other forms of zinc available, including zinc acetate, zinc sulfate, and zinc oxide, but they have not been well studied for acne except at ridiculously high doses that have more potential for short- and long-term side effects, including the loss of taste and smell! Keep in mind that the Recommended Dietary Allowance for zinc is 8 to 12 milligrams per day from the age of 9 and up. Taking high doses like what I'm recommending here can cause a copper deficiency (and possibly anemia), so make sure your multivitamin or zinc supplement also has 1 to 2 milligrams of copper in it if you're taking 30 milligrams of elemental zinc daily.

Keep in mind, it's almost impossible to get 30 milligrams of zinc per day from food unless you like to eat *a lot* of oysters (I love oysters, but every day? No way!), so you are better off sticking with a supplement.

2. Niacinamide (vitamin B₃ or nicotinamide) combination *see dosage information to follow*

Vitamin B₃ can take two forms, niacinamide or niacin (which is also known as nicotinic acid). Only niacinamide has anti-inflammatory properties that may help several dermatologic conditions, including acne and rosacea (see the Rosacea section, page 398). Niacin, which some people take to reduce cholesterol, can cause temporary facial flushing and can make your skin worse, so make sure you don't get them confused when you're perusing store shelves.

In the Nicomide Improvement in Clinical Outcomes Study (also known as NICOS), a dietary supplement containing niacinamide (750 milligrams), zinc (25 milligrams), copper (1.5 milligrams), and folic acid (500 micrograms) reduced the number and severity of acne pimples (and also rosacea) after 4 and 8 weeks of daily use. This is the dosage I recommend. (Some people may experience nausea and stomachache, so take this supplement combo during or right after a meal.)

Additionally, I've had patients see reduced redness and faster skin healing with a 2 percent niacinamide facial moisturizer (use it alone or with oral niacinamide). Although clinical trials with both (alone or in combination) are still ongoing, I wonder why oral and topical niacinamide aren't tested more often for inflammatory skin conditions? Probably because there's no profit in it for drug companies!

The exact product used in the NICOS trial, called Nicomide, is available, but you have to ask your doctor about it, or you can make your own version, which is pretty inexpensive to do. There is also a new prescription dietary supplement known as NicAzel that contains nicotinamide, azelaic acid, zinc, B₆, copper, and folic acid. It reduces acne and scarring and accelerates healing, which shouldn't come as a surprise based on the NICOS results. Ask your doctor about it.

3. (tie) Tea tree oil 5 percent topical gel applied twice a day

This antibacterial oil (from the native Australian tree *Melaleuca alternifolia*) also accelerates skin healing. In one large study, a 5 percent tea tree oil gel significantly reduced both inflammatory and noninflammatory acne lesions after 45 days. It doesn't work as fast as benzoyl peroxide, but I'm always a fan of other options for acne because benzoyl peroxide isn't very effective for a small group of people. Many companies do not report the concentration of tea tree oil they use in their products, but if it's the active or main ingredient, then it should be effective. When applying the gel, leave it on for 20 minutes, then wash it off.

3. (tie) Vitamin A 5,000 to 10,000 IU a day

Oral vitamin A (retinol) has been shown to fight acne, but the doses used in past studies were way too high (300,000 IU daily for women and 400,000 for men). These are potentially toxic levels that can cause dry skin, inflammation of the lips, and liver damage. I suggest you start with a more realistic 5,000 to 10,000 IU dose to see if it's effective. Over-the-counter topical retinol and retinoid prescriptions may also be beneficial. Vitamin A and its derivatives have always been a tale of two cities when it comes to skin health. It's known to improve the appearance and smoothness of the skin (which is why it's also used as an antiwrinkle agent topically), but in some people it can cause dryness and irritation. Bottom line: Never take even slightly more than what's recommended in this book without talking to your physician.

HONORABLE MENTION

A combination of omega-3s and omega-6s may help with mild to moderate acne, according to a recent Korean randomized trial. The benefit in combining them is that they fight inflammation in different ways. Many sources of omega-3s (like flaxseed) also contain some omega-6s and vice versa, however, larger doses are often needed to really see a benefit. If you want to combine them for acne, try taking 2,000 milligrams of fish oil *plus* up to 400 milligrams of gamma-linolenic acid.

WHAT'S WORTHLESS

Protein powder. Look, I love protein powder more than chocolate (that is a lot of love), especially flavored whey protein isolate, but there is some recent evidence that states using higher quantities (25 to 50-plus grams per day) could raise insulin and growth factors, such as IGF-1 (insulin-like growth factor 1), in the body. Both of these can exacerbate acne. If you or your teenager is using huge quantities of whey protein or other protein powders and cannot get acne to go away, try backing off or switching to a protein powder that has no sugar and taking it with water instead of juice or milk. You should get no more than half your weight in grams of protein per day (for example, a 150-pound person should get a maximum of 75 grams per day).

Chromium. Many experts tout chromium for improving skin (it helps with two factors that can exacerbate pimples, blood sugar and weight loss), but it hasn't been studied for treating acne. I'm all for this mineral when it comes to some other problems (like diabetes), though! High doses (more than 1,000 micrograms) can increase the risk of rash (urticaria), which can look like acne.

Selenium. This mineral is found in many supplements. But in large amounts (more than 200 micrograms daily), selenium may increase insulin resistance, which increases the risk of type 2 diabetes. Insulin resistance means you have more sugar in your blood, and bacteria (including those found in acne) thrive on sugar. I tell patients to stay away from selenium in high doses because it can only make your skin worse.

LIFESTYLE CHANGES

Cut back on carbs. Recent research suggests that eating a low-carbohydrate, high-fiber diet rich in omega-3s might reduce the risk of acne, and I suspect this is because it helps normalize blood sugar and insulin and can lead to weight loss. High blood sugar and insulin levels create a bacteria-friendly environment in the body. This is why doctors should not only treat acne but also determine if there are any underlying health problems, especially in moderate to severe cases. Recent research shows that acne may be a signal of something else wrong in the body, such as polycystic ovary syndrome.

WHAT ELSE DO I NEED TO KNOW?

Benzoyl peroxide lotions, like Proactiv (which I love and recommend all the time), are very effective and safe. If you find the right strength, they can work as well as prescription topical and systemic (oral) antibiotics. I'm not a fan of antibiotics in general unless they're absolutely necessary because they can lead to antibiotic resistance and side effects ranging from diarrhea to intestinal infection. I am not a dermatologist and I do not play one on TV; ask your doctor about using multiple treatments (such as benzoyl peroxide and zinc gluconate pills) before doing so.

Acute Bronchitis

Dr. Moyad Secret Although we now know acute bronchitis in adults and children is caused by a virus 95 percent of the time, doctors still prescribe antibiotics in about one-third of cases, which only adds to drug-resistance and sometimes serious toxicity. Frightening!

Pelargonium sidoides. This is a species of South African geranium that's been used for centuries in Zulu medicine (it's also one of my picks for cold symptoms; see the Common Cold and Flu section, page 141). It contains compounds that may protect cells from viral infection. There have been at least two randomized trials with *Pelargonium* showing some improvement of symptoms of acute viral bronchitis, including cough, difficulty breathing, chest pain when coughing, sputum, and others. You can get *Pelargonium sidoides* (a.k.a. EPs 7630) in the United States and other countries in a supplement product called Umcka ColdCare, and the dosage is based on age (so follow the package instructions). The trials with this product used good (not great) methodologies, and they showed some consistent and real potential benefits. There are a number of supplements that have been proven useless for acute bronchitis (and more that will be), so for now, stick with *P. sidoides*.

Vitamin C. In a famous head-to-head study (published in the prestigious journal *Lancet* more than a decade ago) from Cook County Hospital (now John H. Stroger, Jr. Hospital of Cook County) and Rush University Medical Center, both in Chicago, 1,500 milligrams of vitamin C worked as well as azithromycin for acute bronchitis (about 90 percent of the subjects in each group returned to work by day 7 of their illness).

NAC (N-acetylcysteine). This has good evidence for treating chronic bronchitis and chronic obstructive pulmonary disease, or COPD, because it's a mucolytic (breaks up mucus), so I'm confident about its ability to help with acute bronchitis as well.

Acute or Chronic Rhinosinusitis
(Sinusitis)

THE JURY'S STILL OUT

Dr. Moyad Secret *Rhinosinusitis* is the preferred term now because sinusitis is almost always associated with general sinus inflammation and rhinosinusitis refers more specifically to inflammation of the nasal passages, but I use them interchangeably. Antibiotics provide very little, if any, benefit in many cases. Viral sinusitis usually lasts less than 10 days, but acute bacterial sinusitis can last longer.

Pelargonium sidoides. Like with acute bronchitis, use of this supplement for rhinosinusitis has some preliminary data where other supplements have failed. In South Africa, it has been used to treat bronchitis and even tuberculosis (I do not recommend it for the latter) and is traditionally known as Umckaloabo. It has been standardized in Germany as an extract of its root (EPs 7630) and preliminarily appears to lessen sinusitis severity, including reducing headache and nasal discharge. You can find *P. sidoides* in Umcka ColdCare in the United States and other countries (follow the instructions on the label). Beyond this, there just aren't any other supplements with good research.

WHAT'S WORTHLESS

Bromelain. Bromelain data was interesting 50 years ago, but this supplement, which is usually sold as a mixture of enzymes from pineapples, showed minimal clinical impact in both the old and more recent studies. It can also interact with some antibiotics and interfere with the metabolism of other drugs, so I would not use it until a more recent clinical study shows good efficacy and safety.

Acute Otitis Media
(Middle Ear Infection)

A

Dr. Moyad Secret This is an infection of the eustachian tube, which connects the middle ear with the back of the throat. Symptoms usually come on quickly and involve fluid accumulation, inflammation, pain, fever, and irritability. While acute otitis media (AOM) is usually related to a viral (not bacterial) respiratory tract infection (another reason to get your kids vaccinated against the flu), it can set the stage for bacteria to get a foothold. AOM is the most common reason for antibiotic use in children, and there is a need for supplements (or anything) to help reduce antibiotic use in kids who are prone to recurrent infections.

Lactobacillus rhamnosus **GG probiotic (Culturelle).** Four clinical trials (and counting), with more than 1,800 kids in total, suggest that the probiotic *Lactobacillus rhamnosus* GG can reduce the incidence of AOM by 24 percent, upper respiratory infection by 38 percent, and antibiotic use by 20 percent. While this is still preliminary evidence, the fact that the adverse effects were similar to the placebo means it may be an excellent option to try. It appears to work by preventing infectious bacteria from adhering to the middle ear and other locations. Follow the dosage on the box.

Chewing gum with xylitol. In kids up to age 12, chewing gum with xylitol might reduce AOM by up to 25 percent, especially in those attending daycare centers. Xylitol is a natural sugar substitute that not only can reduce tooth decay but also may alter bacterial wall/capsule structure so bacteria cannot adhere and cause infection. Studies had children using it up to five times a day (two pieces of gum after meals for at least 5 minutes), and it worked better than the syrup containing xylitol. It can cause loose stools and abdominal pain in some kids, though.

ADHD (Attention Deficit Hyperactivity Disorder)

Dr. Moyad Secret The primary drug treatments for ADHD are psychostimulants (such as methylphenidate, a.k.a. Ritalin), which have helped many children and adults. They get slammed by some alternative-medicine folks, but the costs of not treating ADHD—increased unemployment, greater drug addiction, poor academic performance, crime, and marital problems—are too great to *not* try everything possible. Conventional medicines have serious side effects—including the potential for abuse; increased blood pressure and heart rate; decreased appetite, weight, and growth rate; and insomnia—but their ability to increase cognitive function and attentiveness and decrease distractibility, hyperactivity, and behavioral issues is remarkable. Many respected associations, like the British Association for Psychopharmacology, suggest some ADHD patients should speak with their doctors about taking periodic "drug holidays" to evaluate the effectiveness of treatment or if there are concerns over side effects. Most supplement studies for ADHD have been poorly done, but there are a few good options that have a low risk-to-benefit ratio.

Daily multivitamin with iron. Prescription stimulants, the conventional treatment option for ADHD, can cause appetite loss and potential nutrient deficiencies, which a multivitamin can help counteract. In fact, your doctor should test for standard nutrient deficiencies if you are taking these drugs. Research from the University of Iowa Medical Center and others suggests that supplementing low iron levels (either with a multivitamin or separate supplement) can increase the response to conventional ADHD medicines.

Omega-3 fatty acids. In more than a dozen clinical trials, these have shown slight to modest reductions in ADHD symptoms, such as hyperactivity/inattention, and suggestions of improvement in literacy/writing. Preliminary research indicates that these benefits could be even stronger when combined with omega-6 supplements. Taking 500 to 1,000 milligrams per day (of mostly omega-3s with 50 to 100 milligrams of that coming from gamma-linolenic acid, or GLA, an omega-6) is a good place to start. (For kids, liquid, flavored options might be more palatable than popping a lot of pills.)

Melatonin or L-theanine. Studies have shown that 3 milligrams of melatonin before bed or 100 to 200 milligrams of L-theanine at breakfast and again after school improves sleep in boys ages 8 to 12, but lower doses could also potentially work. The rationale is that better sleep could reduce ADHD symptoms the following day. Be warned: Melatonin can potentially *increase* the risk of convulsions in some children with epilepsy.

Dimethylaminoethanol (DMAE, Deanol, or dimethylethanolamine). This compound may work by normalizing neurotransmitter (brain chemicals) function. One well-done, older clinical trial of DMAE (500 milligrams) compared with the drug methylphenidate (40 milligrams) or a placebo found that both interventions were more effective than just a placebo with no adverse effects. DMAE is less effective than stimulant drugs but could be an option for those who can't tolerate or refuse medication and have mild symptoms. The biggest problem with this product is that the research on it has been weak over the last decade, and it hasn't done well in trials for other conditions, such as Alzheimer's. Nobody really has a good handle on side effects, but headache, insomnia, increased blood pressure, schizophrenia symptoms, and unwanted movements of the face and mouth have been reported.

Pycnogenol. This extract from the bark of the French maritime pine improved attention and visual-motor coordination and reduced hyperactivity in one study (1 milligram per kilogram of body weight per day). When the participants discontinued the supplement, there was a greater chance of relapse.

***Bacopa monnieri* (Brahmi or bacopa).** Taking 50 milligrams twice daily for 12 weeks might improve memory, learning tasks, and attention. (See the Memory Loss section, page 318, and the Alzheimer's Disease, Dementia, and Mild Cognitive Impairment section, page 65, for more information on this supplement.)

Vitamin B$_6$. A variant of this vitamin, a drug known as metadoxine, has shown some ability to treat inattentive symptoms in adults with ADHD, so many experts theorize that vitamin B$_6$ would also be useful. A clinical trial to test this is needed, though. Be aware that nausea, fatigue, and diarrhea can occur with metadoxine.

WHAT'S WORTHLESS

Acetyl-L-carnitine. In one study, 500 to 1,500 milligrams per day (based on weight) of this amino acid along with conventional medicine worked no better than a placebo for ADHD.

AVOID IT

Food additives. New research suggests synthetic food dyes might make symptoms worse, but the best way to test this is by trying an elimination diet to determine sensitivity. For a few weeks, try to eat only whole foods and additive-free products (stay away from processed food) to see if symptoms change at all. Keep in mind that juice, dietary supplements, and gum can all contain artificial coloring.

Aging (Antiaging)

Dr. Moyad Secret Research has now uncovered the greatest antiaging strategies in the history of medicine, and they don't include supplements. (You can find these strategies in Chapter 2.) Also, if you regularly use sunscreen on your face, lips, and the rest of your body, you can prevent premature aging of the skin better than any pill. Finally, my experience—and the great irony of antiaging pills—is that even if these supplements and drugs help you feel better now, they have the potential to stop making you feel anything in the near future (in other words, they can contribute to disease or early death). Here are two supplements that people commonly use to feel, look, and act younger that are completely worthless.

WHAT'S WORTHLESS

Growth hormone. Any supplement claiming to increase growth hormone (GH) is a waste of money. A lot of folks are getting GH from outside the United States (it's only legally available by prescription in the United States) and injecting themselves with it. These people claim that exercise recovery is faster and day-to-day soreness is reduced and that they just feel better. Do I believe them? Yes! However, the potential downside is huge. And the idea of injecting yourself with anything just seems a bit strange and twisted unless it's a matter of life and death (like with diabetes).

Let's review the research: GH appears to slightly reduce fat mass and slightly improve lean body mass, but it doesn't change bone density or cholesterol levels. In one antiaging study, individuals taking GH (the prescription drug, not the supplement) were more likely to experience joint pain, carpal tunnel syndrome, breast enlargement, and edema (swelling) and have an increased risk of diabetes and high glucose levels. But it's hard to ignore those ads with the 75-year-old who looks like a 25-year-old.

Here's more frightening information: Cancer researchers are studying drugs that can reduce levels of a compound in the body known as insulin-like growth factor 1 (or IGF-1), which increases the risk for multiple cancers. And research continues to show that cancer may be prevented if IGF-1 levels are reduced. Growth hormone *increases* IGF-1 significantly, and we've known this for decades!

The only dietary supplement that has been proven (in a 2-year study with women) to slightly raise growth hormone *safely* is protein powder.

Using 25 grams of whey protein isolate or another protein powder daily may be the smartest thing you can do to build muscle mass and help maintain or slightly raise growth hormone levels.

Resveratrol. This antiaging dietary supplement from the skin of grapes is getting too much hype. I've written about it, lectured about it, and warned about the hype! The large clinical trial testing SRT501 (a formulation of resveratrol) for various conditions was stopped because of lack of activity (it wasn't doing anything) and speculation that it may increase the risk of kidney problems and kidney failure.

Perhaps some clinical study in the future will show some obvious benefit with this supplement, but in the meantime, it's expensive and can cause side effects at higher doses. In fact, resveratrol supplements of 1,000 milligrams or more have the potential to interfere with some prescription drugs by reducing their ability to be metabolized, leading to higher drug exposure than necessary. In addition, the supplement has failed to show benefits in many heart health studies, and according to some preliminary studies (being done at the time I was writing this book), it may even reduce the benefits of exercise.

If you really want resveratrol, have a glass of red wine or some peanuts. The former is arguably the healthiest and safest source of resveratrol in the world (in moderation, of course). Until someone provides some well-done, exciting research, put your resveratrol supplements where they belong: down the drain!

Airplane Travel Health

THE JURY'S STILL OUT

Dr. Moyad Secret When you start to think about all the germs on a plane, it can make you crazy. I know, because I fly almost every week during a large portion of the year. If the person next to you is hacking up a lung, my best advice is to either move or turn on the air nozzle above you to push the particles toward the floor, where they can reenter the filtered air system. (If you do move, to be polite, make up an excuse, like you just won the annual prune juice–drinking contest at the local fair, and then slink to another seat.)

In the early 1980s, in order to enhance fuel efficiency, aircraft makers began to build ventilation systems that recirculated cabin air. Older systems used 100 percent fresh air, which was compressed, humidified, and cooled by the engines in a process that used a lot of energy. Now, the newer airplane models recirculate as much as 50 percent or more of the cabin air. This saves fuel. The recirculated air goes through high-efficiency particulate, or HEPA, filters before mixing with fresh air and reentering the passenger areas. But the filter's ability to catch viruses is limited, and if it's clogged or old, it may be even less efficient. The ventilation system keeps air moving in compartment-like sections in the cabin—it doesn't mix freely from front to back—which means you're sharing the air with the people a few rows behind and in front of you (so if you move away from the sick guy next to you, move several rows away). The good news: Air outside of the plane gets added to the inside air throughout the flight, which keeps it fresh and diluted so that germs aren't able to concentrate.

A bigger concern than germs when flying is the risk of developing a deadly clot, called deep vein thrombosis, or DVT. People with cancer or who are obese or have clotting conditions are at increased risk for DVT. To avoid these clots, get up every 45 to 60 minutes during your flight to stretch your legs.

Do *not* take white willow bark—an aspirin-like dietary supplement that contains salicin—to help thin your blood. It's similar to aspirin, but DVT is very serious, so you don't want to take an untested supplement. White willow bark has quality control issues and a lack of research regarding its ability to thin the blood consistently. Baby aspirin is always the better option, along with staying hydrated. If I had a dime for every time someone passed out on a flight I was on and it was mistaken for a heart problem (understandably) when it was really a hydration problem, I would have 50 cents!

Alcohol Dependence

A

Dr. Moyad Secret Drinking alcohol in excess is a major epidemic, contributing to tens of thousands of deaths each year. Besides the toll on your life, excess alcohol can increase your weight/waist size, blood pressure, allergy symptoms, bone loss, and risk of numerous cancers, plus it's toxic to all your organs, from the liver to the heart. Then, of course, there's the issue of addiction. Alcohol has become the self-medication drug of choice for my generation, next to pain pills. If you think you need help, please seek it.

Kudzu. Puerarin, the active ingredient in kudzu, is mostly made up of isoflavones, and it may have the ability to discourage heavy drinking. It is supposed to help you drink less by giving you that pleasant feeling without reaching for a drink. One of the best preliminary studies on this effect involved taking two 500-milligram capsules of kudzu extract in the morning, afternoon, and evening for a month. Each 500-milligram capsule of kudzu extract contained 125 milligrams of isoflavones, so participants were getting a total of 750 milligrams of isoflavones daily. (The product came from Natural Pharmacia International and is known as Alkontrol-Herbal, or NPI-031.) Taking the isoflavones could impact the brain's reward center faster so you don't have to consume as much alcohol.

Vitamin B$_1$ (thiamin). Excessive alcohol intake can potentially lead to a deficiency of this vitamin, which could lead to temporary or permanent brain damage (Wernicke's encephalopathy and Korsakoff's psychosis).

Acetyl-L-carnitine. It can potentially reduce cravings and the "time to first drink" (at 1,000 milligrams per day), but the results are weak overall.

Alcoholic Hangover

Dr. Moyad Secret According to research, hangover severity is not impacted by many of the factors that were once thought to contribute to it, including hormones, electrolytes, ketone bodies, cortisol, and glucose. One of the best ways to affect a hangover, however, is by inhibiting prostaglandin synthesis. This means taking a pain medication—such as ibuprofen, aspirin, or naproxen—along with hydrating until your urine is clear. Tobacco use, lack of sleep, and overall poor health can make a hangover worse. Most authoritative reviews on alcohol love to ignore the preliminary positive data on supplements. Then they conclude by saying the best thing you can do is drink in moderation or not at all. (I agree with this advice, but a lot of good that does when you've already overindulged!)

My suggestion is to get up, take a naproxen, eat, and then work out a few hours later. I love naproxen because it is even effective at a very low dose (one pill) and has an excellent safety record. I have no research on exercising to help with a hangover, just personal experience and the advice of thousands of people who send me cures after my lectures.

Vitamin B$_6$. Some B$_6$ supplements reduce hangover symptoms, such as headache and vomiting, but there hasn't been much luck using it to treat other effects, like fatigue and drowsiness. There was a promising initial hangover study with a form of vitamin B$_6$ called pyritinol. In it, subjects who were going to a party where they would be drinking took 1,200 milligrams total (400 milligrams before, during, and after the party). The supplement reduced multiple hangover symptoms the next day.

Panax ginseng (containing 4% ginsenosides). When consumed with alcohol, Panax ginseng (up to 3,000 milligrams per 65 kilograms of body weight) cleared blood alcohol faster than controls (alcohol levels in the blood were 32 to 51 percent lower); this has also been observed in laboratory studies. I've seen this study interpreted in two ways: (1) Do not mix Panax ginseng with alcohol because you might not feel the effects, which could lead you to drink more than normal. (2) It might help people who are intoxicated.

Borage oil (gamma-linolenic acid, or GLA) and yeast-derived supplementation. There is some research that taking these supplements after drinking can help with hangover symptoms, but it's old and I'd like to see more supportive data.

Allergies and Allergic Rhinitis

A

Dr. Moyad Secret One of the best theories about why allergies (seasonal or perennial) and autoimmune conditions are at an all-time high is that our current obsession with trying to stay as germ free as possible has kept our immune systems from developing normally. When you finally do get exposed to a potential allergen (and you always will), your immune system is hyperresponsive. This is known as the hygiene hypothesis. Think of it like a soldier who attends some wimpy, nonrigorous boot camp and then gets sent to do hand-to-hand combat in the jungle. He's not prepared, and neither is your wimpy "germ-free" immune system! If you're worried about acquiring new allergies, just hang around other people and pets, allow yourself to get dirty, and spend time outside as much as possible. Immune cells that are not experienced enough to know what's really an enemy will overact and try to take out everything. So getting sick is good for you, and it should be celebrated every once in a while!

WHAT IS IT?

Seasonal allergies simply result from an exposure to airborne particles, like pollens, which can appear at certain times of the year. These pollens or allergens trigger the release of histamine and other compounds (such as leukotrienes) that can cause all those classic allergy symptoms, such as a runny nose, itchy eyes, sneezing, and a scratchy throat. Basically what you're experiencing is an exaggerated immune response. Seasonal allergies generally occur anywhere from early spring to late fall, but in reality, depending on where you live, they can happen all year long (also known as perennial allergies).

Cold, flu, sinusitis, and even bronchitis symptoms can overlap with seasonal allergies, so it's important to get a proper diagnosis before you take anything (how many times have you said, "I don't know if this is a cold or allergies?"). Preventing allergy symptoms is critical because, for many people, they can be draining and exhausting, and dealing with them on a day-to-day basis takes a toll on physical and mental health. There are numerous good conventional prescription and over-the-counter drugs available as well as some simple lifestyle changes and dietary supplements that can make a difference too.

Allergic rhinitis is a form of allergy that primarily has nasal symptoms. Current OTC antihistamines don't do a very good job of treating nasal congestion, which is why there's room for dietary supplements. However, I'm a far bigger fan of conventional medicines for most

61

allergy sufferers because of the availability of inexpensive and effective once-a-day drugs for kids and adults. The supplements ranked here made it for several reasons, including their ability to compete with conventional medicines and in some cases reduce nasal symptoms.

WHAT WORKS

1. Butterbur (*Petasites hybridus*) leaf extract two to four tablets (containing 7.5 to 8 milligrams of total petasins per tablet) a day

Preliminary clinical research suggests butterbur may work as well as some of the conventional antihistamine medications, and the biggest side effect with butterbur has been gastrointestinal problems, such as stomachache. The root and leaf extracts contain petasins (also known as sesquiterpenes), which have been used to treat migraines, asthma, and smooth muscle spasms. Laboratory research suggests petasins may block leukotriene and histamine production and may even prevent mast cells from making allergies worse. One of the most tested extracts was Ze339, which was approved more than a decade ago in Switzerland for the treatment of seasonal allergic rhinitis. In randomized studies,

---

MOYAD FACT: The term *hay fever* is a misnomer because allergy symptoms aren't limited to the summer when hay is grown and harvested and allergies don't usually generate a fever.

Ze339 significantly improved overall symptom scores, and the results were comparable with conventional OTC antihistamines and allergy products (cetirizine and fexofenadine). Other trials haven't been as impressive, though, so I still think the convenience, cost, and safety of conventional OTC medicines make them a better choice if you can tolerate them.

Since it's not always easy to find the Ze339 extract, look for a butterbur product that has at least 7.5 to 8 milligrams of the active compounds isopetasin and petasin (or total petasins). In clinical trials, the average dose of Ze339 was standardized to 8 milligrams of total petasin per tablet and participants used two to four tablets daily (however, you know my rule: start low and go slow; one tablet may be sufficient).

One note: Extracts of raw butterbur contain unsaturated pyrrolizidine alkaloids—UPAs or PAs—that can be toxic to the liver and carcinogenic, but these are removed during processing. Regardless, always check the label to make sure it says "UPA or PA free," even though it's rare today for a company to sell this product without cleaning it up first.

2. Spirulina
1,000 to 2,000 milligrams a day

Spirulina is a dried blue-green algae that is mainly made up of proteins (70 percent of its dry weight) in addition to vitamins, minerals, and essential fatty acids. Laboratory research suggests it may inhibit histamine release from mast cells in the body and may reduce a compound known as interleukin 4 (or IL-4), which is also involved in allergy symptoms. It appears to work better than a placebo for improving nasal discharge, congestion, sneezing, and itching. One fairly well-done study had participants taking up to 2,000 milligrams once per day for 21 weeks. It may take a few weeks to notice a difference, although spirulina seems to work better as a preventive for allergic rhinitis and seasonal allergy symptoms than a treatment.

3. EpiCor yeast extract (dried *Saccharomyces cerevisiae* fermentation product)
500 milligrams a day

EpiCor, or fermented yeast extract, has a history of reducing cold and flu symptoms (including nasal issues) in clinical trials, and this is why it earned a spot in my top three (see the Common Cold and Flu section, page 141). In one study, people who took 500 milligrams per day for 12 weeks had fewer cold and flu symptoms and a shorter duration of symptoms than with a placebo. It has also reduced nasal congestion from seasonal allergies in trials.

Research on this supplement began when workers who were handling this yeast extract had lower rates of sick days (which resulted in lower insurance rates for the company). As a result, the company decided to test it as an immune-modulating supplement. It appears to improve immune surveillance without excessively activating the immune system, which is the desired response. During times of high pollen counts over a 12-week period, it signifi-cantly lowered the severity of congestion, runny nose, and watery eyes. (I've done a lot of research on EpiCor, and I have experience using it with patients as well.)

Eliminating or reducing nasal issues, especially nasal congestion, is the Holy Grail of allergy treatment because not many drugs or supplements can prevent or treat this, apart from nasal steroid sprays. (These are usually safe, but they make many people nervous because of really rare and still unproven side effects, such as immune suppression and bone loss.) So, if a pill could favorably impact nasal symptoms, that would be great news. Another advantage of the EpiCor supplement is that in all of its clinical trials, the side effects have been similar to a placebo. It would be nice to see one more clinical trial replicate these results in individuals with seasonal or perennial allergies.

HONORABLE MENTION

Vitamin C at moderate dosages (approximately 500 milligrams per day) may work as a preventive, reducing mild histamine concentrations and the amount of steroids or other conventional medications needed by both kids and adults. However, the evidence is preliminary and nothing new has been published in a long time.

WHAT'S WORTHLESS

In laboratory studies, using quercetin to reduce histamine release and seasonal allergy symptoms appears promising, but this supplement just doesn't have the clinical research behind it yet. Capsaicin, fish oil, and stinging nettle are often touted for allergy relief, but scientists don't have the research to back these claims up, either.

LIFESTYLE CHANGES

Heart healthy = immune healthy. Okay, I'm not saying that if you reduce your risk of heart disease, you'll definitely reduce your risk of allergies, but I *am* saying that it can keep general body inflammation moderate to low, which could have a positive impact on allergies.

Drink less. Alcohol can activate histamine receptors, and in some cases, it contains histamine-like compounds that can make a mild seasonal allergy much worse. The next time you think your allergies are due to the latest high pollen counts, please ask yourself how much you're drinking and what type of alcohol (beer and wine can trigger allergies). Reducing, eliminating, or changing your beverage of choice could make the difference between having a good day and a stay-the-heck-away-from-me-I'm-miserable day.

Kill tiny triggers. To remove dander and pollens and kill dust mites, wash your laundry in water that is at least 130° to 140°F. In addition:

1. Remove carpeting from the bedroom.

2. Encase mattresses, box springs, and pillows in covers that are allergen-proof.

3. Wash throw rugs and curtains on a regular basis.

4. Vacuum frequently with a model that scored well in independent testing, such as the Kenmore Progressive. Try to wear a dust mask or have someone else vacuum if you're sensitive to allergens.

5. Use a dehumidifier in order to keep humidity under 50 percent, and use the air conditioner.

6. Keep in mind: An air cleaner or filter is not always a good idea because most models do not trap allergens—such as pollen, pet dander, or smoke particles—very well and some can produce high concentrations of ozone, which can actually make allergies and asthma worse. Dust mites and their allergenic droppings don't circulate in the air but stay closer to the surface, so an air cleaner or filter would not work well in this situation either. Check on the latest models and their research to trap these allergens.

Alzheimer's Disease, Dementia, and Mild Cognitive Impairment

Dr. Moyad Secret The conventional medical track record for fighting Alzheimer's, dementia, or even mild cognitive impairment (MCI) is terrible! Despite the hundreds of millions—if not billions—of dollars spent, there are simply no medications that can slow the progression of this devastating disease. In fact, a new Cleveland Clinic report indicated 244 out of 245 Alzheimer's clinical trials over the past decade have failed. (However, there are many medications to treat the symptoms associated with it.) Since there is nothing available, it's always a shame when I meet families of MCI or Alzheimer's patients who have been told by their doctors that there are no supplements worth trying. What is the downside of experimenting with a product that has some evidence and a good safety record? If someone in my family had any form of this disease, I would not hesitate to try one of the supplements recommended in this section. In fact, two FDA-approved drugs that are being used to improve cognitive ability in Alzheimer's patients both came from plants, including galantamine (from the snowdrop or *Galanthus woronowii*) and rivastigmine (from physostigmine derived from the Calabar bean). If you or your family is dealing with Alzheimer's or MCI, review this section with your doctors.

WHAT IS IT?

Alzheimer's disease is the number one cause of dementia (70 percent of cases). Cardiovascular events, including reduced bloodflow to and within the brain, are a leading cause, which is known as vascular dementia (17 percent of cases). MCI is kind of a gray, transition area between "normal" and dementia. It's often defined as having memory or other cognitive problems that are worse than expected for someone's age but not severe enough to be classified as dementia. About 10 to 15 percent of people with MCI will progress to Alzheimer's. Others will see improvement; it's a highly unpredictable condition, so staying heart healthy is critical. MCI may actually have the potential to be reversed in my lifetime through drugs, supplements, and lifestyle changes.

Alzheimer's-related dementia, the primary type of dementia I'll be referring to in this section, and MCI are abnormal brain conditions that can result in acute memory loss. They're caused by aging, genetics, poor heart health, and many unknown reasons. Multiple changes can occur with dementia, including:

1. **Cognitive differences** (new forgetfulness, difficulty finding words,

65

disorientation, not knowing common facts, like the name of the president)

2. **A reduction in daily functioning** (difficulty driving, getting lost, and neglecting self-care or household chores)

3. **Personality changes** (social withdrawal, easy frustration, disinterest, and explosive outbursts)

4. **Problem behaviors** (nighttime restlessness, obsessive/compulsive behaviors, and wandering)

5. **Mental health issues** (depression, paranoia, abnormal beliefs, anxiety, fearfulness, and suspiciousness)

Alzheimer's is now the sixth leading cause of death in Americans and the fifth leading cause of death in people over 65. And a recently released report from the Centers for Disease Control is suggesting that in one out of every three deaths there is some form of dementia present (it may be undiagnosed). This doesn't mean it was the cause of death, just that it's very common. Survival time after a diagnosis of dementia has historically been fewer than 5 years, but with so many clinical trials of new medicines right now, this could be changing soon.

Alzheimer's risk factors include older age (the biggest risk factor); family history; poor performance on cognitive tests; having the apolipoprotein E, or ApoE, gene (you can ask your doctor about a test for this); abnormal brain MRI findings; thicker carotid or neck artery measurements; slowness in buttoning shirts; and a history of cardiovascular disease. The bottom line for prevention is that heart healthy = brain healthy, even when it comes to Alzheimer's!

Whatever the potential cause, dementia results in profound memory loss that can be difficult to understand from the outside. Here's a common example: Many folks forget where they put their car keys; people with dementia often forget what car keys are used for. In many cases, long-term memory stays intact so someone with dementia might remember things from childhood, but that person won't be able to recall a conversation from 15 minutes ago.

WHAT WORKS

Note: The supplements mentioned here may hopefully have some ability to slow the disease or improve some aspects of the condition, such as memory loss or maintaining independence.

1. Vitamin E (as dl-alpha-tocopheryl acetate) 1,000 IU twice a day

As I was writing this book, the encouraging results of a new clinical trial were published in the *Journal of the American Medical Association*. The 5-year study, called the TEAM-AD VA Cooperative Randomized Trial, was conducted at 14 Veterans Affairs medical centers and followed patients with mild to moderate Alzheimer's disease. More than 600 participants—

in what is now one of the largest and longest clinical trials in patients with Alzheimer's—took 2,000 IU of vitamin E, 20 milligrams of a well-known prescription drug used in some Alzheimer's patients (memantine), a combination of the two, or a placebo daily. (The patients in this clinical trial were already on an acetylcholinesterase inhibitor, a standard drug treatment for Alzheimer's.) The results: The vitamin E group experienced a significant delay (more than 6 months) in the progression of the disease compared to the other groups. Caregiver time also decreased by 2 hours each day in the vitamin E group (and that's *huge* if you're a caregiver)! There was no difference among the treatment groups in safety or mortality; in fact, the patients taking vitamin E had the lowest risk of mortality. This is critical because for more than a decade high-dose vitamin E has been hampered by the suggestion from many experts that it increases the risk of death.

Although a previous clinical trial with moderately severe Alzheimer's patients found that 2,000 IU of vitamin E daily resulted in a delay in clinical progression of approximately 7 months, more testing is still needed. Regardless, these results are worth discussing with your doctor immediately, especially in mild to moderate Alzheimer's cases. This is another classic example of how vitamin E and other supplements should not be painted with such a broad brush; the decision to use a supplement should be based on the individual disease and situation. Vitamin E could delay the loss of independence that occurs with these patients (such as dressing or bathing themselves) by 6 months or more, which would not only improve quality of life but save large amounts of health care dollars— and all this with a supplement that costs pennies a day.

Note: This recommendation is *only* for Alzheimer's patients. It did not work for people with MCI.

2. Huperzine A (*Huperzia serrata*)
400 micrograms twice a day for 16 weeks

Derived from club moss (a well known Chinese herb), huperzine A is used to treat Alzheimer's disease in China and other countries. More studies are still needed, but there have been at least 20 randomized clinical trials with this herb, so it's worth looking at. Researchers believe it works in a variety of ways, including increasing acetylcholine levels in the brain, which is also how some of the Alzheimer's prescription drugs work (that's also why it's been called a natural cholinesterase inhibitor). Preliminary results in Alzheimer's clinical studies from China suggest that at dosages of up to 400 micrograms per day, huperzine A does improve mental health, including memory, and maybe even the ability to carry out activities of daily living.

The Alzheimer's Disease Cooperative Study (comprising a diverse group of experts from around the United States) did one of the best studies of this compound. In the large, 16-week Phase 2 clinical trial, huperzine A (200 or 400 micrograms twice

67

a day, or 400 to 800 micrograms total) was compared with a placebo in 177 patients with Alzheimer's. The primary measure the researchers used was the well-known Alzheimer's Disease Assessment Scale (ADAS), but they also looked at many other secondary parameters to determine if the herb would have any impact. At 200 micrograms twice daily, huperzine A did not work better than placebo; in the group that took 400 micrograms twice daily, there was significant improvement on the ADAS as well as some improvement on a mental health questionnaire called the MMSE (Mini Mental State Exam). Therefore, these results suggest there's a short-term benefit in symptoms or cognitive improvement.

Many of the study subjects had stopped taking their conventional cholinesterase inhibitor drugs, and the responses to huperzine A were no different between those who had used or never used these drugs. Still, about 11 percent of the people taking huperzine A could not tolerate it, primarily due to nausea. Since a large, rigorous study (in addition to the Chinese studies) has shown a preliminary benefit, I had to rank this number two for now. It's certainly worth sharing with your doctor. It's possible that this herbal product works no better or worse than what is available today by prescription, but the research is exciting. One word of caution: This herb should not be combined with FDA-approved cholinesterase inhibitors (donepezil, galantamine, rivastigmine) because the side effects in combination could be serious.

3. (tie) Panax ginseng or Korean red ginseng 4,500 to 9,000 milligrams a day in divided doses

The primary active ingredients in ginseng are ginsenosides, and there are seven main ones found in many dietary supplements: Rb1, Rb2, Rc, Rd, Re, Rf, and Rg1. Some of them have shown an ability in the laboratory to reduce levels of a compound called amyloid beta peptide, which is found in the brains of Alzheimer's patients. Ginsenosides can also cut the production of some inflammatory compounds and improve bloodflow. One trial using 4,500 milligrams per day of Panax ginseng (ginsenoside content of about 8 to 8.5 percent) showed cognitive improvements in Alzheimer's patients within 12 weeks that were significantly better than a placebo. A smaller trial with Korean red ginseng, a special form of Panax ginseng, found that 9,000 milligrams per day over 12 weeks improved cognition better than 4,500 milligrams per day. Since Panax ginseng has a good safety record overall, the trials are promising. (American ginseng, which is somewhat similar in structure, has been shown to improve energy levels in patients with severe fatigue.)

Research is ongoing, so it's always best to copy exactly what worked in clinical trials. If you find a product with a higher concentration (17 percent, for example) then you want to take a lower dose because the potency is higher. You should also divide your daily dose and take it with food to reduce gastrointestinal problems. Also, start low with 1,000 to 2,000 milligrams a day and build up (and always talk to your doctor).

Keep in mind: This supplement seems to have a slight stimulant effect (that's why it increases energy), so taking it late in the afternoon or in the evening could cause sleep problems. (See the section on Memory Loss, page 318, for a ginseng product that can help improve memory.)

3. (tie) *Bacopa monnieri* (Brahmi or bacopa) 150–450 milligrams a day

This is an alternative Ayurvedic medicine that in preliminary clinical trials has reduced stress and anxiety better than a placebo. That's one reason I like it for Alzheimer's, but the other is its potential for memory enhancement.

Many of the components of bacopa were isolated years ago and include alkaloids, saponins, sterols, bacopa saponins, and bacosides. The latter appear to be involved in nerve cell repair, production, and signaling, and they also appear to have some antioxidant benefit in different areas of the brain, including the hippocampus, frontal cortex, and striatum. The compounds garnering attention and research for their effects on the brain are bacosides A and B.

In one 12-week trial, a 300-milligram daily dose (55 percent combined bacosides, meaning a combo of A and B) resulted in a significant improvement in memory, learning, and speed of information processing. The results were observed in the final weeks of the study, suggesting you need to take it long term to potentially see

a benefit; no real benefits have been seen in studies lasting fewer than 12 weeks. In the *Journal of Alternative and Complementary Medicine*, Australian researchers reviewed six clinical studies and found that bacopa extract at 300 to 450 milligrams per day (40 to 55 percent bacoside content) appeared to improve memory, but not other areas of cognition. (Always look for a product that has been standardized to a minimum of 25 percent bacoside A or ideally 50 percent bacosides.) The most common side effect, especially at higher doses, is mild gastrointestinal upset, such as abdominal cramps, increased stool frequency, and nausea, so I recommend taking bacopa with a meal.

The only real problem with this supplement is that all of the impressive clinical research has been in people who don't have dementia. There is a desperate need to test this product in individuals with MCI and Alzheimer's. So why did I include it, you ask? The preliminary results with memory in older adults are encouraging, and they make this a supplement to keep on the radar and discuss with your doctor. Laboratory studies of dementia suggest bacopa can improve bloodflow in the brain and perhaps even raise brain levels of neurotransmitters that are believed to be involved in enhancing the memory process. In fact, at the time of this book's publication, I learned of a small study in Alzheimer's patients using 300 milligrams of bacopa twice daily for 6 months. The researchers reported improved cognitive performance in regard to time, places, and people as well as an improved quality of life because of less irritability and better sleep. Stay tuned!

HONORABLE MENTIONS

Omega-3 supplements may improve appetite and weight gain in people with Alzheimer's (1.7 grams of DHA and 600 milligrams of EPA for 6 to 12 months). They do *not* appear to help with memory overall, but the research hints that they might help reduce depression symptoms.

Saffron (*Crocus sativus*) extract (15 milligrams twice a day) may have some antidepressant benefits, and preliminary studies are showing it might be able to enhance cognition in mild to moderate Alzheimer's patients. Larger studies are needed, and if they show the same thing, this will definitely be worth trying.

WHAT'S WORTHLESS

Ginkgo biloba. I know what you're thinking: How can I reject the *number one* supplement used around the world for memory, MCI, and dementia? (That was what you were thinking, right?) In my "salad days," I wanted to believe that ginkgo or an extract from ginkgo could help people with Alzheimer's, but now I'm incredibly skeptical—for three reasons. First, researchers have learned just how difficult it is to really make any kind of serious impact on this disease. Second, there are serious quality control issues. And third, as the clinical trials have

become more rigorous, the results with ginkgo have become less impressive.

The largest US study on this supplement, called the Ginkgo Evaluation of Memory (GEM) trial, which was very well done, found *no* impact despite using one of the finest ginkgo products available in terms of quality control and research. Subjects with either normal cognition or MCI took 120 milligrams of ginkgo biloba extract (EGb 761, from Schwabe Pharmaceuticals) or a placebo twice daily. The researchers were trying to determine if the supplement could reduce the risk of being diagnosed with dementia or Alzheimer's disease. The median follow-up was just over 6 years, and out of 1,500 subjects, 277 developed dementia in the ginkgo group and 246 in the placebo group. The overall dementia rate was 3.3 per 100 person-years in participants taking ginkgo and 2.9 in the placebo group. Plus, there were *twice* the number of hemorrhagic strokes (16 versus 8) in the ginkgo group. Even though this was not statistically significant, it emphasizes a point about this supplement that definitely worries me: It has extreme blood-thinning potential. Researchers saw similar results (including the increased incidence of strokes) in the second-largest ginkgo and memory study, known as GuidAge, which was conducted with patients reporting memory problems; it also failed to show a reduced risk of progression to Alzheimer's disease with this herb.

High doses of B vitamins. These actually made depression worse in patients with Alzheimer's in the large Alzheimer's Disease Cooperative Study, which was published in the *Journal of the American Medical Association*. Researchers tested 5 milligrams of folic acid, 25 milligrams of vitamin B_6, and 1 milligram of vitamin B_{12} over 18 months and found that the combination reduced a blood marker called homocysteine, which has been associated with cognitive decline (when it's at high levels). However, this is a case where improving the blood test results doesn't necessarily translate to improving the actual symptoms (i.e., your number may go down, but it doesn't mean your symptoms will change). It was also concerning that almost 28 percent of patients in the B-vitamin group experienced depression, compared to 18 percent who took a placebo.

Curcumin. This compound in the spice turmeric is being studied for its anti-inflammatory properties. It has not shown any benefit in long, rigorous studies, but I believe that curcumin may have better potential in the *prevention* of Alzheimer's, if it works at all.

Resveratrol. It's still in the superhyped stage and entering clinical trials now. I want to believe it can do something for dementia, but I'm not betting on it. (I hope I'm wrong.)

Melatonin. In the vast majority of well-done clinical trials, melatonin (at both low and high doses) didn't work much better than a placebo to improve sleep in Alzheimer's patients. In my experience, low doses have provided some small benefit as reported by caregivers, so it may still be an option to consider. And there is some hint that melatonin might not only improve sleep but also reduce the risk of MCI progressing to Alzheimer's if used early enough, so stay tuned.

Phosphatidylserine. Lots of the "experts" recommend this dietary supplement for improving memory, but based on my experience and the lack of really good research, I say save your money.

LIFESTYLE CHANGES

Heart healthy = brain healthy. Experts believe that anything that has been found to reduce the risk of cardiovascular disease (exercising and maintaining a healthy weight and normal cholesterol, blood sugar, and blood pressure levels) can also help lower the risk of Alzheimer's disease and dementia. We know that a leading cause of dementia is reduced bloodflow to the brain, so lowering your risk of stroke (a cardiovascular problem) is hugely important.

Find the right protein, fat, and carb balance. New studies are suggesting that a diet high in lean protein and healthy fats may protect against mild cognitive impairment, while a high-carbohydrate diet may promote MCI. I think what's really going on is that people who have problems controlling their blood sugar, those with pre-diabetes and diabetes, may have a greater risk of Alzheimer's. There is a theory that the brain may experience its own diabetes-like condition, where its ability to absorb sugar (your noggin's number one fuel source) is compromised. This may increase the risk of Alzheimer's disease. (New research is looking at giving inhaled insulin to MCI patients to see if it works, so stay tuned!)

Flex your mental muscles. Cognitively demanding exercises—such as crossword puzzles, Sudoku, playing cards, and reading—appear to reduce the risk of MCI and Alzheimer's in some people. Activities that challenge the mind help strengthen and protect the mind. In fact, that "use it or lose it" saying was initially coined in this area of research.

Take time to de-stress. Chronic stress can increase the amount of stress steroids produced in the body, which can block brain activity and may increase the risk of Alzheimer's disease, based on recent laboratory research from Umeå University in Sweden. Whether this turns out to be true is not so much the issue because it is already known that chronic stress is damaging to the human body in general, so you should minimize it as much as possible.

Anorexia Nervosa and Bulimia Nervosa

A

Dr. Moyad Secret Anorexia nervosa, bulimia nervosa, and other eating disorders are as much mental disorders as they are physical disorders. Complications of all eating disorders potentially include osteoporosis, cardiovascular problems, and even kidney failure. (In fact, some studies indicate that up to 80 percent of chronic anorexia patients have cardiovascular problems.) Higher cortisol levels, an indicator of increased internal and external body stress, are common in eating disorders, as are low levels of one or more of the following nutrients: sodium, potassium, magnesium, phosphorus, calcium, iron, zinc, and vitamins A, B_1, B_2, B_6, B_9, B_{12}, C, and D. It's crucial to test for these and other deficiencies *before* you take any supplements to try to treat eating disorders.

Some people with eating disorders will use supplements to replace nutrients from food (self-medicate) rather than seek professional treatment, but this is obviously not the answer. Overall, there is a lack of research on supplements for anorexia and other eating disorders, but I encourage you to peruse all of the sections in this book that deal with related issues these individuals may experience, from depression to osteoporosis.

Zinc gluconate. In a preliminary double-blind trial with females hospitalized for anorexia, 100 milligrams of zinc gluconate (containing 14 milligrams of elemental zinc) taken for 2 months significantly improved the rate of weight gain in participants compared to a placebo. It's possible that zinc has a role in improving taste perception and reducing anxiety and depression during the recovery period.

Protein powder. To reduce compulsive eating, people with bulimia are often encouraged to consume protein powder (not pills), which helps increase feelings of satiety. Protein, the most satiating macronutrient, can increase the release of the hormone cholecystokinin from the gut, sending feelings of fullness to the brain; 25 to 50 grams is the average daily dose for bulimia patients. People with other eating disorders, such as anorexia, should speak with their doctors about using protein powder to combat the muscle loss that frequently accompanies severe weight loss.

Antibiotic- and *Clostridium difficile*–Associated Diarrhea

THE JURY'S STILL OUT

Dr. Moyad Secret Diarrhea triggered by antibiotic use (antibiotic-associated diarrhea, or AAD) is one of the primary reasons people quit taking their antibiotics. One of the largest reviews ever conducted on randomized trials with probiotics (82 trials in total) found that they could reduce the incidence of AAD significantly. Lactobacillus interventions (*Lactobacillus rhamnosus* and *L. casei*) reduced risk by about 42 percent, and they appear to work by restoring gut flora or creating a more hospitable environment for friendly bacteria. Look for a pill that contains at least 1 billion colony-forming units, or CFUs, of *L. rhamnosus* or *L. casei*.

Saccharomyces boulardii is a probiotic that could help to prevent and possibly even treat AAD. It's typically used for several days and even for up to 2 weeks after antibiotics are completed. If diarrhea occurs, it can help shorten the duration. Dosages in pill form vary from 250 to 1,000 milligrams daily or 5 billion CFUs once or twice daily.

The only consistency in dosages of these supplements, especially lactobacillus, is that greater or equal to 5 billion CFUs per day appeared to be more effective than fewer pills. That doesn't mean it *is* more effective, and I don't want readers taking too much. In other words, I would look for *L. rhamnosus* GG (found in Culturelle) or *S. boulardii* (found in Florastor and others) when starting antibiotics and start low. Apparently the benefits of probiotics did not differ for adults versus children and inpatients versus outpatients or based on duration of the antibiotic treatment.

Now for the catch! AAD does not occur in the majority of individuals on antibiotics, and when it does, it's usually self-limiting (it goes away on its own). So you have to decide if you want to spend the money to possibly prevent something that probably won't happen. Do not take probiotic supplements if you have a weakened immune system or are pregnant or nursing. Older studies have reported some isolated cases of bacterial sepsis (a life-threatening bacterial infection in the blood), and there are some concerns over fungemia (increasing infections with probiotics in rare cases), but, in general, researchers have not monitored side effects well with probiotics.

Stick with me here. *Clostridium difficile* (a.k.a. C diff) is a nasty bacterium that is commonly picked up in hospitals, but it can be acquired at home as well. Any time your gut bacteria are compromised, like during AAD, you run the risk of picking up C diff, and the diarrhea *it* causes is really bad (it also causes general inflammation of the colon). Think of it this way: Getting C diff is the worst-case outcome of having AAD. Some patients can be infected over and over again to the point where it becomes life-threatening. What's worse, the bug is getting more aggressive and more resistant to most antibiotics. And up to one-third of patients cannot tolerate antibiotics for C diff, so alternatives are needed. This is where probiotics may be very beneficial.

It's incredibly exciting that there have been more than 30 randomized trials of probiotics for the prevention of diarrhea caused by C diff. In studies, when researchers gave probiotics with antibiotics, it reduced the risk of diarrhea by up to 64 percent; results are preliminary but encouraging. Side effects were also reduced with probiotics, including abdominal pain, nausea, fever, soft stools, gas, and taste changes. In sum: I'm not going to take a probiotic to prevent AAD, but I *will* take one to prevent getting C diff.

Preliminary research on probiotic drinks (*L. casei*, *L. bulgaricus*, and *Streptococcus thermophilus*) to reduce AAD and C diff in hospitalized geriatric patients shows they may be just as beneficial as taking probiotic pills. Researchers believe live culture yogurts may work just as well (look for one that contains bifidobacterium or lactobacillus).

WHAT ELSE DO I NEED TO KNOW?

The most interesting thing happening in this area of medicine by far is "fecal transplantation" (FT, or FMT for fecal microbiota therapy—why not just call it PT, or poop transfer? This humor is what kept me out of the good schools, by the way). It's pretty much just what it sounds like: Feces from a healthy donor (it's screened for infectious organisms) are homogenized and placed in the recipient's gastrointestinal tract. This may be done through a nose tube—what I call the front door approach—or anally via colonoscopy or enema, the back door approach. New research suggests oral FT via a pill might also be effective (what is this, the mail slot approach?). Despite the yuck factor, there's so much excitement about FT because it's cheap, it directly tackles the reason for the problem (antibiotics don't do this), and no serious side effects have been observed. Currently, it has an 80 to 100 percent cure rate in preliminary clinical trials, which beats any other therapy at the moment. Does it work like a perfect probiotic to colonize or take over an area of the intestine so the nasty bacteria can't find a place to live, or does it provide an immune system boost—or both? Researchers do not know, but they do know it works. Talk to your doctor and don't be shy about it.

Asthma and Exercise-Induced Bronchoconstriction

THE JURY'S STILL OUT

Dr. Moyad Secret Heart healthy = lung healthy, which I have to admit is surprising to me. I wouldn't have thought they would be that connected. But the consensus now is that obesity and weight gain, both of which have been linked to heart disease, may increase the risk of asthma. There is no "home run" supplement for asthma or exercise-induced bronchoconstriction (EIB), but there are some interesting trials taking place that could be helpful for people who have trouble tolerating conventional medications.

Kampo extract. This Japanese herbal combination of gardenia fruit, licorice root, and cinnamon root is popular on the Internet. However, there are so many versions of it with different combinations of herbs that you don't know what you're getting and the risk exceeds the benefit. Researchers are testing it to reduce airway inflammation in asthma patients, so there may be some promising use in the future.

Pycnogenol. This extract from the French maritime pine tree may block some anti-inflammatory compounds (leukotrienes) at 200 milligrams per day.

Vitamin C. Taking 500 milligrams per day could reduce hyperactive airways, but it shouldn't be used as a treatment during exercise. And taking 1,000 milligrams daily may reduce steroid use without making symptoms worse.

Fish oil. It might help improve lung function in people with EIB, but the dosages used in studies were large (up to 5,000 milligrams per day). However, other medications for EIB, such as montelukast, offer a more consistent benefit. And when both were used together, there was no additive effect, so they probably both work through the same pathways. If you have trouble tolerating conventional medications, this may be an option.

Pelargonium sidoides. It may prevent asthma attacks during a viral upper respiratory infection.

Vitamin D. Taking as much as 1,200 IU per day may reduce asthma attacks in schoolchildren who have very low levels of vitamin D. This is indirect evidence from clinical trials, but it's impressive.

Magnesium. Good clinical research is suggesting this may have a preventive effect. Stay tuned!

Athletic Enhancement

Dr. Moyad Secret So many parents and college and professional athletes have thanked me over the last 30 years for a very simple and legal performance-enhancing tip: Take a few sips (4 ounces) of Diet Mountain Dew before an athletic activity, a few sips during a break or at half-time, and another hit after the activity is over. Forget the deer antler spray (remember that supposed source of steroids?)! Caffeine increases energy and focus and may also reduce muscle fatigue and pain, so a little of it before, during, and after exercise can be helpful. (Caffeine may reduce muscle pain because it blocks the activity of a compound called adenosine, which is released as part of the inflammatory response and can activate pain receptors in the body.) Here's another tip to try before a big game or athletic event: Avoid caffeine for 1 or 2 days beforehand and then use it that day for an enhanced reaction.

WHAT IS IT?

During regular or high-intensity exercise, blood and muscle levels of several compounds, including ammonia and lactate, increase and pH drops (you become more acidic), which reduces muscle strength and can accelerate fatigue. As we age, sarcopenia, or age-related muscle loss, sets in, and it may be a primary reason why many in my generation will require long-term nursing home care. Therefore, anything that can enhance your ability to exercise or help maintain or improve your muscle mass is beneficial.

WHAT WORKS

1. Whey protein concentrate, hydrolysate, or isolate 25 grams a day (containing 3 to 5 grams of the amino acid leucine)

There have been more than 50 clinical trials of whey protein powder to improve muscle protein synthesis—in everyone from teenagers to nonagenarians—so it will always be one of my top choices. Still, as we get older and muscle becomes less responsive to amino acids, using these protein powders soon after exercise appears to allow muscle tissue to repair itself and grow in much the same way it does in a teenager or twenty-something. New clinical research suggests just 6 grams of whey protein along with 5 grams of leucine (an amino acid found in whey and also available as an individual supplement) may promote muscle building and growth; the same goes for taking up to 25 grams of whey protein

77

powder that contains 3 to 5 grams of leucine, but a few more studies to further support this surprise finding would be nice.

The great thing about whey protein powder is that it tastes good when mixed in water, smoothies, or almost any other fluid (many other protein powders have flavor issues). Whey has the most research, but in the future we'll be seeing more positive studies with other animal- and plant-based protein powders, including casein, egg white, soy, hemp, pea, and brown rice.

Protein isolates have little to no carbs (sugar) or fat and almost no lactose, and they can be an integral part of any weight loss plan, from Atkins to Paleo. The hydrolysate form is partially broken down, so it is easier to digest and may be more readily used by muscle tissue but often contains carbs, fat, and lactose. The concentrate form contains less protein than isolates and generally contains more lactose, carbs, and fat as well. Be careful with taking too much, though; in excess, whey protein can increase the risk of acne in younger men and women by slightly increasing insulin-like growth factor 1. In addition, getting more than 50 grams of whey protein per day *or* more than half your body weight in grams of total protein (through diet and supplements) daily can tax the kidneys, so people with kidney disease need to check with their doctors.

2. L-citrulline malate or L-citrulline
1,500 to 6,000 milligrams a day in divided doses

L-citrulline malate and L-citrulline are known ammonia detoxifiers (they clear it from the blood), and they may also reduce lactate and increase blood supply to skeletal muscle tissue. (When ammonia accumulates in muscles, it accelerates fatigue.) L-citrulline increases nitric oxide levels, which helps with glucose uptake (muscle fuel) and contractile functions and plays many other roles in skeletal muscle, including repair. Trials have used moderate doses of 1,500 to 6,000 milligrams of L-citrulline and L-citrulline malate per day, but I've seen benefits with as little as 500 milligrams. My biggest concern is that it could also drop blood pressure, but I love taking some of this stuff before a long run. (Interestingly, L-citrulline malate has been used in countries like Spain in prescription form—the product is Stimol—for asthenia or weakness at 1,000 milligrams three times a day.) To sum up, L-citrulline can give some people a burst of energy and may improve muscle function, especially during higher-intensity workouts.

3. Creatine monohydrate 5 to 10 grams a day

Creatine is a naturally occurring amino acid–like compound produced in the liver, kidneys, and pancreas from the amino acids arginine, glycine, and methionine. More than 95 percent of your body's creatine is found in skeletal muscle, though, and it's an alternate energy source. There have been approximately 100 clinical trials with creatine, and the primary benefit so far has been for short, repeated bursts of high-intensity exercise (in other words, use this on your interval days). Creatine is receiving some new research in people with neuromuscular disorders, and it's being investigated to reduce side effects of cholesterol-lowering drugs as well.

When you take creatine, you usually do a "loading phase"—20 to 30 grams of powder per day (in 5-gram doses) for 5 to 7 days—and then take 5 to 10 grams a day for maintenance. However, you can also just take 5 grams about an hour before or right after exercise.

Creatine may be one of the best supplements to improve muscle size based on the benefit-to-risk ratio. Some argue it works by bringing more water into cells, which may reduce the breakdown of protein in the cells and increase protein synthesis. If your muscles are retaining water, you can expect to notice some weight gain with creatine.

Researchers have found it to be safe for the kidneys, and excessive amounts of protein in the urine have not been found with this supplement (any additional creatine in the body gets converted to creatinine and excreted in the urine). Yet, I would argue that the majority of studies on creatine involved young and completely healthy men. If you have any kidney issues, be careful and check with your doctor. Also, creatine is dehydrating, so drink a glass or more of water with your supplement. Finally, meat, fish, and poultry are good sources of creatine, which is why vegetarians have the most to potentially gain from taking this supplement.

HONORABLE MENTION

Beta-alanine, a nonessential amino acid, is a popular supplement that has shown mixed results for high-intensity exercise performance. Beta-alanine and L-histidine in combination create carnosine (a dipeptide), which is found in high concentrations in skeletal muscle. Researchers believe carnosine can potentially boost athletic performance. Beta-alanine acts as a buffer to soak up compounds that can drop the pH of the muscles and cause fatigue. But since beta-alanine amounts in muscles are low and L-histidine amounts are high, the theory is supplementing with beta-alanine (3 to 6 grams per day) means there's more available to combine with L-histidine, which makes more carnosine and improves performance. It can cause temporary paresthesia (tingling sensation of the skin), but a sustained-release form can reduce this.

WHAT'S WORTHLESS

HMB (hydroxymethylbutyrate). This is a metabolite of the branched-chain amino acid leucine, and the more HMB you have, the more leucine you get, supposedly. But leucine supplements themselves have far more data here.

Bitter orange. This compound became popular when ephedra was removed from the market. It can increase blood pressure and can interfere with prescription drugs, so I say skip it.

Chromium picolinate. Since it can

improve insulin sensitivity, the most impressive research has been in prediabetes and diabetes. The studies on performance have been mixed, and I don't recommend it.

Vitamin C. High doses (1,000 milligrams or more) have not been found to enhance exercise performance, and some studies even show that they may hurt it. *However,* I take 500 milligrams daily when I'm training for a marathon and doing high mileage because it can have a profound effect on reducing the risk of colds and treating them, based on numerous clinical trials.

Taurine. Many athletic and energy drinks contain a compound called taurine. Although it resembles an amino acid, it isn't one. The data recommending it for performance or recovery is weak, and new research suggests that even if you ingest megaquantities of taurine, it still doesn't get incorporated into skeletal muscle. To me that means the idea that it can enhance muscle activity and boost athletic performance takes another hit (ouch!). Plus, there are safety questions that still need to be answered, so skip this one.

LIFESTYLE CHANGES

Heart healthy = athletic performance and muscle healthy. Maintaining a healthy weight and normal cholesterol, blood pressure, and blood sugar levels keeps body inflammation to a minimum and allows you to maximize athletic performance and muscle enhancement.

It's that simple, folks! And the more athletic you are, the more heart healthy you are (in most cases), so it's a win-win.

Stay hydrated. Dehydration slows down all of the body's recovery functions after a workout, so drink plenty of water and get some electrolytes (use a zero-calorie sports drink or several ounces of coconut water), which help regulate body temperature and enhance recovery.

Chill out. Taking a cold bath or shower for 5 minutes post-workout might reduce delayed-onset muscle soreness, but adding heat to certain muscles may also work. Similarly, spot icing for 5 to 10 minutes makes more sense to me for relieving pain and inflammation.

Roll on. Massage or using a foam roller reduces the activity of proinflammatory proteins and stimulates cells to enhance recovery.

Tart it up. Many studies have shown tart cherry juice can reduce muscle soreness or pain and inflammation when consumed for a few days before and on the day of an athletic event. The catch is that there are 150 calories in 8 ounces of juice (and some trials recommend drinking more than that). Not to be a downer, but I'm not the biggest fan of ingesting tons of calories to reduce postexercise pain, even if it does work.

Eat the right mix. Within 1 to 2 hours of exercising, eating a 3:1 or 4:1 ratio of carbs to protein helps with recovery (it increases glycogen stores), but again, be careful with calories. Some people like to recommend chocolate milk, but if you're going to go this route, I suggest drinking the 100-calorie (reduced-sugar) chocolate milk packs. Getting too much sugar can cause insulin spikes and weight gain.

Walk it off. Stretching is overrated and controversial. If you stretch too much before a workout, you might increase the risk of injury, and if you overdo it postexercise, it won't help reduce soreness much (the research on this benefit isn't strong to start with). Warming up with some light activity that mimics the movements you'll be doing before you hit it hard is the best way to prepare for exercise, and an easy walk afterward works just as well to cool you down. If you are hell-bent on stretching, then always do it after your muscles are warm (ideally, after your session).

Give yourself time to recover. Your muscles recover during your downtime. If you're working out hard day after day, your muscles don't get a chance to repair themselves and you won't get stronger. Cross-training, where you do workouts that use different muscle groups, is one way to switch it up. (Instead of running daily, try cycling, skating, yoga, etc.) Fact: Older Olympic athletes tend to spend as much time recovering from exercise as they do exercising. This brings me to high-intensity interval training, or HIIT, which is all the rage across the country. This is where you alternate going hard with exercising at an easier intensity (for example, sprinting for 30 seconds followed by 30 seconds to a minute of "recovery," repeated several times). It's a great way to improve your fitness in a short amount of time, but I'm starting to see more injuries from it, especially in older men and women. I'm not warning you to stay away from it; you just need to do it in moderation, as with everything else in life. Two or three HIIT workouts a week are plenty.

Get your z's. Sleep is the best way to recover. During slumber your body releases growth hormone, which helps repair tissues. If you don't sleep, you don't get the maximum amount of repair. If you're an athlete, I suggest eating a low-calorie protein snack before bed to further stimulate overnight muscle repair. Resistance exercise, such as weight training, and protein powder are two other ways to promote the release of growth hormone.

WHAT ELSE DO I NEED TO KNOW?

Taking NSAIDs (nonsteroidal anti-inflammatory drugs) or pain killers before a workout can actually impair muscle growth and dull signals that your body is injured or fatigued. If you're using NSAIDs daily for pain, you should go to your doctor to address the source of the problem.

Atopic Dermatitis (Eczema) in Children

THE JURY'S STILL OUT

Dr. Moyad Secret Atopic dermatitis (AD, a.k.a. eczema) is the most common chronic inflammatory skin disease in infants, and it is on the rise for unknown reasons, with 20 percent of infants, and young children experiencing symptoms. Infant AD is also associated with lung diseases, such as hay fever and asthma.

Probiotics are everywhere these days, but arguably one of the most tested products in children and adults—for a variety of conditions—is *Lactobacillus rhamnosus* GG (found in Culturelle, for example). When it comes to kids, this is the product I'm most comfortable discussing with parents.

Probiotics. The best evidence for preventing and reducing the severity of AD is for probiotic supplementation in mothers and infants. *L. rhamnosus* GG has shown to be effective in long-term prevention of AD development. (Follow package dosing instructions based on weight.)

Gamma-linolenic acid (GLA). This looks interesting for reducing the severity of AD, but more studies are needed. A combination of prebiotics and black currant seed oil with GLA and omega-3s also appeared to be effective in reducing the development of AD, but this needs more research, too.

Protein powder. Partially hydrolyzed whey formula and extensively hydrolyzed casein formula have been associated with reducing AD development, especially in infants without a family history of AD.

Atrial Fibrillation

Dr. Moyad Secret Atrial fibrillation (a.k.a. A-fib or AF) is the most common cardiac arrhythmia. It causes abnormal heart function and increases the risk of stroke. Age, heavy alcohol use, drug abuse, sleep apnea, stress, medical procedures (surgery), and even obesity increase the risk of this condition. Heart disease can cause AF as well, so reducing your risk is one of the smartest things you can do.

Red yeast rice. Statins and other cholesterol-lowering drugs appear to reduce the risk of AF, so it would be wise to study red yeast rice supplements for this same purpose! (See the High Cholesterol section, page 234.)

Vitamin C and E. There is preliminary data suggesting that taking 1,000 to 2,000 milligrams of vitamin C the day before surgery and continuing for a week after surgery might reduce the stress and free-radical production associated with cardiac procedures, thereby reducing the risk of postoperative atrial fibrillation. And at least five randomized trials have shown that vitamin E (400 IU), especially in older patients (60 and above), may reduce the risk of postoperative atrial fibrillation by half. These supplements may decrease the length of your hospital stay as well. The bad news is that these trials do not score very high on the Moyad scale (see the Appendix for an explanation of how I evaluate studies), but the good news is that your doctor may be open to trying one of these options because postoperative atrial fibrillation is such a problem (and in most clinical trials the supplements were combined with conventional medicine, so it's not like you're taking one or the other).

NAC (N-acetylcysteine). This is a precursor of L-cysteine and glutathione and helps prevent free radical damage. NAC is used for acetaminophen overdose and to break up mucus in chronic pulmonary disease, so perhaps it has a role in preventing damage to different tissues of the body. More than eight clinical trials found an almost 38 percent reduction in postoperative atrial fibrillation with NAC, and some studies reported an almost 80 percent reduction (but only one of them was good enough to pass the Moyad test for scoring studies discussed in the Appendix). Still, this is another interesting approach to discuss with your doctor before valve or cardiac surgery. Most studies gave NAC as an IV infusion, but one study used 600 milligrams per day, which is a standard dose in other areas of medicine. It appears that NAC does not reduce the length of hospital stay at this time.

Magnesium. This is used by some doctors in European countries for postoperative atrial fibrillation, and it's usually given as an infusion. Higher-quality studies have not shown as consistent a benefit as with conventional medicines, but the greater lesson here is that you should talk to your doctor about increasing or normalizing your intake of magnesium and potassium before and after procedures that increase the risk of AF. These two electrolytes are critical to maintaining healthy heart function, and most individuals do not get close to the recommended daily allowance (4,700 milligrams per day for potassium and 320 to 420 milligrams per day for magnesium).

WHAT'S WORTHLESS

Omega-3s. In arguably the largest randomized trial ever conducted to prevent postoperative AF (the OPERA study), no benefit was found for moderate to large doses of these supplements compared to a placebo. The trial included more than 1,600 patients scheduled for cardiac surgery in 28 medical centers in the US, Italy, and Argentina and was published in the *Journal of the American Medical Association*.

Miscellaneous. There are more supplements that can cause AF than can control or cure it, including aloe vera, bitter orange, echinacea, ginkgo biloba, ginseng products containing added stimulants, gossypol, guarana, hawthorn, horny goat weed, licorice, oleander, and St. John's wort.

Autism Spectrum Disorders

Dr. Moyad Secret Experts now estimate that one in 68 children in the United States—and 1 percent of children globally—have autism. I think we can do better here in terms of research, especially when it comes to diet, lifestyle, and supplement studies (not just drug interventions). I wasn't sure there was enough research out there to warrant writing a full section on autism, but I hear from so many parents who are frustrated and looking for anything that might help their situation (or looking to identify anything that could potentially aggravate it). After a little digging, I realized there was enough preliminary evidence for parents right now in the areas of prevention and dietary supplement treatment combined with conventional therapies.

WHAT IS IT?

Autism is one of a group of pervasive developmental disorders. It's characterized by impairments in communication and social skills and by repetitive behaviors (often referred to as stereotypy). This group of disorders also includes Asperger's syndrome, Rett's syndrome, childhood disintegrative disorder, and pervasive developmental disorder not otherwise specified (that is, PDD-NOS or atypical autism). Autism, Asperger's, and PDD-NOS are frequently referred to as autism spectrum disorders (ASDs). Autism is the most serious ASD because it can involve an intellectual disability and a range of behavioral, medical, and psychiatric issues.

Risk factors for autism are unknown, but there are many theories as to what's causing the increased prevalence, including environmental factors, older parents at conception, a shrinking supportive family unit, an expanded medical definition of ASD, and better diagnosing.

In my experience, more children with ASD should be taking supplements. Doctors often put these kids on restrictive (gluten- or casein-free) or elimination diets, which could increase the need for a multivitamin. It's also important to get periodic (every few years) nutrition checkups. There have been some reported cases of vision loss and other serious health issues due to deficiencies of vitamin A and other nutrients.

WHAT WORKS

1. (tie) Folic acid 400 micrograms a day for all women of reproductive age for prevention; 800 micrograms a day if you're trying to conceive

85

Folic acid is an essential vitamin, especially in the first trimester of pregnancy, because it's involved in the formation of major organ systems, including the brain and spinal cord. Fifty percent of pregnancies are unplanned, which is why folic acid should be on every woman's nutrient list if she's of childbearing age. Preliminary research from Norway (published in the *Journal of the American Medical Association*) suggests that taking folic acid during pregnancy may reduce the risk of autism by as much as 40 percent. Clinical research should test higher doses—such as the 4 milligrams (or 4,000 micrograms) that has been shown to dramatically reduce the risk of neural tube defects in high-risk pregnancies—in couples believed to be at higher risk of having an autistic child. There is preliminary evidence from several studies that a dose of 800 micrograms of folic acid could be more effective than 400 micrograms because lifestyle behaviors—drinking, weight gain, certain medications, and exposure to pollutants (such as secondhand smoke)—can reduce B-vitamin levels.

There is no concrete evidence that folic acid can really prevent autism, but the research is interesting enough to keep investigating. Although there are some authoritative voices out there suggesting overexposure to folic acid might contribute to autism—and you know I am a firm believer that some of us are being overexposed to antioxidants and other nutrients—the opposite (underexposure) appears to have more data. Men might also want to supplement if they're trying to conceive (ask your doctor about this).

1. (tie) BH4 (tetrahydrobiopterin)
1 to 20 milligrams per kilogram of body weight for treatment

BH4 is involved in the degradation of the amino acid phenylalanine (too much phenylalanine can cause mental problems and seizures). But it turns out that BH4 may operate in other human pathways, including metabolizing cellular by-products that might be harmful to neural connections in the brain and producing certain neurotransmitters and even nitric oxide. Abnormal changes in all of these pathways may increase the risk of ASD, and low concentrations of BH4 in the central nervous system have been found in individuals with ASD.

There has been a minimal amount of preliminary research with BH4 in children with autism at a dosage of 1 to 3 milligrams per kilogram of body weight, and a hint of improvement in social interaction and IQ over 3 to 6 months was seen. I initially had trouble jumping on this bandwagon until a better, but small, randomized trial from Emory School of Medicine came out. In it, children with ASD (ages 3 to 7) were given 20 milligrams per kilogram of body weight of BH4 per day or a placebo for 16 weeks. Although there was no difference in overall improvement between the groups by the end, the investigators did find significant improvements in the BH4 group in the areas of social awareness, autism mannerisms, hyperactivity, and inappropriate speech. Best of all, the side effects were similar to the placebo. Another small study from the Arkansas Children's Hospital Research Institute using sapropterin (a synthetic form of BH4) also found benefits at 20 milligrams per kilogram a day.

2. NAC (N-acetylcysteine)

1,200 milligrams a day in two divided doses titrated up over 2 weeks for treatment, or 900 to 2,700 milligrams in divided doses titrated up over 12 weeks

NAC works on multiple pathways that impact mental health disorders. It increases levels of the antioxidant glutathione, reduces inflammation, and normalizes glutamate concentration and transmission, which in combination improves nerve cell health and cellular energy function. This is exemplified by some evidence showing it can help with drug addiction, schizophrenia, and bipolar disorder, and it's also being tested for Alzheimer's and Parkinson's.

A recent well-done but small trial with 40 children and adolescents with ASD found that 1,200 milligrams of effervescent NAC per day along with the drug risperidone resulted in decreased levels of irritability after 8 weeks. Side effects were low and similar between the two groups tested, but the risperidone-plus-NAC cohort had more incidences of constipation, increased appetite, nervousness, and daytime drowsiness than the risperidone-plus-placebo group. This study backed up

an earlier 12-week study from Stanford University where 31 children (ages 3 to 11) with autism were given 900 milligrams of NAC or placebo once daily for 4 weeks, then 900 milligrams twice a day for 4 weeks, and then 900 milligrams three times a day for 4 more weeks. The researchers found significant improvements in irritability in the NAC group with no significant side effect difference compared to the placebo (nausea, vomiting, diarrhea, and increased appetite occurred in just two or three more cases in the NAC group).

3. Melatonin starting dosage of 1 to 3 milligrams a day (with weekly increases of 1 to 2 milligrams if not effective) for treatment of sleep issues

The research with melatonin is exciting because up to 80 percent of children with ASD have problems with sleep (difficulty falling asleep, frequent waking, and restless sleep), compared to just 20 percent of children without ASD. Researchers speculate that problems with internal melatonin production or use could be triggering the sleep issues.

Melatonin usually works quickly—within a week—and may improve both the duration of sleep and the ability to fall asleep by as much as 60 minutes; additionally it may reduce the number of night awakenings, behavioral problems (such as hyperactivity), and parent stress. Controlled-release melatonin may be an option for children who have trouble staying asleep as well. In my experience, most kids respond to 1 to 3 milligrams, which is also reflected in the research, but the ultimate optimal dose does not appear to be related to weight or age, so you may have to experiment. Dosages of 0.5 to 15 milligrams a day have been used in clinical studies, with 3 to 6 milligrams (30 to 60 minutes before bedtime) being the most common. One of the largest Phase 3–like multicenter trials of melatonin involving children (ages 3 to 16) with ASD and other neurodevelopmental disorders who have sleep issues showed that more than half of the subjects responded to doses of 6 milligrams or less. Clinical studies have tested melatonin from 14 days to 4 years, so it appears safe to use long term.

Side effects were similar to placebo in most studies, but melatonin can rarely cause morning sleepiness, enuresis (involuntary urination), diarrhea, headache, dizziness, hypothermia, and rash. When it comes to ASD, drug interactions need to be considered. Drugs like cimetidine, tricyclic antidepressants, fluvoxamine, and ciprofloxacin can increase blood concentrations of melatonin; likewise, melatonin may lead to increased concentrations of certain drugs. In addition, melatonin may reduce blood pressure or glucose levels, so children taking drugs for these conditions should be monitored closely.

HONORABLE MENTIONS

Note: The need for other supplements should be addressed on a case-by-case basis. It should be based on legitimate nutrient testing (e.g., vitamin D, iron, B_{12}) and reviewed with a dietitian or other health care professional who specializes in this area of medicine.

Vitamin D deficiency during pregnancy and childhood might increase the risk of autism, based on very preliminary research. ASD children have an unusually high rate of vitamin D deficiency; normalizing intake won't necessarily improve symptoms, but it will improve nutritional status.

Iron supplements can improve iron-deficiency anemia for kids, but they may cause constipation and abdominal discomfort (dosage should be determined by a physician based on laboratory tests).

Vitamin B_{12} (cobalamin) deficiency is not uncommon in ASD cases. Many kids eat restricted diets that eliminate meat, which is one of the primary sources of B_{12}.

WHAT'S WORTHLESS

Other supplements for ASD really have weak data: L-carnitine (50 milligrams per kilogram of body weight a day) may improve cellular (mitochondrial) dysfunction in ASD; vitamin C in high doses (8 grams per 70 kilograms of weight a day) showed some reduction in symptom severity, but nothing further has been published in more than 20 years (which makes me nervous); omega-3 supplements (1,000 to 1,500 milligrams a day) have some weak—and overhyped—data on reducing hyperactivity, but I think this is more applicable to ADHD, and I think it's smarter to get plant or marine sources of omega-3s from diet first. Overall the studies have not been well done and have not found benefits in social interaction, communication, stereotypy (repetitive behaviors), or hyperactivity. Some so-called experts recommend omega-6s, including evening primrose oil (EPO), but EPO can lower the seizure threshold and also cause lipoid pneumonia. Until the benefit outweighs the risk in ASD, I cannot recommend these products.

LIFESTYLE CHANGES

Adjust diet. Gluten- or casein-free diets provided a mild benefit in a small study, but keep in mind that restrictive diets can be difficult and expensive for families— who are already burdened—so there needs to be more evidence. That said, I think the benefit of trying a variety of diets outweighs the risk here. For example, a high-fat, or ketogenic, diet might be beneficial. Seizures are commonly associated with ASD, and following a ketogenic diet (90 percent fat) or modified Atkins diet (70 percent fat) can help control seizures, especially for kids who aren't responding to standard antiseizure medications. You can use medium-chain triglycerides (coconut oil and palm kernel oil) instead of butter and cream as the main source of fat if necessary. I think there should be more research to determine this diet's impact on other ASD symptoms. There was a wonderful case study done at Massachusetts General Hospital in Boston where the patient became almost seizure free and saw other ASD symptoms reduced to nonautistic levels (this was only a single published case study, but the ketogenic approach has had well-documented success for epilepsy).

WHAT ELSE DO I NEED TO KNOW?

The drug methylphenidate can reduce hyperactivity and impulsive behavior better than any dietary supplement right now, but it has some minor side effects that require monitoring. It can inhibit growth, raise blood pressure, increase social withdrawal and irritability, reduce appetite, and cause difficulty sleeping and abdominal discomfort. Still, for many children with ASD, the benefits greatly outweigh the drawbacks.

Bariatric Surgery

Dr. Moyad Secret Bariatric, or weight loss, surgery would be a disaster if it weren't for dietary supplements. Physicians commonly recommend them before and especially after the procedure to reduce complications, such as anemia and bone, neurologic, and even vision problems. If your doctor puts you on supplements after your procedure without running blood tests to check for nutrient deficiencies, I recommend asking her to do so, or possibly finding another doctor. As a general rule of thumb, I recommend the same comprehensive series of nutrient deficiency blood tests for bariatric surgery patients that I do for Crohn's disease, celiac disease, irritable bowel syndrome, and so on. (See "Your Nutrient Testing Checklist" on page 92. It's about as comprehensive as you can get without going completely overboard.)

WHAT IS IT?

Bariatric surgery includes a number of procedures that restrict the size of the stomach to reduce food intake and nutrient absorption as a way to achieve weight loss in obese individuals. The number of bariatric surgeries performed in the United States has increased twelvefold over the past decade, and these procedures are increasing worldwide as well (the United States and Canada account for about 66 percent of the procedures being performed). In three out of four individuals with a body mass index (BMI) of 35 or higher, bariatric surgery can reduce or completely eliminate the need for type 2 diabetes medications.

Bariatric surgical procedures are typically classified as **completely restrictive** (common), **completely malabsorptive** (not very common), or a **combination** (common and the most well known). They reduce food intake (restrictive) and impact calorie and nutrient absorption by either delivering food to a point lower in the intestine than usual or limiting the amount of intestine that is available for absorption of nutrients (malabsorptive). Nutrient deficiencies requiring dietary supplementation are more common with malabsorptive or combo procedures.

The most common bariatric surgeries performed today are as follows:

Laparoscopic adjustable gastric banding. In this type of bariatric surgery, the surgeon places a flexible, hollow silicone band (commonly referred to as a lap band) around the upper part of the stomach to reduce its size and expandability. This way you feel full quickly and can't overeat without feeling extremely uncomfortable. Postsurgery, a below-the-skin port (lateral to the belly button) allows your doctor to inject saline into the band to tighten it further if needed. This is a completely restrictive procedure; the intestines and nutrient absorption are not affected. Any postsurgical dietary deficiencies that weren't there before the procedure are usually due to the reduced intake of food.

Laparoscopic sleeve gastrectomy. For this procedure, surgeons remove most of the body of the stomach, creating a long, narrow, tubular organ. Laparoscopic sleeve gastrectomy is usually a completely restrictive procedure with the intestines left intact. Again, any nutrient deficiencies that did not exist prior to the procedure are usually due to reduced food intake. *Note:* Some centers perform this surgery with a duodenal switch, which is an intestinal (malabsorptive) procedure. This combination creates problems with nutrient absorption, which means supplementation will be key.

Roux-en-Y gastric bypass. In this combination procedure, the surgeon divides the upper stomach, which creates a small pouch (restrictive component) and then joins the upper stomach with the middle part of the small intestine (malabsorptive component). As a result, food bypasses most of the stomach and upper small intestine, which creates nutrient absorption issues. It's the most common bariatric procedure in the world today.

Biliopancreatic diversion and **biliopancreatic diversion with duodenal switch.** Both of these are malabsorptive procedures with a restrictive component, so there will be nutrient absorption issues. Most physicians won't do a duodenal switch unless the patient is severely obese (a BMI of more than 50). For a biliopancreatic diversion procedure, the surgeon removes part of the stomach and connects the remaining section to the lower part of the small intestine. Biliopancreatic diversion with duodenal switch involves taking a different part of the stomach so that the pyloric valve, which controls food drainage from the stomach into the first part of the small intestine (duodenum), is left intact. Then the surgeon connects the duodenum to the lower part of the small intestine so that the food you eat bypasses most of the small intestine, resulting in fewer calories and nutrients getting absorbed. Any type of biliopancreatic diversion procedure results in a greater need for higher doses of supplements postsurgery to prevent deficiencies (except for calcium, because you still retain some absorption of this mineral in the small intestine).

CURRENT CLINICAL GUIDELINES

The American Association of Clinical Endocrinologists, the Obesity Society, and the American Society for Metabolic and Bariatric Surgery are the authorities on bariatric surgery, and I follow them closely. They recently issued comprehensive clinical guidelines for people preparing for or recovering from these procedures. Now,

91

the following tests and recommendations are a minimum. Based on the procedure, you might need more, less, or something different. See "Your Nutrient Testing Checklist" below for additional information on nutrient screenings to discuss with your doctor.

1. Get a clinical nutrition evaluation from a registered dietitian specializing in bariatric patients before and after the procedure to evaluate your dietary habits and identify areas for improvement and supplementation postsurgery.

2. Arrange for preoperative blood tests for these nutrients, at a minimum (see "Your Nutrient Testing Checklist" below, for more details on nutrients to potentially test for): iron, vitamin B_{12}, folate, and vitamin D (specifically the serum 25-OH vitamin D test). You should also get a urine analysis (more on that later). Patients having a malabsorptive procedure should consider more extensive testing based on symptoms and risk.

3. Early postoperative nutrient care should include the following, regardless of your nutrient test results.

   ▪ At least one daily multivitamin tablet for laparoscopic adjustable gastric banding and two daily tablets for all other types of bariatric surgeries

   ▪ Calcium citrate (1,200 to 1,500 milligrams per day, with further discussion needed in the case of

biliopancreatic diversion with duodenal switch because there is no consensus)

   ▪ Vitamin D (at least 3,000 IU per day to reach more than 30 ng/mL)

   ▪ Vitamin B_{12} as needed to reach normal levels

   ▪ Maintain proper hydration

4. Follow-up tests should include: B_{12} (methylmalonic acid and homocysteine tests optional); folate (red blood cell folate test optional); iron; vitamin D with intact PTH (parathyroid hormone check); vitamin A (especially in biliopancreatic diversion with duodenal switch); copper, zinc, and selenium (all three recommended with Roux-en-Y gastric bypass and biliopancreatic diversion with duodenal switch; other procedures on a case-by-case basis); and vitamin B_1. A bone mineral density test should be conducted at 2 years, and a 24-hour urinary calcium excretion test is recommended at 6 months and then annually. (Remember, these recommendations can change based on the procedure and surgeon, so make sure you know exactly what tests you need and when.)

YOUR NUTRIENT TESTING CHECKLIST

Before taking any supplements related to bariatric surgery, you should get pre- and postoperative nutrient testing, as mentioned earlier. In addition to adhering to

NUTRIENT VOCABULARY

You may hear these classifications thrown around a lot pre- and postsurgery. Here are the vitamins that fall under each.

- Water-soluble vitamins: B_1 (thiamin), B_2 (riboflavin), B_3 (niacin), B_5 (pantothenic acid), B_6 (pyridoxine or pyridoxal-5'-phosphate), B_7 (biotin), B_9 (folic acid), B_{12} (cobalamin)

- Fat-soluble vitamins: A, D, E, K

- Essential minerals: calcium, iodine, iron

- Trace elements: chromium, copper, manganese, selenium, zinc

the clinical guidelines (pages 91–92), discuss the following nutrients with your doctor or dietitian to see if you need blood tests for them and to figure out how you will get adequate amounts of them going forward. (Anyone with Crohn's or celiac disease or following an extreme diet may want to consider tests for these as well.)

1. **Calcium.** Calcium citrate is the preferred calcium supplement for bariatric patients. It helps prevent bone loss and reduces the risk of kidney stones (calcium carbonate won't do that). Rapid weight loss results in oxalate levels in the urine increasing substantially, which can increase the risk of kidney stones.

2. **Copper.** This mineral, when deficient, can create another type of anemia. And too much zinc can lower copper absorption. Many weight loss centers recommend extra copper if needed (usually as gluconate for better absorption).

3. **Folate** (three potential tests: red blood cell, serum folate, and homocysteine). Folate is absorbed throughout the small intestine, though, so deficiencies are less likely after bariatric surgery because there's always some part of the small intestine left intact. Some doctors recommend prenatal vitamins for folate, while others believe a multivitamin provides sufficient amounts. Just remember that the homocysteine blood test along with the serum folate test will give you a more accurate picture of any potential deficiency.

4. **Iron** (three potential tests: iron, ferritin, and CBC or complete blood count). Elemental iron is crucial for patients who've had a Roux-en-Y gastric bypass or a laparoscopic sleeve gastrectomy (a minimum of 20 to 30 milligrams per day taken at least 2 hours apart from food or a supplement containing calcium), but it always comes

93

WHAT GOES WHERE DOWN THERE

Nutrient absorption occurs primarily in the stomach and small intestine. When you inhibit it through surgery, you aren't able to get the full benefit of vitamins and minerals from your diet. This table explains the nutrients that are absorbed in the stomach and small intestine.

SECTION OF GI TRACT	NUTRIENTS ABSORBED
Stomach	Copper, iodine
Duodenum (first part of the small intestine)	Calcium; copper; iron; selenium; vitamins A, B_1, B_2, B_3 (niacin), B_7 (biotin), B_9 (folate), D, E, K
Jejunum (middle section of the small intestine)	Calcium; chromium; iron; manganese; zinc; selenium; vitamins A, B_1, B_2, B_3 (niacin), B_5 (pantothenate), B_6 (pyridoxine or pyridoxal-5'-phosphate), B_9 (folate), D, E, K
Ileum (final section of the small intestine)	Vitamins B_9 (folate), B_{12}, C, D, K

down to your blood levels. These procedures will reduce both heme (meat) and nonheme (plant sources) iron absorption. Ferrous sulfate is the best option as it tends to have the highest amount of elemental iron per dose (about 65 milligrams of elemental iron per 324-milligram dose), but ferrous fumarate (with 33 milligrams per 100-milligram dose) and ferrous gluconate (with 36 milligrams per 300-milligram dose) have also been used. Keep in mind: Iron supplements should be taken between meals or at bedtime to avoid the alkalinizing effect of food and to take advantage of the peak gastric acid production that occurs late at night.

5. **Selenium.** A deficiency of this nutrient is rare—especially if you're taking one or two multivitamins daily—except with biliopancreatic diversion procedures.

6. **Vitamin A.** You'll usually get a sufficient dose in a multivitamin.

7. **Vitamin B_1 (thiamin).** Thiamin deficiency can appear quickly in the first few weeks to months after surgery. Additionally, neuropathy (nerve problems) can occur in the first year after surgery, so some experts recommend taking a separate B_1 supplement for the first year.

8. **Vitamin B_6 (pyridoxal-5-phosphate or pyridoxine).** A deficiency is uncom-

mon, and B_6 is usually plentiful in a multivitamin.

9. **Vitamin B_{12}** (three potential tests: serum B_{12}, holotranscobalamin, and methylmalonic acid). This is one of the most common deficiencies after weight loss surgery, with a third of patients being deficient a year post-op. Some doctors may offer intramuscular B_{12} injections or an intranasal form.

10. **Vitamin C (ascorbic acid).** A deficiency is not common after weight loss surgery, and I don't recommend taking a separate C supplement unless there's a documented deficiency or your doctor instructs you to take it to help with iron absorption. Remember, weight loss increases kidney stone risk and vitamin C supplements by themselves can increase the risk of a calcium oxalate kidney stone. The calcium ascorbate form of C might not raise your risk as much as plain vitamin C, so talk to your doctor about this alternative.

11. **Vitamin D** (three potential tests: serum 25-OH vitamin D, 1,25-dihydroxyvitamin D, and PTH to determine efficacy of vitamin D). At a minimum you should get 800 to 1,000 IU per day (even if your levels are fine) and approximately 1,000 to 2,000 IU with a Roux-en-Y gastric bypass. (A normal blood test is 30 to 40 ng/mL.) Some medical centers like to give large initial amounts of vitamin D for patients who've had malabsorptive procedures.

12. **Vitamin E.** A deficiency is rare. Some doctors recommend 10 times the recommended daily allowance (100 to 150 IU) for patients having biliopancreatic diversion with duodenal switch.

13. **Vitamin K.** A deficiency has been observed in patients who have any type of biliopancreatic diversion. The bacteria in your large intestine produce vitamin K—along with what you get in your diet—and this is usually not affected in other types of weight loss surgery.

14. **Zinc.** It's only absorbed well in the middle part of the small intestine (the jejunum), so it's not unusual to experience zinc deficiencies after some procedures.

15. **Miscellaneous blood tests based on your medical history** (for electrolytes, such as magnesium and potassium, and albumin to check overall nutritional and protein status, for example). Magnesium and potassium deficiencies in the general population are on the rise, and I expect to see them more in bariatric patients as well. Look for foods that are high in magnesium and potassium (think heart-healthy foods, such as avocado and spinach). One problem with potassium is that the daily recommendation (4,700 milligrams per day) is high, so it's hard to get enough from your diet or even a multivitamin. The intake for magnesium is 320 milligrams daily for women and 420 milligrams for men.

Other vitamin, mineral, and trace element deficiencies—such as B_7 (biotin), chromium, iodine, manganese, B_3 (niacin), and B_5 (pantothenic acid)—are rare after a bariatric procedure.

16. **Urinary test** for calcium, citrate, oxalate, and other nutrients as suggested by your physician to evaluate the risk of kidney stones.

THE IMPORTANCE OF POSTOPERATIVE TESTING

As mentioned earlier, the American Society for Metabolic and Bariatric Surgery, the American Association of Clinical Endocrinologists, and the Obesity Society all recommend regular nutritional testing after weight loss surgery. It's usually done within 1 month of the procedure, and most patients will have to continue to get testing for the rest of their lives. How critical is it?

Here's what can happen when nutrients are not normalized after surgery.

- Vision problems, such as night blindness, can result from a deficiency of vitamins A and E. (Biliopancreatic diversion procedures can cause very low vitamin A levels.)

- Congestive heart failure and even brain abnormalities can occur with a severe vitamin B_1 deficiency.

- Diseases of the heart—and even heart failure—can occur from a selenium deficiency.

- Skin changes—such as dermatitis, rash, and itching—can occur from a deficiency of B vitamins; vitamins A, C, and E; and zinc. (Even a year post-op, 90 percent of patients who had biliopancreatic diversion with duodenal switch suffer from a zinc deficiency.)

- Neurologic problems can occur from B_{12}, B_1, B_3 (niacin), copper, and many other deficiencies.

- Bone pain, bone loss, muscle pain and cramping, and fatigue can occur from vitamin D deficiency.

- Low blood counts (anemia) can occur with a deficiency of copper, folate, iron, and B_{12}.

- Younger women who want to become pregnant after a bariatric procedure need to pay special attention to nutrient testing because deficiencies can endanger the fetus as well as the mother. Check levels of calcium; folate; iron; and vitamins A, B_{12}, and K. (Vitamin K deficiency can increase the risk of internal bleeding in the fetus.)

MOYAD FACT: Pre-op nutrient testing and supplementation can help you recover from your procedure. Nutrients such as selenium, vitamin C, and zinc play a role in wound healing, and people who are malnourished have a higher rate of postsurgery complications. Arguably, the biggest concern after weight loss surgery is an internal leak (called an anastomotic leak) around sutures in the stomach or intestine. There is some indirect research suggesting that normal nutrient blood levels may speed healing at the internal suture sites and may even reduce the risk of this kind of leak.

WHAT'S WORTHLESS

Trying to determine the exact dosage of the supplements you need after surgery without working with a physician, dietitian, and medical team specializing in bariatric surgery is very dangerous. Dosages are based on experience and regular blood testing for deficiencies and insufficiencies. Any nutrients not discussed here—such as probiotics or exotic herbal products—provide no benefit.

LIFESTYLE CHANGES

Create a network. In postsurgery studies, patients most commonly cited a need for more dietary and psychological support. Seek out a dietitian or weight loss group and ask for referrals to a therapist who has experience working with bariatric patients.

Take your time. Eat slowly, chew thoroughly, and avoid fluids for about 15 to 30 minutes before, during, and right after meals. Food can pass quickly through the stomach before you get the signal that you're full, which can lead to diarrhea.

Start with protein. It reduces the risk of muscle loss (very common in bariatric patients) and improves feelings of fullness; if you wait to eat it until later in the meal, you may be full already. Getting 60 to 120 grams of protein per day (from a variety of sources) has been shown to reduce muscle loss as you're losing weight. The more muscle you have, the more calories you'll burn every minute of every day. Protein powders (not pills) are an excellent way to reach your daily protein needs. Look for one with around 25 grams of protein for every 100 calories and no sugar (the isolate form).

Watch what you eat. More than half of bariatric patients who've had a Roux-en-Y gastric bypass report experiencing "dumping syndrome"—stomach pain, nausea, diarrhea, light-headedness, flushing, and rapid heart beat after eating certain foods. You can avoid it by reducing or eliminating the intake of simple sugars (including fruit), increasing protein intake, and eating small and frequent meals.

Remember that Hydration is your friend. The new clinical guidelines suggest drinking more than 1½ liters of fluid per day postsurgery. When you cut back on calories from food, you get less water, and when you lose weight, you lose water, so it's very easy to become dangerously dehydrated.

97

B Benign Prostatic Hyperplasia

Dr. Moyad Secret What kind of cruel joke is being played on aging men? Everything with our bodies gets smaller or shorter (muscles, height, penis) or thinner (hair, bones) with time *except* our stomachs and our prostate glands, which continue to grow bigger every year! Benign prostatic hyperplasia (BPH) is the most common male-specific health condition in the United States, and while there are a ton of supplements out there that claim to be able to help, I believe the most successful ones work by simply lowering cholesterol, which improves your heart health, and because of a large placebo effect (33 to 50 percent in some studies!). As you'll learn throughout this book, reducing your cardiovascular disease risk can make a difference with all kinds of health conditions, from BPH to varicose veins.

WHAT IS IT?

BPH is a noncancerous enlargement of the prostate gland, a walnut-size organ that surrounds the urethra (the tube that carries urine from the bladder out through the penis) and secretes fluid that helps make up semen. BPH increases the risk of erectile dysfunction, but there is *no* relationship between BPH and the risk of prostate cancer. This is good news! Your age *is* directly related to your risk of BPH, though. You have a 40 percent risk in your forties, a 50 percent risk in your fifties, and so on. If you're lucky enough to live to be 100, well, you'll have to deal with BPH.

The incidence of BPH is on the rise thanks to the baby boomers. But it's also due to heart-unhealthy lifestyle choices. Men who are obese, don't exercise, or have high "bad" cholesterol, low "good" cholesterol, and high blood pressure also have a higher risk of BPH.

Because the gland surrounds the urethra, when it gets bigger, it can affect the flow of urine. That's why common symptoms include frequent urination (especially at night), increased urgency, weak stream, dribbling, starting and stopping, and a feeling that your bladder hasn't emptied. (These are sometimes referred to as lower urinary tract symptoms, or LUTS.) If you're experiencing these, go online and download the American Urological Association (AUA) Symptom Score or the International Prostate Symptom Score (I-PSS) questionnaire, fill it out, and take it to your primary care doctor or urologist. They're both very short (they take less than 2 minutes), and the higher your score, the higher the chance that you have BPH. Your score also provides a baseline so that when you get treated, you can retake the test and see if you've improved. In addition to asking about the previous symptoms, the AUA Symptom Score questionnaire also inquires about how BPH symptoms affect your quality of life, which is hugely important.

Size does not always matter when it comes to BPH. Some men with tiny prostates have terrible symptoms of BPH, and others with gigantic prostates have few to no symptoms. What matters is whether the urethra is being pinched or squeezed.

Prescription BPH medications either relax the prostate (alpha-blockers) or shrink it (5-alpha-reductase inhibitors). Due to multiple side effects and cost, BPH prescriptions have wildly varying compliance rates, from 10 to 60 percent. The alpha-blockers can cause retrograde ejaculation (it goes up into the bladder instead of out the urethra—ouch!), orthostatic hypotension (you get dizzy when you stand up), and an increased risk of falls. The 5-alpha-reductase inhibitors can reduce libido and increase erectile dysfunction. So as you can see, there's plenty of room (and need) for a safe, effective, over-the-counter, research-based dietary supplement.

WHAT WORKS

Note: These supplements can be used with conventional BPH treatment options.

1. (tie) Beta-sitosterol and other plant sterols 60 to 195 milligrams a day in divided doses (or up to 2,000 to 3,000 milligrams a day in divided doses potentially)

Phytosterols, or plant sterols, are found in a variety of plants and plant oils, and this is the only way we can get them (we can't make them ourselves). They block the uptake of cholesterol from dietary and bile sources in the intestinal tract. They also reduce LDL (bad) cholesterol, but do not impact HDL (good) and triglycerides. (This is somewhat similar to how some healthy dietary fats, such as those found in almonds or pistachios, may also reduce LDL.) The main phytosterols found in our diets are sitosterol, stigmasterol, campesterol, and beta-sitosterol.

Since plants arguably contain more beta-sitosterols than the other phytosterols, they've been the subject of many studies, but there are only four that I consider to be high quality. (No well-done studies have been published in the past 10 years, by the way.) One of the four showed beta-sitosterol did not work better than a placebo, but the other three showed a big improvement in urinary flow and frequency in patients with moderate BPH taking beta-sitosterol. These studies used higher dosages (20 to 65 milligrams three times a day, or 60 to 195 milligrams total) within a mixture of phytosterols. The beta-sitosterol used in these studies is called Harzol, or Azuprostat, which is usually derived from South African star grass. Since it's very tough to get these products in the United States today, you can look for beta-sitosterol as a stand-alone ingredient. The studies used products with at least a 50 percent concentration of beta-sitosterol and in the form nonglucosidic beta-sitosterol. (It's interesting that the single study that did not work used a different form of beta-sitosterol.)

Overall, there were no differences in withdrawal rates in the beta-sitosterol group compared to the placebo group (both were around 8 percent). Gastrointestinal side effects were the most common complaint (1.6 percent) and erectile dysfunction was another side effect, but only in approximately 0.5 percent of men.

I've talked about making heart-healthy changes to impact BPH because improving cholesterol levels and exercising does improve symptoms in some men. There have been more than 50 clinical trials using phytosterols for lowering LDL cholesterol. As a result, plant sterols have even been added to some foods, including yogurt, margarine, orange juice, mayonnaise, olive oil, and milk. The typical phytosterol dose to reduce LDL by 6 to 15 percent, based on research, is 2,000 to 3,000 milligrams a day. This is 10 times higher than the dose that worked in the BPH trials! But I have seen it work for BPH patients many times throughout my career, so taking this much plant sterol to reduce BPH could also reduce your cholesterol and may be an option if lower doses do not work. You can get it by taking one or two caplets twice a day with a glass of water right before your largest meals (so you can block cholesterol absorption). You can also just buy the enhanced food products. (For more information on supplements for lowering cholesterol, see the High Cholesterol section, page 234.)

1. (tie) *Pygeum africanum* 75 to 200 milligrams a day in divided doses

Most of the active substances in *Pygeum africanum* (bark of the African plum tree) are triterpenes, ferulic acid esters, and phytosterols, including beta-sitosterols, which could have anti-BPH properties, although beta-sitosterol is the most researched, as previously mentioned. *Pygeum africanum* has been used in Europe since 1969 for the treatment of mild to moderate BPH, and it arguably has the largest number of consistently positive clinical trials to date compared to almost any other dietary supplement product for BPH right now. Laboratory research suggests that it can lower some growth factors that could impact the prostate, and it may also have anti-inflammatory effects.

An analysis of 18 *Pygeum africanum* clinical trials involving 1,562 men suggested a potential benefit with this supplement. The majority of the studies looked at the effects of taking 75 to 200 milligrams a day (usually standardized to 14 percent sterol content or higher, which is what you should look for when you're buying a product) divided into two doses. The average age of participants was 66, and the average study duration was 64 days. Out of 13 placebo-controlled trials, 12 reported a positive impact on at least one measure of symptoms (such as flow rate or frequency) with Pygeum; men taking it were more than twice as likely to report an improvement in overall symptoms compared to the placebo groups. Nocturia, or getting up at night to pee, was reduced by almost one episode per night (this failed to reach statistical significance, but for most men this is still a big improvement!). The withdrawal rate was similar to the placebo (12 percent), as were side effects, which were usually GI-related.

However, there are two big problems with Pygeum. First, there has not been a well-done study in more than a decade (similar to beta-sitosterol). Second, it comes from an endangered tree and the demand, as you would expect, is high. Year after year, the supply appears to wane. (This is not the case with most other BPH nutraceuticals, such as pumpkin seed, which you'll read about in the next column.) As a result, there are quality-control issues. Whether companies are selling the actual Pygeum used in studies or a new or altered version of it usually isn't clear from the packaging alone. So check with the manufacturer to find out where its Pygeum came from (the company is obligated to tell you).

2. (tie) Flaxseed and SDG 300 to 600 milligrams a day

I'm a big advocate of flaxseed for BPH simply because, if nothing else, it's heart healthy and low cost. Not to mention, both preliminary clinical research and my own experience with it have been positive. In one clinical trial with 87 patients, 300 to

600 milligrams daily of a flaxseed-derived supplement called secoisolariciresinol diglucoside (SDG), made of purified lignan (phytoestrogen) extract, significantly improved urinary symptoms compared to the placebo. Similar SDG products have also been found to significantly reduce cholesterol and glucose levels. Whether ingesting inexpensive ground flaxseed powder (2 to 3 tablespoons per day) will reduce BPH symptoms as well as an SDG supplement has not been well studied, but it should be. Preliminary research from Duke University suggests taking 3 tablespoons of ground flaxseed a day has an anti-inflammatory effect on BPH tissue, which could potentially improve flow and reduce frequency in some men.

2. (tie) Pumpkin seed (*Cucurbita pepo*) oil 320 milligrams a day

It's used as a salad oil in countries such as Austria, and maybe we should take a cue from them! The majority of the fatty acids in pumpkin seeds are monounsaturated and polyunsaturated, both healthy fats. The seeds are also high in alpha- and gamma-tocopherol and tocotrienol (vitamin E), carotenoids (including lutein and zeaxanthin), and plant sterols. To sum up, they're loaded with heart-healthy compounds, which might as well be prostate-healthy compounds.

There has been some preliminary lab data showing that pumpkin seed oil may slow BPH growth by reducing prostate weight, protein content, and prostatic acid phosphatase levels and by altering cholesterol metabolism. This data also suggest, similar to beta-sitosterol and Pygeum, a potential preventive role for pumpkin seed oil when it comes to BPH. Clinical studies have been either small or not that well done, but they're still impressive: One randomized, double-blind, placebo-controlled trial with 47 patients who had moderate to severe BPH saw improved flow and reduced frequency with 320 milligrams per day of pumpkin seed oil in pill form over 12 months. But if you have to take more than one or two pills daily, or if cost is an issue, then I'm not so excited about it.

HONORABLE MENTION

Cernilton (a pollen extract mixture) is fairly well known for prostate health because it has been shown to significantly improve quality of life and reduce pain in men with chronic prostatitis/chronic pelvic pain syndrome (see the Chronic Prostatitis/Chronic Pelvic Pain Syndrome section, page 135). Study results have suggested it has anti-inflammatory and muscle relaxation effects in the prostate and maybe even in the bladder and urethra, which may explain why it has shown preliminary positive results in BPH research.

In two past meta-analyses (which are essentially reviews of clinical studies), published in the *Cochrane Database of Systematic Reviews* and *BJU International*, that included 444 men from four different clinical trials, 63 milligrams of Cernilton twice daily improved self-rated symptoms, such as the number of times the subjects got up to urinate (about one less time); side effects were mild and rare.

In another study of 240 patients with moderate BPH, researchers compared two doses: 350 and 750 milligrams of Cernilton twice a day for 4 years. The higher dose group showed more rapid improvement as well as a more significant reduction of prostate size and urinary symptoms, including less urine left in the bladder after urinating and improved urinary flow rates. The high-dose subjects also required less surgery. However, there hasn't been any good, positive research done recently, and there are quality control issues with Cernilton, so buyer beware.

WHAT'S WORTHLESS

Saw palmetto. I'm rejecting the most popular dietary supplement for BPH in the world? Yes! I'm not a fan because of two very well-done US government–funded trials: STEP (Saw Palmetto for Treatment of Enlarged Prostates) and CAMUS (Complementary and Alternative Medicine for Urological Symptoms). Plus, patients I've worked with over the years tend to see minimal or reduced efficacy over time, which suggests more of a placebo effect. Anyhow, back to the research.

The STEP trial was one of the better herbal studies ever completed. It was funded by the National Institute of Diabetes and Digestive and Kidney Diseases and by the National Center for Complementary and Alternative Medicine. A total of 225 men with moderate to severe BPH symptoms were randomized to saw palmetto extract at a dosage of 160 milligrams twice a day (320 milligrams total) or a placebo. After 12 months of treatment, there was no difference between saw palmetto and the placebo. (The herbal extract used in this trial was one of the best.)

The CAMUS trial was a double-blind, multicenter, placebo-controlled randomized study conducted at 11 North American clinics with 369 patients. The CAMUS researchers found that low (320 milligrams), moderate (640 milligrams), and high doses (960 milligrams) of saw palmetto given over 72 weeks did not work better than a placebo for BPH or LUTS. Again, the saw palmetto used was outstanding quality.

By the way, these big trials were originally designed to compare supplements to standard prescription drugs, but no companies offered up their drugs for testing! Makes you wonder.

Stinging nettle. Different parts of this plant have different effects. Apparently, the roots are used for BPH, but the bulk of the studies were completed long ago, they weren't well designed, and the results weren't impressive. Plus, there is potential for numerous diverse side effects.

Zinc. High doses (80 to 100 milligrams or more) of this mineral have been associated with increased BPH severity and an increased risk of prostate cancer, respectively. One of the largest studies of zinc supplements showed that megadoses of zinc actually *cause* megaprostate problems!

LIFESTYLE CHANGES

Heart healthy = prostate healthy. Virtually any lifestyle change found to be heart healthy has been shown to reduce the risk or progression of BPH, including maintaining normal blood pressure, blood sugar, and cholesterol levels and a healthy weight or waist size, eating a healthy diet, and exercising. Alpha-blockers are the top-selling drug class used to treat BPH; they work by relaxing the prostate. They were originally derived from blood pressure–lowering medicines because men reported peeing better when their high blood pressure was reduced. Bam!

Drink in moderation. This has been consistently associated with a lower risk of BPH and reduced symptoms associated with BPH, probably due to the anti-inflammatory effects or the heart-healthy benefits of moderate alcohol consumption. Of course, this doesn't mean you should *start* drinking if you don't currently imbibe.

Work up a sweat. One of the best ways to prevent BPH or reduce the progression of it is to exercise regularly, about 30 minutes a day. In a famous Harvard study, regular physical activity was even associated with a lower risk of getting surgery for BPH! Patients tell me all the time that after a good, long aerobic workout, their urinary stream seems stronger, and this is further proof of how exercise relaxes the prostate and helps improve urinary function.

103

B Bipolar Disorder

THE JURY'S STILL OUT

Dr. Moyad Secret Heart healthy = bipolar disorder healthy? Yes! Individuals with bipolar disorder tend to also have a higher incidence of metabolic syndrome and other cardiovascular risk factors, such as high cholesterol, high blood pressure, obesity, and diabetes. In addition, a lack of physical activity and less than optimal eating habits are more likely with this disorder, which only further impact physical and mental health. Interestingly, preliminary studies of exercise have shown it can potentially lower the risk of depression, anxiety, and stress and should be added to any treatment regimen. And even though conventional treatment can improve this condition dramatically, more than 50 percent of patients continue to have what are known as subthreshold symptoms, such as low-level depression. A similar percentage have difficulty adhering to medications because of side effects, so you should explore adding anything with a high benefit-to-risk scenario.

NAC (N-acetylcysteine). Taking 1,000 milligrams of NAC twice daily may improve depression because glutathione (one of the main internally produced antioxidants) metabolism appears to be disrupted in multiple mental health disorders, and NAC is a precursor of glutathione. In a 6-month, multisite Australian study, 75 participants reported significantly improved depression when using NAC along with conventional treatment (called add on NAC). It didn't impact cognition in bipolar disorder, but the reduction in depression was significant enough to warrant a discussion with your physician.

A small pilot trial in Brazil of 1,000 milligrams of NAC twice a day over 24 weeks (in bipolar II disorder patients) found a significant reduction in depression. These research groups (the Australian and Brazilian) are also seeing some improvement in mania symptoms at these same NAC dosages. This is still preliminary, but since treatment for bipolar disorder is resistant to many medications, NAC could be helpful for some people.

Omega-3 fatty acids. Researchers are evaluating a reduction in depression in children and adults with bipolar disorder with approximately 1,000 to 2,000 milligrams of omega-3 fatty acids from marine sources. It may help by reducing the overactivity of cellular signals transmitted in the brain.

Chromium picolinate (500 to 1,000 micrograms per day). This supplement appears to improve the metabolism of glucose and fat, which could enhance neurotransmitter production, and preliminary research suggests it may improve depression. Some studies with this supplement have shown large dropout rates, though, which is concerning.

Folic acid. Folate depletion also appears to occur in the severe depression phase of some bipolar disorders, and it's worth supplementing (500 micrograms of folic acid or more) to reduce depression.

Inositol. This vitamin-like substance is present in all body tissues, with the highest concentrations being in the brain and heart. Supplementation may modulate serotonin activity, and it's also being tested for depression in bipolar disorder. The only issue I have with this supplement is large doses—as high as 12 grams—have been used in some successful preliminary studies, which can be hard to take.

Magnesium oxide. Taking 300 to 400 milligrams per day may improve the conversion of 5-HTP to serotonin, a calming neurotransmitter, and 5-HTP supplementation may do the same, but dosages must be worked out on an individual basis.

Choline. Supplementation modulates high-energy phosphate metabolism and is also being studied to improve mania in bipolar disorder, but preliminary clinical data hasn't shown any benefit. Since it's receiving more large-scale research and derivatives of it are showing potential promise, I think this supplement is worth discussing with your doctor.

Ketogenic diet. A ketogenic diet (high in fat) may help some patients by altering cellular signaling in a beneficial way (it may restore or reboot more healthy brainwave activity). Doctors use these diets to treat seizures in kids and adults who don't respond to medications or cannot tolerate antiepileptic drugs. And since some antiepileptic drugs have been used to treat bipolar disorder, it's worth discussing with a specialist. There are some small studies of ketogenic dieting in bipolar II disorder under way, and I'm keeping an eye on them.

B Bladder Cancer

Dr. Moyad Secret Probiotics are touted for so many medical conditions—digestive health, colds, weight loss, autoimmune disorders—but what you never hear "experts" telling the public is that the strongest area of clinical research with probiotics in medicine is for bladder cancer (during and after conventional treatment), where they have been used for several decades. If you've been diagnosed with bladder cancer, you should have a mandatory discussion with your physician about including probiotics in your treatment regimen. In my experience, very few doctors who treat bladder cancer have been educated about the benefits of probiotics in this situation, but no other supplements have anywhere near the data that probiotics do for this condition.

WHAT IS IT?

Each year almost 400,000 people worldwide are diagnosed with bladder cancer, and about 75,000 of those are in the United States. Blood in the urine (hematuria) is the most common symptom that leads to testing and a diagnosis. Nonmuscle invasive (or superficial) bladder cancer accounts for 80 percent of cases. In general, this type has a good prognosis because it usually stays localized (it doesn't leave the bladder), although bladder cancer does have a reputation for coming back over and over again. When you're diagnosed, your doctor will tell you if your cancer is low grade (not that aggressive), high grade (more aggressive), or muscle invasive (very aggressive, needing surgery as well as chemo or radiation in most cases).

Besides tobacco use, other risk factors for bladder cancer include a family history, previous pelvic radiation to the bladder, a history of inflammation of the bladder, occupational exposure to chemicals (such as in the synthetic dye manufacturing industry), and contaminated drinking water (including high arsenic levels in well water).

WHAT WORKS

Note: All of the supplements recommended in this section were studied either for prevention or in individuals with nonmuscle invasive bladder cancer.

1. *Lactobacillus casei* Shirota probiotic 3,000 milligrams a day for at least 1 year following conventional treatment, or Yakult drink for prevention or treatment

Researchers are not positive, but they think this probiotic appears to improve the body's immune response to bladder tumors, possibly by activating so-called natural killer cells within the immune system and inducing cancer cell death. There's a milklike product called Yakult that contains a high concentration of this probiotic strain, and it may also be associated with a reduced risk of bladder cancer (meaning it may help prevent cancer). Researchers believe the probiotic may detoxify carcinogens or other toxins when they hit the bladder, preventing them from taking up residence there. Drinking a serving (approximately 3 ounces) of Yakult several times a week if you're at high risk is a good preventive strategy, or if you don't want to take the lactobacillus pills posttreatment, this is an adequate replacement.

So let's talk research: Randomized trials with this probiotic strain were first completed more than 25 years ago. Two older trials were conducted in individuals with superficial localized transitional cell cancer of the bladder to determine the effect of taking 3 grams of oral *L. casei* Shirota (biolactis powder) daily. Researchers specifically hoped to determine whether the cancer would return after being removed. Both trials showed a significant reduction in the risk of bladder cancer recurrence 1 to 2 years posttreatment. (Mild diarrhea was the primary side effect in 5 percent of the study subjects.) Another trial with patients who had surgery for superficial bladder cancer compared recurrence rates with the drug epirubicin (an intravesical chemotherapy treatment)

alone and with the drug along with *L. casei* Shirota. The combination group had a significantly greater chance (75 percent) of going 3 years posttreatment without recurrence versus the drug-alone group (60 percent).

You can purchase the same probiotic agent used in these patients in capsule form (although it's easier to just use the Yakult; one 2.7-ounce serving is one dose). Each dose, which may be one to two capsules, contains about 1×10^{10} cells of *L. casei* Shirota strain per gram (the dosage used in the research is 3,000 milligrams or 3 grams per day). The capsule form has been tested in several clinical trials now with positive results, and side effects have been similar to a placebo. It has been used as an "add on" (during or after conventional treatment) for bladder cancer in Japan for 25 to 30 years, so I'm comfortable with the benefit-to-risk ratio here. You should definitely talk to your doctor about this one. Again, the research appears to show a benefit for low-grade bladder cancers treated by resection only (not tested with BCG treatment) and in some cases chemotherapy.

2. Centrum Silver or an equivalent multivitamin one capsule daily for prevention and after conventional treatment

I know multivitamins have been under a lot of scrutiny in the last few years, and it's partly deserved because some companies have made them so complicated (you have to take multiple pills and they're expensive) without having research to back them up. Low-dose multivitamins, such as Centrum Silver, have very good research and safety records and deserve more respect. In fact, Centrum Silver was tested in one of the largest and best studies in the history of dietary supplement medicine to determine if it could reduce the risk of cancer. This study, known as the Physicians' Healthy Study II (a.k.a. PHS II), was a randomized, double-blind, placebo-controlled trial with more than 14,000 super-healthy male doctors ages 50 or older at baseline (some had a history of cancer). The study began in 1997 and follow-up was completed in 2011. At that point, 2,669 men had been diagnosed with cancer. Men who took a daily multivitamin had a statistically significant (8 percent) reduction in the risk of cancer, but those men who had a baseline history of cancer, meaning they had a higher risk of getting cancer, experienced a 27 percent decrease in the risk of being diagnosed with cancer. There was also a statistically nonsignificant (12 percent) reduction in cancer deaths in the multivitamin group compared to the placebo. Researchers did see a large (28 percent), albeit statistically insignificant, reduction in bladder cancer risk compared to other cancers and a reduction in bladder cancer deaths. If the trial had been allowed to go a bit longer, I believe these stats would have reached significance (it was close).

The side effects were similar to a placebo, except for a higher number of rashes in the supplement group. This is exciting! A basic low-dose adult multivitamin daily may reduce the risk of bladder cancer by providing enough nutrients to allow for optimal immune function, keeping bladder cancer as well as other types from forming. No supplements have been tested for this long and have shown this kind of safety and efficacy against cancer, especially bladder cancer.

HONORABLE MENTION

Selenium is currently being tested in a large clinical trial called SELEBLAT (Selenium and Bladder Cancer Trial) that is testing a dose of 200 micrograms of selenium (from a yeast source) a day to determine if it can reduce the risk of bladder cancer returning after conventional treatment. It's being conducted at 18 hospitals in Belgium. In other studies, such high dosages of selenium have shown some scary side effects, including increased risk of diabetes and recurrence of skin cancer. I don't recommend going this route until the results of the SELEBLAT study are in. Even then, will it be worth the risk? I'm skeptical, but we shall know soon enough.

WHAT'S WORTHLESS

High doses of vitamins and minerals. A multi appears to work, so wouldn't a "turbocharged" multi work even better? No! But this is how the thinking got started: In 1994, a small (67 patients) trial published in the *Journal of Urology* found bladder cancer patients appeared to have a reduced risk of recurrence after conventional treatment when taking large doses of certain supplements. This study obviously required larger randomized trials to confirm its findings, but the initial result was so promising that many patients started taking the supplement that was tested (a product called Oncovit). Megadoses of nutrients were used with conventional bladder cancer treatment (BCG).

Finally, a larger, more definitive study (670 patients from 75 medical centers) was published in 2010 in the same journal showing the large doses below did not work better than a standard multivitamin supplement.

- Vitamin A (36,000 IU per day)
- Vitamin B$_6$ (100 milligrams per day)
- Vitamin C (2,000 milligrams per day)
- Vitamin D$_3$ (1,600 IU per day)
- Folic acid (1,600 micrograms or 1.6 milligrams per day)
- Vitamin E (400 IU per day)
- Zinc (30.4 milligrams per day)

My guess is that the original study subjects had a variety of vitamin and mineral deficiencies, so the megadoses probably did reduce the risk of recurrence. But today, most patients are not deficient. We're getting oversupplemented with antioxidants from foods, beverages, and supplements. And as we all know, too much of a good thing isn't always good. In some cases—like vitamin E—it can increase cancer growth.

Vitamin B$_6$. This important vitamin impacts the metabolism of numerous compounds in the body, and there used to be some research suggesting that it could favorably reduce the amount of toxic compounds affecting the bladder. But a large study known as EORTC (European Organization for Research and Treatment of Cancer), done by the Genitourinary Tract Cancer Cooperative Group, found no significant difference in recurrence rates between vitamin B$_6$ and a placebo. This study, published in 1995, shows just how long bladder cancer researchers have been doing large studies on dietary supplements.

Exotic herbal products with no quality control. I will never understand why some people are willing to take the risk on products like these. For instance, some herbal supplements contain a compound called aristolochic acid that occurs naturally in specific plants. But it belongs to a family of carcinogenic compounds, and it can increase the risk of permanent kidney damage and bladder cancer! Even herbalists who've handled it in Asia have a higher risk of getting these medical conditions. It's illegal in the United States, but we all know that you can buy products from all over the world these days. Know what you're buying and whom you're buying it from. You have to do your research!

LIFESTYLE CHANGES

Heart healthy = bladder healthy. Some factors that are associated with an

MOYAD FACT: The same vaccine that's used to prevent tuberculosis (BCG) is used to treat bladder cancer! Your doctor inserts it into the bladder via the urethra, which causes an immune reaction that can clear superficial bladder tumors. And it's generally very safe. Amazing!

increased risk of heart disease are also associated with a higher risk of bladder cancer, especially smoking and tobacco use. (Some preliminary studies suggest—and I agree with them—that smokeless tobacco also increases risk.) Other factors, such as weight gain, have not been linked to bladder cancer, but controlling your weight and adopting heart-healthy habits—such as eating a healthy diet and maintaining normal cholesterol, blood sugar, and blood pressure levels—is a no-brainer since not doing so contributes to so many other diseases and conditions.

Hydrate—but not too much. Here's the rule: Clear colored urine is healthy urine. Fluid consumption may reduce the risk of bladder cancer by reducing the ability of carcinogens to attach for long periods to the inside of the bladder, but it does not appear to treat bladder cancer or benefit conventional treatment. In fact, drinking too much water reduces blood sodium levels and can be life threatening, but this is rare.

Check your water supply. Inorganic arsenic in drinking water has been found to be a potential carcinogen to the skin and lungs, and I am convinced it increases the risk of bladder cancer as well. Arsenic occurs naturally throughout the environment, and it's primarily transported through water. Municipal water systems routinely check for arsenic (you can request the testing results) and are generally safe, but private water supplies are at risk and should be tested.

Chew gum. What? No, chomping on a stick of gum does not prevent or treat bladder cancer, but it may speed recovery after surgery: Recent evidence suggests that patients who chew gum several times a day after bladder cancer–removal surgery are more likely to get their bowels moving again, which speeds recovery time. Chewing sends a message to the gastrointestinal tract to get ready for food, so the bowels begin their natural movement. Get your doctor's permission though, and only do it if you're sitting upright.

Get more omega-3s from plants. An interesting US study found that people who regularly consumed omega-3 fatty acids (alpha-linolenic acid or ALA) from plants had an almost 75 percent reduction in the risk of bladder cancer. Certain foods—such as walnuts, canola oil, flaxseed, and chia seeds—are loaded with ALA and have been shown to potentially reduce the risk of heart disease as well.

Load up on veggies. Cruciferous veggies (broccoli, cauliflower, Brussels sprouts, kale, cabbage, and bok choy, to name a handful) reduce the risk of bladder cancer. They're also low in calories and high in fiber and nutrients.

Breast Cancer

B

Dr. Moyad Secret This topic is near and dear to me (like prostate cancer) because my beautiful cousin died at age 38 from this disease. Even with all the money that has been devoted to cancer research and treatment, most cases cannot be tracked to a particular cause. Age is one of the biggest risk factors, and genetics play a strong role as well. The good news is that research has quite clearly shown that exercising and maintaining a normal weight/waist size (especially after menopause) are two of the best ways to prevent this disease. So—you know I'm going to say it—heart healthy = breast healthy! The smartest thing a woman can do to reduce her risk of breast cancer is to reduce her risk of cardiovascular disease to as close to zero as possible.

WHAT IS IT?

Breast cancer can occur in various structures within the breast, but especially the milk ducts and glands. It's the second most common cancer (after skin cancer) in women; approximately 1 percent of cases occur in men. While there may be no early signs, common symptoms once a tumor takes hold include puckering or dimpling of the breast; a fixed, painless nodule or lump (although there can be pain and tenderness); unusual nipple discharge or a change in appearance of the nipple; and redness or a change in color of the breast.

Risk factors include:

- Age (risk increases as you get older)
- Benign breast disease (hyperplasia, or extra cells, increases risk)
- Breast density (the denser the tissue, the higher the risk)
- Early menstruation (before 12) and late menopause (after 55); menstruation involves regular hormonal stimulation, which can encourage the growth of abnormal breast cells
- Family history, especially if it involves early diagnosis (fifties or younger)
- Genes (5 to 10 percent of cases can be traced to a gene, such as BRCA1 and BRCA2)
- Giving birth later (giving birth before age 30, especially, might normalize breast cells and lower risk)
- Height (the taller you are, the higher the risk, perhaps due to greater exposure to growth factors at earlier ages)
- Jewish ethnicity (those of Ashkenazi or European descent have a higher risk, probably due to gene mutations)
- Postmenopausal obesity

WHAT WORKS

Note: I don't recommend any supplements to prevent breast cancer or help with conventional treatment. In fact, there is some evidence to suggest that, similar to prostate cancer, overexposure to certain supplements could increase risk and block the effects of conventional treatment. However, there are some incredible supplements to discuss with your doctor that can help you deal with the side effects of treatment, and some researchers believe they may also have some anticancer properties.

1. (tie) American ginseng (*Panax quinquefolius*) 2,000 milligrams a day (1,000 milligrams around breakfast and 1,000 milligrams around lunch) for at least 2 months, especially right before or during cancer treatment for cancer-related fatigue

Ginseng may reduce the inflammatory process associated with cancer, which in turn impacts cortisol levels and reduces stress and fatigue. In a very well-done Mayo Clinic–directed study (contrary to what some "experts" in alternative medicine suggest, most of the best medical centers in the United States embrace evidence-based dietary supplements) with 364 cancer patients at different stages of treatment, participants took either 2,000 milligrams of Wisconsin ginseng, a common type of American ginseng, or a placebo. (Approximately 60 percent of the participants had breast cancer.) By the end of the first month, both groups were experiencing a reduction in cancer-related fatigue. After about 2 months, twice as many ginseng patients reported a decrease in fatigue. Side effects were similar to a placebo. After further analysis, patients receiving radiation or chemotherapy had significantly better results at 4 and 8 weeks with the ginseng compared to the placebo. People who were just starting conventional treatment—and perhaps didn't have as much fatigue yet—responded better than those who were further on in the process (who would be expected to have more severe fatigue). As a result, researchers speculated that ginseng could be better for preventing fatigue—or keeping it from getting worse—than for treating severe fatigue. (As I was preparing this section, a preliminary clinical trial from MD Anderson Cancer Center found similar benefits in cancer patients with Panax ginseng at similar dosages.)

The ginseng used consisted of pure ground root from one production lot (manufactured by Beehive Botanicals) and contained 3 percent ginsenosides, which researchers believe are the active ingredients. Most ginseng products on the market have at least 3 percent; some go as high as 50 percent. The higher the concentration of ginsenosides, the lower the dose you should start with. The same research group at the

Mayo Clinic saw some benefits for cancer-related fatigue at 1,000 milligrams per day with a 5 percent ginsenoside product in a previous clinical trial.

It's so encouraging that there were no side effects beyond what the placebo group experienced, and American ginseng has been found to have no strong drug interactions so far either. One interesting thing to keep in mind: The researchers at the Mayo Clinic made it clear that certain extraction properties (the purifying process to isolate the active ingredient) with ginseng and its ginsenosides could theoretically disrupt treatment. For example, ginseng from methanol extraction may have some estrogenic properties, which could be harmful for some breast cancer patients. Ginseng derived from water extraction or from pure ground root has not demonstrated estrogenic characteristics, and it may even have cancer cell–inhibiting properties. Regardless, discuss this with your doctor ASAP because there is currently no safe, effective pharmaceutical option for cancer-related fatigue (just a lot of off-label stimulants).

the nausea. This is only a theory, but I agree with it. Arguably, the best study was done by the University of Rochester Cancer Center and the National Cancer Institute's Community Clinical Oncology Program, which is known as URCC CCOP. In this study of 576 patients (93 percent female), participants took a purified liquid extract of ginger root with 8.5 milligrams of concentrated combined gingerol, zingerone, and shogaol, equivalent to 250 milligrams of ginger root, in extra virgin olive oil (made by Aphios Corporation). Almost 75 percent were being treated for breast cancer (others had gastrointestinal or lung cancers). Ginger reduced nausea 40 percent more than the placebo. Higher dosages (2,000 milligrams a day) did not work better than lower dosages (1,000 milligrams). Side effects are rare with ginger but can include heartburn, bruising/flushing, and rash. *Note:* There is some preliminary evidence that consuming a high-protein diet with ginger could potentially be even more beneficial for nausea. (See the Nausea and Vomiting section, page 333.)

1. (tie) Ginger (*Zingiber officinale*)

500 to 1,000 milligrams 3 days before receiving chemotherapy and 3 days after chemotherapy (repeat at next cycle) for chemotherapy-induced nausea along with conventional drug treatment for nausea

Researchers believe ginger might prepare the gut for chemotherapy-induced nausea by sending a message to the brain to ignore

2. Guarana (*Paullinia cupana*)

50 milligrams twice a day for cancer-related fatigue and various other symptoms

This plant from the Amazon River basin has been used as a stimulant for ages because it contains caffeine, but it also has a high saponin and tannin content, which may also contribute to reducing fatigue and improving focus. The most famous study with cancer-related fatigue and guarana was done in Brazil. Researchers used a standardized extract with a 6.46 percent caffeine content (not much) and 1.7 percent tannin content. Essentially, patients in this study received only about 5 milligrams of caffeine a day from guarana (a standard cup of coffee has 50 to 100 milligrams). More than 70 patients took either a 50-milligram supplement or a placebo for 3 weeks, then took nothing for a week, and then crossed over to the other group (placebo subjects took the supplement and vice versa). After 21 days, half of the guarana patients reported significantly reduced fatigue compared to about 10 percent of the placebo group.

Most other trials have also used guarana with a fairly low caffeine content. When I (and others) have tried it, the effects seem to go beyond what you'd expect with just caffeine; it doesn't make you jittery, and it allows you to maintain your concentration and focus. Instead of a roller-coaster effect—with higher energy and then a crash—it's more of a consistent merry-go-round feel. This is why guarana is also being studied for other symptoms of breast cancer treatment, such as depression and the memory, mood, and attention disruptions associated with so-called chemo brain. While the participants in the breast cancer (and most) studies did not report anxiety and insomnia (as you might expect with products containing caffeine), I wouldn't take it in the late afternoon because it could be too stimulating for some people.

3. Calcium up to 1,000 to 1,200 milligrams a day and **vitamin D** 600 to 800 IU a day or enough to normalize the 25-OH vitamin D blood test (30 to 40 ng/mL)

Bone loss is a major problem with many breast cancer treatments, and calcium and vitamin D have been a part of almost every successful clinical study of an osteoporosis drug for bone loss. They maximize the effects of these drugs. Even if you don't need an osteoporosis medication, calcium and vitamin D can still support bone health. And you don't necessarily need to take them in supplement form: There is so much calcium in various food and beverages today that it's easy to get your daily 1,000- to 1,200-milligram dose from diet alone.

The Institute of Medicine recommends 600 to 800 IU of vitamin D a day (many of the low-dose multivitamins have 400 to 1,000 IU per pill), but every breast cancer patient should get a 25-OH vitamin D test to check for any profound D deficiency (less than 10 ng/mL), which would require higher doses. Vitamin D_3 (usually derived from an animal source) and vitamin D_2 (plant source) supplements are both effective; the human body makes vitamin D_3 when exposed to sunlight, and it's the form that has been used in more clinical trials, so it may be slightly more potent. In reality, I think both are fine.

There is a lot of talk about calcium and especially vitamin D to reduce breast cancer risk, but the data is weak. It's not weak in the area of preventing bone loss and arthralgia, though, which is important especially when one of the primary and most effective treatments in breast cancer is to eliminate estrogen or reduce the effects of it. Estrogen is the primary hormone responsible for maintaining or improving bone mineral density; when you take it away or decrease the effects of it, bone loss accelerates. There's also concern over calcium and heart disease risk, but this is more for people who get more than 1,000 to 1,200 milligrams per day. Finally, calcium and vitamin D results may even be more profound when combined with resistance exercise (always check with your doctor to make sure this is allowed during or after treatment). Synergy!

HONORABLE MENTION

Diosmin or oxerutin (rutin), both types of flavonoids, may be beneficial for severe lymphedema (see the Varicose Veins and Chronic Venous Insufficiency section, page 442, and the Hemorrhoids section, page 226). Lymphedema of the arms after breast cancer treatment is a major problem, and there really aren't any good conventional or alternative solutions, with the exception of specialized massage therapy. However, an older study of women with breast cancer who took 1,000 milligrams a day (in two 500-milligram doses) of diosmin for 6 months showed it may improve lymphatic drainage and swelling. I think it has more promise as a preventive therapy than as a treatment; it's worth discussing with your doctor, regardless.

Oxerutin, a cousin of diosmin, is also used for varicose veins and hemorrhoids. When taken for 6 months (up to 3,000 milligrams a day), it could reduce swelling, immobility, and discomfort from lymphedema caused by breast cancer treatment.

WHAT'S WORTHLESS?

Magnesium oxide. No supplement has consistently worked for reducing hot flashes in breast cancer patients, but I had my fingers crossed for this because it is inexpensive and had shown preliminary promise. (It's also being studied for other hot flash–related symptoms, such as fatigue and sweating.) The biggest problem with any hot flash remedy is that the placebo response rate is consistently high, so it's difficult for anything to beat it on a consistent basis. Study results just came out on this, and it failed to beat the placebo. Of course, since it worked as well as placebo and is safe, you could try it if you wanted to.

Miscellaneous. L-carnitine and CoQ10 have not been able to reduce fatigue in cancer patients better than a placebo; soy pills and most others do not reduce hot flashes more than a placebo in breast cancer; horse chestnut seed extract does not appear to reduce lymphedema; and taking higher doses of folic acid (more than 400 micrograms) is unnecessary and could interfere with some breast cancer treatments and encourage breast cancer growth.

THE SOY CONTROVERSY

Soy is a very heart-healthy and high-quality plant protein that gets a lot of positive and negative attention, mainly due to compounds called isoflavones, which are also known as plant estrogens. They're similar to the hormone estrogen but too weak to really cause an increase in estrogen levels in women or men (I have never seen this happen with food or beverage sources), unless you take megadoses on a daily basis. Still, because of these isoflavones, there has always been a concern that consuming soy products may increase the risk of breast cancer returning or may reduce the ability of conventional medicine to treat it. Until recently, this had never been adequately studied, and the idea was to be safe rather than sorry and avoid it (which is completely understandable).

However, a 2009 Chinese study (published in the *Journal of the American Medical Association*) looked at soy consumption in more than 5,000 surgically treated breast cancer survivors. The women were divided into four groups based on how much soy they consumed: The low-dose group got about $1/2$ cup of soy milk a day and the high-dose group ingested about 3 cups daily (the other two were in-between). After 4 years, 7.4 percent of those who ate the most soy died compared to 10.3 percent of those who ate the least soy. In other words, there was approximately a 30 to 40 percent reduction in the risk of dying earlier or of cancer coming back in the high-soy group. The more amazing finding in this study is that the reduction in risk was not just in women with estrogen receptor–positive breast cancer and tamoxifen users; those with estrogen receptor–negative or more aggressive breast cancers and pre- and post-menopausal women benefited as well. A recent California study of breast cancer survivors found somewhat similar results, especially for estrogen

LIFESTYLE CHANGES

Heart healthy = breast healthy! The most important thing you can do to reduce your risk of breast cancer, especially after menopause, is to avoid gaining weight or to try to drop pounds if you're overweight. Exercise—both aerobic and resistance training—is extremely important as well (it can reduce both your risk of breast cancer and the risk of recurrence after treatment). Premenopausal women who are heavy have a slightly lower risk of breast cancer, and they tend to have lower levels of estrogen for reasons that are not clear.

receptor–positive breast cancers. Some researchers believe soy may partially work like a breast cancer drug, preventing estrogen from stimulating breast cancer cells.

These larger studies suggest that eating a little more than 10 grams of soy protein a day—from milk, edamame, protein powder, tofu, miso, tempeh, and more—is safe and enough to potentially see a benefit. Bonus: Soy might also reduce your cholesterol levels (I love this kind of twofer)! However, this does *not* mean that soy dietary supplements are safe, and I wouldn't recommend them.

Perhaps the reason dietary soy is so beneficial is because it's so heart healthy; it contains fiber, omega-3s, B vitamins, and calcium, and it's low in saturated fat and cholesterol. However, you should know that the women who consumed the most soy in the Chinese study also exercised more; consumed more cruciferous vegetables (broccoli, Brussels sprouts, kale), fish, and meat; drank tea; and used vitamin supplements. People who ate more soy tended to have healthier lifestyles. Also, in many Asian countries, people start consuming soy at a young age, so there may be benefits from lifelong consumption, versus recent consumption. Perhaps this is why we see the strongest positive effects for soy and breast cancer prevention coming from Asian population studies; the results have not been as impressive in Western trials.

Obviously, nobody on prescription breast cancer medications should read this and stop taking them, but it could prompt you to add soy to your diet. Still, talk to your doctor about the latest research. Finally, I always receive questions about soy's impact on thyroid levels. My answer: This is just hype. Soy consumed in moderation has minimal to no impact on thyroid levels.

As you get older, though, the main source of estrogen is fat cells; the more fat cells you have, the more estrogen you can make, and many breast cancers grow better with estrogen around. Being overweight or obese also increases your risk of colon, endometrial, esophageal, gall bladder, kidney, liver, pancreatic, thyroid, and probably ovarian and other cancers.

According to the Women's Intervention Nutrition Study (WINS)—which was the first large, randomized trial to investigate dietary changes and breast cancer recurrence in postmenopausal women—it would take 38 women adopting a more heart-healthy lifestyle to prevent one recurrence of breast cancer. I realize these aren't great odds (that's a 2.6 percent chance of benefiting), but following a heart-healthy diet and lifestyle helps *everyone* (100 percent) win by lowering the risk of heart and multiple other diseases, improving quality of life, and reducing side effects from cancer treatment.

Avoid hormones. If you do have to take them, use a low dose and only for a short time. In studies, hormone replacement therapy, or HRT, increased the risk of cardiovascular events and showed a negative impact on memory and other mental abilities. It also decreased the risk of colon cancer and hip fractures. In the years after these results came out, hormone sales dropped almost 40 percent. A couple of years after that, breast cancer rates dropped about 11 percent in postmenopausal women—the first time they had significantly fallen since 1945! There was a huge drop in estrogen-positive tumors as well. Weight gain and hormones may account for half of breast cancer deaths, based on the Nurses' Health Study from Harvard. The good news: The risk from HRT drops quickly after women go off it.

MOYAD FACT: Artificial sweeteners, breast implants, pesticides, power lines, underarm deodorant, and underwire bras *do not* increase breast cancer risk, but these conspiracies certainly help sell a lot of books from health "experts."

Limit alcohol. Even in moderation, drinking slightly raises breast cancer risk as well as the risk of mouth, throat, voice box, and gastrointestinal cancers. Alcohol also acts like weak estrogen, stimulating cancer cell growth and suppressing immune function.

Add some seeds. Ground flaxseed (25 grams per day from food, not pills) may help reduce breast cancer risk and enhance treatment response. Bonus: It's heart healthy (high in fiber and low in calories).

WHAT ELSE DO I NEED TO KNOW?

I think the controversy surrounding breast cancer screening (that is, doing it less often)—similar to prostate, thyroid, and some other screenings—is somewhat justified. There is clear evidence that some of the tumors caught by tests will not progress and be fatal; some could even naturally regress. There is no question that screening saves lives, but that's not the issue. The issue is how many individuals will be harmed by potentially saving a single life. I think the screening debate is ultimately healthy because it will force us to spend more money on research to determine who benefits from screening and under what circumstances. Regardless, you should discuss your options with the doctor you trust the most.

Brittle Nail Syndrome

B

Dr. Moyad Secret There are so many supplements being touted for dry skin, brittle hair, and brittle nails these days. And people think that because skin, hair, and nails all contain keratin, what works for one must work for all three. But the truth is that only a few supplements have been tested for treating all three problems in humans—and without much success—so I'm tackling each condition individually. One caveat: If your nails, hair, and skin are healthy but you want them to look even better, supplements won't help. You may see claims that vitamins C and D, gelatin, amino acids, essential fatty acids, and even biotin can help make a difference, but there's simply no research that these supplements work with already healthy tissue. Many of the claims are based on rare deficiency syndromes that when corrected can improve nails, hair, and skin.

WHAT IS IT?

Brittle nail syndrome, or BNS, is characterized by rough, ragged, and peeling nails. Approximately 30 percent of women and 15 percent of men experience it, and it's more common with age. In BNS, the nails become soft, dry, and weak and they chip, peel, and break easily. The nail tips may split (a condition called onychoschizia) or the nail plate—the rest of the visible part that sits on top of your skin—may form longitudinal ridges (a condition called onychorrhexis, or senile nail).

Most cases of BNS are idiopathic, which means doctors are stumped about the cause. Aging may be the biggest risk factor, simply because our bodies aren't as productive and efficient as they used to be at keeping all of our tissues healthy, and one of the areas where this shows up is the nails (and hair). In rare cases, BNS can be caused by an iron or zinc deficiency. It can also be a side effect of underlying problems, such as gout, osteoporosis, peripheral artery disease, and gastrointestinal and eating disorders; basically any medical issue that affects the entire body will also impact the nails.

WHAT WORKS

Note: It generally takes 2 to 3 months to see an improvement in nails, and the condition can return if you stop taking the supplement.

1. Silicon (the ch-OSA form)
10 milligrams daily (5 milligrams in the morning and evening)

119

This mineral is found throughout the body, and it helps with the formation of proteins in your hair, nails, and skin. Studies have shown that taking 10 milligrams daily of a form of silicon called choline-stabilized orthosilicic acid (ch-OSA) for 20 weeks reduced nail (and hair) brittleness and might even reduce skin roughness caused by the sun. (*Note:* This is the rare supplement that may be beneficial for all three conditions.) Other forms of silicon might deliver results as well, but there hasn't been enough human testing yet to give them my official stamp of approval, so I recommend the ch-OSA form. One word of warning: Excessive amounts of silicon from supplements can increase the risk of kidney stones, so more is not better.

2. Biotin (B$_7$) 1 to 3 milligrams daily (1,000 to 3,000 micrograms)

Farmers and ranchers have used biotin for years to treat abnormal horse hooves and pig claws, so researchers decided to test its effectiveness in several small human studies and noticed a benefit. Based on the research, daily supplementation for 6 to 15 months with doses ranging from 1 to 3 milligrams (1,000 to 3,000 micrograms) resulted in stronger, thicker, and smoother nails with fewer ridges. Brittleness generally returned within about 10 weeks after quitting, and the only side effect most subjects experienced was mild stomach upset. In horses and pigs, biotin supplements correct a nutrient deficiency, but researchers aren't sure if it works the same way in humans. Biotin deficiency is rare today, but it can be caused by a limited diet, regular consumption of large amounts of raw eggs (a compound in uncooked egg whites binds to biotin so it doesn't get absorbed), intestinal absorption problems, and some medications (like antibiotics and anticonvulsants). Keep in mind that all the good research has been conducted with oral dietary supplements; topical biotin has not been proven to work.

3. Iron only as directed by your physician

It's somewhat rare for people to suffer true nutrient deficiencies that can lead to BNS or brittle hair syndrome (BHS), but iron is the one exception. Iron helps the blood carry oxygen throughout the body, and it's also used in all the cells. Low iron stores can easily cause brittle nails and even hair loss because the cells aren't getting sufficient nutrition and oxygen to grow. While iron deficiency is arguably the most common nutrient shortage in the world, you should only supplement this mineral if directed by your doctor since getting too much iron is just as dangerous as not getting enough.

Certain foods can hinder or improve absorption of iron, but I always just recommend taking it by itself between meals (an hour before or a couple of hours after) or at bedtime, when your gastric juices are most active, which is better for absorption. Work with your doctor to find the correct dose for you because iron can cause stomach upset, constipation, and other problems (don't be surprised if your stools turn dark; this is common and harmless). Like most supplements, iron comes in various forms; some of the most common are ferrous sulfate, ferrous gluconate, ferrous fumarate, and ferrous lactate. You may find that you tolerate one better than another, so don't give up after trying one type. Also, some people prefer enteric-coated supplements because they cause fewer stomach problems, but I've found that they're less effective, primarily because the coating prevents the iron from being fully absorbed in the small intestine.

WHAT'S WORTHLESS

Selenium. People take this for a variety of reasons, but in high dosages (more than 200 micrograms per day), selenium can actually cause weak or brittle nails or nail loss and brittle and discolored hair and hair loss.

Calcium and vitamins A and D. I can't tell you how many times during the past 20 years someone has come up to me and sworn that calcium supplements can improve brittle nails or hair. They think that because calcium is good for bones, it must help nails and hair as well, but this is a myth. Calcium does not make nails harder. And since there is so much calcium in our diets today, getting too much of it from supplementation can increase the risk of kidney stones or potentially cause calcification of the arteries. There's no research showing any nail or hair benefits from vitamins A and D either.

LIFESTYLE CHANGES

There is a small amount of clinical research suggesting that our food and water intake diminishes as we age, which can make BNS worse, so a healthy diet and adequate hydration are key. Also, one study showed that overwashing and overdrying hands and nails can increase the risk of BNS (germaphobes, consider yourself warned). Other tips for reducing your risk of BNS include: filing nails in one direction only, wearing gloves to reduce trauma to the nails or exposure to harsh chemicals, keeping nails short, and limiting the use of nail polish removers and artificial nails.

WHAT ELSE DO I NEED TO KNOW?

There aren't really any effective drugs (over the counter or prescription) for BNS—and none have yet proven to be better than dietary supplements—but tazarotene cream (0.1 percent) applied twice daily for 24 weeks is showing promise in preliminary research.

MOYAD TIP: When I moisturize (yes, I am an adult man and I just used the word *moisturize*—my wife taught me) in the morning, I use a lotion with sunscreen and rub some of it on my hands and nails.

Cachexia/Underweight

THE JURY'S STILL OUT

Dr. Moyad Secret Cachexia is unintended weight loss, despite eating sufficient calories. It's a serious condition that can be caused by many things, including cancer, drug addiction, and certain diseases (such as multiple sclerosis and HIV/AIDS). Cancer treatments often result in substantial weight loss and muscle atrophy due to reduced appetite, physical inactivity, or simply because of the cancer itself. As they grow, some tumors or cancers release compounds that accelerate the metabolism (known as a hypercatabolic state). Besides losing weight, you begin to lose muscle mass and your organs even lose protein and suffer injury. Cachexia can be fatal if left untreated.

Less serious, but still important to address, is being underweight or unable to gain weight. Most people look at obesity as being a huge health risk (and it is), but those who are underweight face a potentially higher risk of dying compared to obese individuals, according to new findings published in the *Journal of Epidemiology and Public Health.* Being underweight may be due to excess drug, tobacco, and alcohol use; malnourishment; poverty; and mental health issues. Finally, if you just can't gain weight through lifestyle changes and supplements, talk to your doctor about a variety of drugs, including hormones and marijuana, that are available to stimulate weight gain.

Protein powder. In small amounts, these powders can suppress appetite, but in larger quantities they help to maintain muscle mass and provide a large source of calories. I recommend taking one to two servings between breakfast and lunch, lunch and dinner, and again before bedtime (three doses of 10 to 15 grams, depending on your weight, a day are ideal). The amino acid leucine in these powders appears to be one of the most important stimulators of muscle protein synthesis (muscle building) and maintenance. In fact, researchers are currently looking at patients who are taking 500 to 1,000 milligrams or more of leucine as a dietary supplement capsule *in addition to* the leucine they're getting from a protein powder. I believe taking additional leucine outside of a protein powder is worth a try. (You can find animal-based as well as vegetarian/vegan powders.)

Creatine monohydrate. Creatine dietary supplements are a safe way to spur muscle building in people who are losing weight but still able to exercise. Creatine monohydrate increases the energy capacity of the muscles during times of muscle loss and inactivity, which means it could improve workouts or at least help to maintain muscle. Add 5 grams of creatine powder to the protein powder recommendations mentioned above (with meals or on its own).

LIFESTYLE CHANGES

Start resistance training. Targeting your upper and lower body with weights two or three times a week can increase muscle mass within 1 month. When combined with a high protein intake, the results can be profound.

Add healthy fat to your diet. Dietary fat has the most calories per gram (over twice that of carbs and protein), so look for healthy sources of fat from certain oils (such as olive, coconut, flaxseed, or fish oil), nuts, and avocado to incorporate into daily meals.

Canker Sores

Dr. Moyad Secret Canker sores (a.k.a. mouth or aphthous ulcers or stomatitis) affect 20 percent of the population, and while the exact cause is unknown, possible triggers include stress, hormones, genetics, nutritional issues, tobacco use, bacterial and viral agents, and even some systemic immune diseases. In the largest review of conventional and alternative medicine in canker sore history, no single treatment was found to be effective. However, multiple nutritional deficiencies (caused by anemia, gluten intolerance, or malabsorption problems) may play a role in canker sores, so if you get frequent sores, you should work with a nutritionist and doctor to get tested. Basically, anything that is safe and might help even a little is worth trying, folks! The goal of any treatment is to impact one or more of the following: pain and ulcer size, rate of healing, and risk of recurrence. Keep your eye out for ongoing studies on hyaluronic acid gel. Also, zinc sulfate in high dosages (150 milligrams twice daily) has shown some preliminary promise for speeding ulcer healing times.

Deglycyrrhizinated licorice (DGL). A mouthwash with DGL has preliminary data showing it might improve recovery time for canker sores, but the product is hard to find. You can mix the supplement with water, though, swish it around, and then spit it out a few times a day (you can find a DIY version on YouTube).

Berberine. There's also early data for the herbal product berberine when applied topically in gelatin form to the sore four times a day over 5 days; it reduced both ulcer size and pain. Laboratory research with this compound suggests it has immune-modulating, anti-inflammatory, and antimicrobial properties, which makes it a natural for canker sores.

Omega-3 fatty acids. In one study, taking 1,500 milligrams daily of the active ingredients in fish oil (the omega-3 fatty acids EPA and DHA) over 6 months led to a significant reduction in the number of ulcer outbreaks, average level of pain, and the duration of ulcer episodes per month, starting in the third month of treatment. The anti-inflammatory effects of omega-3s may be the key. I think this would be a good option to try for people with an increased risk of short-term recurrence.

Vitamin B$_{12}$. In a preliminary trial, 1,000 micrograms of sublingual B$_{12}$ over 6 months reduced ulcer duration, number of ulcers, and pain. What's more, initial vitamin B$_{12}$ blood levels did not impact the results—meaning you don't have to be deficient in B$_{12}$ to try it. This is an option for anyone suffering from regular canker sore outbreaks.

Eupatorium laevigatum. A paste made from this Brazilian plant improved 5-day cure rates and pain relief more than a comparative steroid, but this herbal is hard to find outside of Brazil.

WHAT'S WORTHLESS

Multivitamins. These have proven worthless for canker sores in clinical trials, which is why I'm skeptical about just solving nutritional deficiencies to prevent or treat these sores when there are so many other potential causes.

MOYAD TIP: One of my favorite old-time home remedies for canker sores is an aspirin mouth rinse to reduce inflammation. Crush one or two aspirin, mix with 8 ounces of water, and swish the mixture in your mouth for 15 to 20 seconds morning, noon, and night.

Carpal Tunnel Syndrome

Dr. Moyad Secret Carpal tunnel syndrome (CTS) is the most common entrapment neuropathy, or peripheral nerve-pinching medical condition, and it results from a combination of compression and traction on the median nerve at the wrist. Pills rarely serve as a solution, and while surgical treatment for CTS has an 80 to 90 percent satisfaction rate, many people don't opt for surgery. The bottom line: You do not want to see this nerve die because of lack of treatment. My favorite advice to prevent CTS is to adopt heart-healthy behaviors (heart healthy = wrist healthy!). Shocker, I know. People with diabetes and obesity have a higher risk of CTS. There's a theory that fat tissue in the arm can compress the median nerve, which makes sense.

   Alpha-lipoic acid (ALA). ALA at 600 milligrams per day has a history of reducing nerve injury (see the Peripheral Neuropathy section, page 364) in people with diabetes and possibly cancer patients. And because of these results, ALA is now getting some preliminary research as a neuroprotectant early in the course of CTS or before and after surgery. Talk to your doctor about the latest research. Just be warned: It can cause a harmless malodorous urine smell (like asparagus does) and increase the risk of rash and itching, and it can also increase insulin levels and drastically drop blood sugar levels in very rare cases.

WHAT'S WORTHLESS

Vitamin B_6. Some experts still recommend vitamin B_6 (pyridoxine), but I don't think it works. There was an early theory that CTS may be due to a B_6 deficiency, but well-done clinical trials have shown that it doesn't work better than a placebo. Plus, taking high doses of B_6 (300 milligrams or more per day) can cause sensory peripheral nerve injury (a loss of sensation that increases your risk of falling or losing your balance) and tingling or numbness, and it can increase the risk of an unsteady gait. I believe the reason some people still think B_6 can help is related to the fact that a minority of CTS patients get better on their own (the body's own repair mechanisms are amazing). So when this happens in people taking B_6, their recovery is attributed to the supplement. If you and your doctor believe it will work, then taking 200 milligrams or less for several months may be a good placebo.

Cataracts

C

Dr. Moyad Secret Cataracts are the number one cause of blindness in the world (50 percent of cases). Cataract extraction and artificial lens replacement is the most commonly performed surgical procedure in the United States, accounting for more than 10 percent of the annual Medicare budget and 60 percent of annual eye-related spending. If there was a way to delay surgery by just 10 years, half as many people would need the surgery and that money could be spent on other important health concerns. An inexpensive supplement may be the way to do that: There is clear evidence now that a multivitamin can reduce the risk of cataracts and perhaps even cataract surgery. But this hasn't been embraced by many in conventional medicine circles because the results didn't come from an official Phase 3 clinical trial, even though the results are equivalent. I am dumbfounded by this, especially when you consider that patients routinely report loss of sight as one of their biggest health-related fears! (*Note:* Please see the Macular Degeneration section, page 311; both conditions have similar advice.)

WHAT IS IT?

The lens of the eye is normally transparent, but due to age, unhealthy lifestyle habits, or UV exposure, proteins clump together and create cloudy, opaque areas that are known as cataracts. Common symptoms include blurry vision, double vision, seeing "halos" around lights, sensitivity, glare or floaters, and decreased depth perception. Eventually the cataract can completely obstruct vision, leading to blindness. Cataract risk doubles every 10 years after the age of 40, to the point where most people walking the planet in their eighties and nineties will be affected. However, not everyone with cataracts needs surgery, especially if you can still read, drive, or watch TV; it's an individual decision.

Now for a little anatomy lesson! The lens of the eye is made up of four layers of crystalline tissue: the cortex, nucleus, capsule, and subcapsular epithelium. In this section, I'm going to discuss three types of cataracts that can potentially cause visual problems as we age, and these are named for the layer they impact.

- Cortical cataracts
- Nuclear cataracts (the most common type)
- Posterior subcapsular cataracts (PSC)

Each type of cataract is given a grade from 1 to 4, with a higher number typically indicating a more severe cataract.

WHAT WORKS

1. Low-dose multivitamin, such as Centrum or Centrum Silver
one tablet daily

The Age-Related Eye Disease Study (a.k.a. AREDS 1—there were two trials) was the largest randomized trial ever conducted with a daily combination dietary supplement versus a placebo for macular degeneration. The results showed a significant reduction in the risk of macular disease progression (for those with intermediate to advanced stages of the disease) over the 6-year study using a product that contained 500 milligrams vitamin C, 400 IU vitamin E, 15 milligrams beta-carotene, 80 milligrams zinc, and 2 milligrams copper. However, the supplement did not have any effect on cataract development or progression. But the researchers did a smart thing at the beginning of this study: They knew many of the participants wanted to either keep taking or start taking a multivitamin, and in order to make sure everyone took the same one, they provided Centrum, a simple multivitamin/mineral supplement (see table, opposite), in addition to the AREDS 1 pill and placebo.

Here's where it gets really interesting, I swear: Researchers followed 4,590 individuals who had at least one natural lens for about 6.3 years to check for the development or progression of cataracts. They found that Centrum was associated with a significant (16 percent) decrease in the progression of any type of cataract, but it was especially protective (a 25 percent reduction) against the progression of nuclear cataracts.

Because these results were so promising, the National Eye Institute supported a randomized placebo trial at the University of Parma in Italy to determine the impact of Centrum use on the development and progression of any type of cataract. This trial, known officially as the Italian-American Clinical Trial of Nutritional Supplements and Age-Related Cataract (CTNS), had 1,020 participants (average age of 68), and the follow-up was at about 9 years at the time this book was being written. Researchers found a significant 18 percent reduction in the risk of any lens event (geek speak for cataract) compared to the placebo. Nuclear cataracts were significantly reduced by 34 percent, but the risk for posterior subcapsular cataracts was significantly increased in the participants taking the multivitamins (keep reading, though)! There was a nonsignificant 22 percent reduction in cortical cataracts, and no difference in moderate visual acuity loss or in the need for cataract surgery. There was also no difference in side effects between the placebo and the multivitamin group. It is possible the increase in PSC cataracts was a chance finding. In fact, the most recent and largest review of clinical studies and trials (14 in all), published in the journal *Nutrients,* found no increased risk of PSC cataracts or cataract surgery and significant reductions in

VITAMINS AND MINERALS CONTENT IN CENTRUM IN AREDS 1 AND CTNS TRIALS

VITAMIN/MINERAL	AMOUNT PER PILL
Vitamin A	5,000 IU
Vitamin E	30 IU
Vitamin C	60 mg
Folic Acid	400 mcg
Vitamin B$_1$ (thiamin)	1.5 mg
Vitamin B$_2$ (riboflavin)	1.7 mg
Vitamin B$_3$ (niacinamide)	20 mg
Vitamin B$_6$	2 mg
Vitamin B$_{12}$	6 mcg
Vitamin D	400 IU
Biotin	30 mcg
Pantothenic acid	10 mg
Calcium	162 mg
Phosphorus	125 mg
Iodine	150 mcg
Iron	18 mg
Magnesium	100 mg
Copper	2 mg
Zinc	15 mg
Other compounds with no RDA: Boron, chlorine, chromium, manganese, molybdenum, nickel, potassium, selenium, silicon, tin, vanadium, vitamin K	Trace/minimal amounts

the risk of nuclear, cortical, and any cataracts in well-nourished individuals. Hmm, interesting.

Additionally, the Physicians' Health Study II, one of the best and most recent studies to address cataracts, found significantly fewer cataracts and a significantly lower chance of having cataract surgery when taking a daily Centrum Silver multivitamin. All of this for just pennies a day! Despite all of this data, there are boneheaded (I could have used worse language) "experts" who continue to tell the public that multivitamins are worthless and do not prevent chronic diseases! This is absurd and an embarrassment. If an inexpensive pharmaceutical had similar data with minimal side effects, there's no way any expert would reject it.

2. N-acetylcarnosine drops dosage varies; follow package instructions

Carnosine is an antioxidant that's found throughout the body, including the eye lens. It's composed of two amino acids (beta-alanine and histidine), and when it gets converted to N-acetylcarnosine, it may be more resistant to enzymes that could break down and damage the lens. A randomized, placebo-controlled study with patients who had cataracts in one or both eyes but had not undergone surgery compared subjects who received N-acetyl-carnosine drops (1 percent; sold as Can-C from Innovative Vision Products in Great Britain), placebo drops, and no drops. Vision improved (including clarity, glare sensitivity, and color perception) with the N-acetylcarnosine drops after 6 months, and the results were sustained over 2 years, which makes this the only antioxidant preliminarily proven to help patients in the early stage of cataract formation, regardless of the type of cataract. (Side effects appeared similar to the placebo.)

3. Lutein 10 milligrams a day and zeaxanthin 2 milligrams a day

The macula of the eye contains high concentrations of these two carotenoids, which offer photoprotection, meaning they help filter or absorb potentially damaging light rays as they enter the eye. The body cannot make lutein or zeaxanthin, so you have to get them from your diet or supplements. Experts believe if you can increase the macular pigment of the eye with lutein and zeaxanthin, then you can reduce the risk of age-related eye diseases, such as cataracts and macular degeneration. However, this still needs some more research.

In the AREDS 2 clinical trial, a follow-up to the first one, researchers found that lutein and zeaxanthin supplements can help prevent cataracts, primarily in people with lower intakes of these nutrients. There was a significant reduction in the risk of being diagnosed with any type of cataract, any severe cataract, and of having cataract surgery for participants with lower dietary intakes of these nutrients who also took the basic AREDS 2 supplements (500 milligrams vitamin C, 400 IU vitamin E, 25 to 80 milligrams zinc oxide, and 2 milligrams cupric oxide).

The "free form" (non-esterified version) of lutein is getting the most attention compared to bound lutein (an esterified form), but the form does not matter that much in terms of absorption. (The AREDS 2 trial used a water-soluable triglyceride form.) You can increase absorption by taking these with a meal that has some fat in it. Naturally then, any medications that block the absorption of fat (such as the weight loss drug Orlistat) may reduce uptake of lutein and zeaxanthin. Do not take these supplements if pregnant or breastfeeding since this has not been studied.

Be warned that lutein can cause a harmless yellowing of the skin. It's temporary and should go away when blood levels of the carotenoids drop. The safety of these two carotenoids has been outstanding so far in 1- to 2-year-long studies, but it's still early.

WHAT'S WORTHLESS

High doses of some supplements. As mentioned earlier, the high-dose combination of vitamins and minerals used in the AREDS 1 trial did not work for cataracts. This just provides further evidence that megadoses of supplements are not usually any better for prevention or treatment than low or regular doses.

Omega-3 fatty acids. The supplement forms of omega-3 fatty acids (EPA and DHA) have not been found to slow the progression of macular degeneration, so I'm skeptical as to whether they'll impact cataracts either. Dietary (plant *and* marine) sources of omega-3s—salmon, sardines, tuna, trout, walnuts, flaxseed, and chia seeds—may be beneficial, though, based on preliminary research. Some studies suggest fish high in mercury might increase the risk of cataracts, but the research is preliminary and I have not bought into it yet.

Blueberry and bilberry extracts. These supplements have not been adequately tested for cataracts outside of the laboratory, so stick with eating real berries for now. The same holds true for bilberry, which contains high levels of

antioxidant compounds called anthocyanins. If you're a mouse or a rat, however, I believe these supplements can cure all of your eye diseases.

Vitamin D. I believe any relationship between higher vitamin D blood levels and lower risk of eye disease has more to do with weight than anything else. As you gain weight, your vitamin D level goes down and your risk of eye disease goes up. When you lose weight, vitamin D in the blood rises and your risk drops. In other words, vitamin D supplements are getting way too much credit!

Astaxanthin. This carotenoid (it contributes to the red color of cooked shellfish and salmon) is being studied and getting a lot of hype, but I believe it will end up being one of the most overrated supplements—along with resveratrol—of my time! It has been combined with lutein and zeaxanthin in a few studies, but I don't see how the results are any better or cannot just be improved by changing the dose of lutein and zeaxanthin.

LIFESTYLE CHANGES

Heart healthy = eye healthy. Virtually all of the factors associated with a higher risk of heart disease increase the risk of cataracts, including smoking (a major risk factor that also increases the severity of the disease quickly), diabetes, weight gain, and heavy alcohol consumption. Again, your goal is to reduce your risk of heart disease to as close to zero as possible.

Wear shades. Sunglasses reduce the risk of cataracts. Look for a wraparound pair that blocks UVA and UVB light.

Add eye-boosting nutrients to your diet. Multiple studies have suggested that getting more lutein and zeaxanthin from food (6 milligrams or higher total) can lower the risk of cataracts and age-related macular degeneration. The following foods contain high quantities of both nutrients (they're usually found together).

FOODS HIGH IN LUTEIN AND ZEAXANTHIN

FOOD SOURCE	APPROXIMATE LUTEIN AND ZEAXANTHIN AMOUNT (MG PER SINGLE SERVING)
Kale (1 cup cooked or raw)	20 to 24
Spinach ($1/2$ cup cooked)	15 to 20
Lettuce (1 cup raw)	2.5 to 3
Broccoli ($1/2$ cup cooked)	2.2 to 2.5
Sweet corn ($1/2$ cup cooked)	1.5 to 2
Green peas ($1/2$ cup cooked)	1 to 1.5
Brussels sprouts ($1/2$ cup cooked)	1 to 1.3
Egg yolk (one yolk)	0.5 (actually one of the best sources because absorption is so efficient)
White cabbage (1 cup raw)	0.3 to 0.5

Note: Other respectable sources of lutein and zeaxanthin include arugula, basil, collard greens, parsley, radicchio, and watercress.

Celiac Disease

C

Dr. Moyad Secret Celiac disease is an intolerance to gluten, a protein found primarily in wheat, barley, and rye (and potentially oats, depending on their source and whether they've been contaminated by wheat products). It's critical to understand that people can be sensitive to gluten without having celiac disease. While those with the disease *have* to give up gluten, people who are sensitive to it have the option of cutting it out or living with the side effects (there are major pros and cons to consider before you take the leap to being gluten free, though). Many patients tell me they just feel better going gluten free; they have more energy and less fatigue. Turns out, what they had simply accepted as "normal"—in terms of how they felt on a daily basis and how they reacted to food—wasn't normal at all! This happens all the time. Then there are the people who don't have celiac disease or a gluten sensitivity but get a good placebo response from going gluten free. At times, eating less gluten means you eat less food—often less junk food—which can also lead to weight loss and feeling better.

A blood test (called a tTG test) can help determine if you have celiac disease, and if the test is positive, your doctor may want to take a biopsy of the lining of the small intestine. If that is positive as well, then you can be sure you have celiac disease (you don't want to cut out a huge part of your diet without being absolutely sure you have it!). The blood test and biopsy aren't reliable if you're already gluten free, so get tested before you make a change. (The odds of having celiac if your blood test for it is negative are about one in 300, which is a very small chance.)

In people with celiac disease, gluten causes an autoimmune reaction that damages the small intestine and leads to nutrient absorption problems. Up to 1 in 100 people in the United States have it, and when a first-degree relative has the condition, the incidence increases to 1 in 22. The only treatment is avoiding foods made from wheat, barley, rye, and possibly some oats. (Many surprising products contain gluten, including some prescription medications, dietary supplements, tomato sauce, chips, and lipstick.) In children with celiac disease, the small intestine can heal within 3 to 6 months after being exposed

---

MOYAD FACT: People with celiac disease have a higher risk of being diagnosed with thyroid disease and lactose intolerance, and their immune systems are less effective, so they're susceptible to more serious effects from infectious agents, like the flu.

---

to gluten, but in adults the damage can take years to heal (although symptoms may improve within days or weeks).

Symptoms include abdominal bloating or pain; chronic diarrhea; vomiting; constipation; pale, smelly, or fatty stools; and weight loss. Adults may have unexplained anemia (low red blood cell count), fatigue, bone or joint pain, arthritis, bone loss/osteoporosis, anxiety or depression, numbness or tingling in the hands and feet, or an itchy rash called dermatitis herpetiformis.

There aren't really many supplements I would recommend for celiac disease, unless deficiencies exist. That's why the smartest thing to do if you're diagnosed with celiac disease is to get tested for basic vitamin and mineral deficiencies: Fat soluble vitamins (A, D, E, and K); folic acid; vitamins B_1, B_2, B_6, and B_{12}; iron; calcium; and magnesium should be high on the list. It's also important to meet with a dietitian who specializes in this area and to ask your doctor about getting a dual-energy x-ray absorptiometry, or DEXA, scan for osteoporosis since people with celiac disease often have a higher rate of bone loss.

Probiotics. This is the one promising area in terms of celiac disease supplements. Probiotics are finally receiving good clinical trials (they're being initiated as we publish), including common strains such as *Bifidobacterium infantis.* A commercial probiotic called VSL#3, which contains eight different bacteria, has preliminary results that it may reduce gluten toxicity (for example, from accidental ingestion), so it's worth discussing with your doctor. In time, taking a probiotic may even help people who are extremely sensitive to even a minute amount of gluten because it has the potential to digest the gluten protein. (Those sufferers who may have a negative response to even 1 milligram of gluten; one slice of bread can have as much as 4,000 milligrams of gluten, to give you some perspective.)

MOYAD FACT : "Safe" grains for those with celiac disease include rice, amaranth, buckwheat, corn, millet, quinoa, sorghum, teff (an Ethiopian cereal grain), and oats that haven't been contaminated by other grains. There are so many gluten-free foods now, including gluten-free peanut butter and bread, and the options continue to grow exponentially. However, be aware that a "gluten-free" claim is not synonymous with "healthy." The product could be loaded with fat, sodium, chemicals, sugar, and so on.

Chronic Prostatitis/Chronic Pelvic Pain Syndrome

C

Dr. Moyad Secret Chronic nonbacterial prostatitis, which is also known as chronic prostatitis/chronic pelvic pain syndrome (CP/CPPS), accounts for 90 to 95 percent of all prostatitis cases, yet it doesn't get much attention. In fact, the average CP/CPPS patient generally deals with symptoms for years before receiving an accurate diagnosis and treatment. There is no FDA-approved drug for this condition, but leading experts and specialists in this area do recommend dietary supplements. Combining them with conventional prescription medication (used off-label) has also become part of the standard of care.

WHAT IS IT?

Prostatitis is inflammation of the prostate, the small gland that surrounds the urethra. Due to its location, inflammation can lead to urinary problems and pain, significantly impacting quality of life. Prostatitis can be caused by bacteria, but more commonly it's not (and the cause is often unknown). Category III (types a and b) is the most common form, and it is commonly referred to as chronic pelvic pain syndrome, or CPPS. However, this is really an umbrella term since CPPS can include other diseases like interstitial cystitis, and we'll see it used more that way in the future.

People with CP/CPPS can experience a variety of symptoms beyond urinary problems. Experts have developed a clinical guide called UPOINT (see page 136) to address different groups of symptoms and treatment options that are commonly used.

WHAT WORKS

1. Cernilton (a pollen extract mixture) dosages vary

Cernilton, which is a pollen extract, has anti-inflammatory effects, and it's been tested in a variety of trials for CP/CPPS. Cernilton from the latest clinical trial was a microbial digestion of a mixture of the pollen extracts (called cernitins) *Secale cereale* (cereal rye or grass), *Phleum pratense* (Timothy grass), and *Zea mays* (corn). The largest and one of the most well-done studies with this supplement for CP/CPPS followed 139 men who took either Cernilton or a placebo. Approximately 45 percent of the subjects were on prior prescription medications for CP/CPPS or a related condition. Researchers found significant reductions in pain and significant improvements in quality of life and total symptoms after 12 weeks with

135

CP/CPPS UPOINT SYMPTOMS

<u>U</u>rinary symptoms (pain during urination, difficulty starting or stopping, urgency, and frequency): Alpha-blockers and antimuscarinic prescription drugs are commonly used.

<u>P</u>sychosocial symptoms (depression, stress, and verbalizing helplessness and hopelessness): Psychological and cognitive behavioral therapy are options.

<u>O</u>rgan specific (bladder or prostate), including prostate tenderness, blood in the semen, or symptom relief with urination: Quercetin or pollen extract supplements (for example, Prosta-Q, Q-Urol, or Cernilton) and prescription medications such as pentosan polysulfate are options.

<u>I</u>nfection (positive cultures of prostatic fluid without a urinary tract infection or concomitant urethritis that may be contributing to CP/CPPS): Antibiotics are an option.

<u>N</u>eurologic/systemic (pain outside the pelvis or systemic pain syndrome): Pregabalin or amitriptyline prescription drugs are options.

<u>T</u>enderness (pelvic floor spasm or muscle trigger points): Pelvic floor physical therapy or myofascial release (massage or stretch the area to reduce tension) are options.

Cernilton compared to the placebo. Approximately 70 percent of the patients on Cernilton had a large (25 percent) reduction in symptoms, compared to 49 percent of those on the placebo (there is a large placebo response rate in these studies, which is why placebo-controlled trials are so crucial to prove efficacy). Urinary scores or function did not improve, and side effects were similar to the placebo. Participants in this trial took two Cernilton capsules every 8 hours; the active ingredient in each capsule was 60 milligrams of Cernitin T60 (water-soluble) and 3 milligrams Cernitin GBX (fat-soluble). This is one of the most impressive clinical trials performed to date

with a dietary supplement for CP/CPPS. Currently, there have been seven positive human clinical studies with pollen extract and CP/CPPS—six with Cernilton and one with a product known as Prostat/Poltit. Clinical efficacy with the supplements ranged from 63 to 87 percent, compared to 36 to 49 percent for the placebo.

The issue with Cernilton is that it has a long history with multiple companies, which can be quite difficult to sort through when you're trying to order this or a similar product. (For example, Cernilton started with AB Cernelle in Sweden, and then it was also licensed in the United States by Cernitin America and discontinued. Graminex currently sells one option, and the most recent randomized clinical trial was supported by Strathmann AG & Co. and AB Cernelle, both in Europe.) Always look for the three active pollen ingredients (page 135).

Dosages in studies varied based on the product, so you may have to experiment with it. I find it interesting that these supplements help reduce pain and improve quality of life but do not improve urinary function, which is similar to other effective supplements for CP/CPPS. This is why most patients take a combination of supplements and prescription medication. In my experience, some men do see an improvement in urinary function or flow with Cernilton and other supplements mentioned in this section, but they're in the minority.

2. Quercetin and quercetin complex
500 milligrams twice a day

Quercetin is an anti-inflammatory compound found in green tea, red wine, and onions. It seems to block cell cytokine release, which may help reduce inflammatory reactions. In an impressive but small randomized, placebo-controlled trial at UCLA, 67 percent of CP/CPPS patients who took 500 milligrams of quercetin twice daily for 4 weeks experienced a large improvement in pain and quality of life (but not urinary function). Only 20 percent in the placebo group experienced improvements. Also, white blood cells in prostatic secretions (a measure of inflammation) dropped by 66 percent in the quercetin group (no significant change in the placebo-takers). A third group (not placebo controlled) of 17 patients received

quercetin with bromelain and papain (digestive enzymes found in pineapple and papaya, respectively)—known as a quercetin complex—to enhance absorption, and 82 percent experienced a significant improvement in symptoms after 1 month (the product used is called Prosta-Q).

3. SAM-e (S-adenosylmethionine)
600 to 1,200 milligrams a day

SAM-e is widely used as a prescription drug in Europe for a variety of conditions, especially osteoarthritis and depression (see the Osteoarthritis and Joint Pain section, page 344, and the Depression section, page 166), and as a result it's receiving more attention in the United States. Researchers are not sure how it controls pain, but it does play a primary role in several neurotransmitter pathways in the body, which basically means it likes to impact multiple areas.

A recent review of numerous clinical trials with SAM-e versus a placebo or NSAIDs (most over-the-counter pain relievers and some prescription anti-inflammatory medications, including Celebrex) concluded that the existing evidence indicates SAM-e is at least as effective as NSAIDs (nonsteroidal anti-inflammatory drugs) at reducing pain but with a lower rate of side effects. In fact, people taking SAM-e were almost 60 percent less likely to experience a side effect compared to NSAID users. SAM-e has a slower onset of action for pain reduction, but by the end of the first or second month of use, the efficacy is similar to many popular NSAIDs. Dosages range from 600 to 1,200 milligrams per day for at least 30 to 90 days. It can be ridiculously expensive, but if you're willing to shop around, you can find some good deals.

The problem with SAM-e or any other supplement for CP/CPPS (apart from Cernilton and quercetin) is that there is no adequate clinical trial suggesting it helps. However, in my experience, SAM-e does help reduce CP/CPPS-related pain and improve mood. This is one of the only sections of the book where I rank something without a clinical trial. I just can't ignore the pain-reducing effects of SAM-e.

WHAT'S WORTHLESS

Saw palmetto. It has essentially failed as a supplement for prostate enlargement, which is why it has shown little ability to reduce CP/CPPS symptoms.

Stinging nettle. This supplement and most others touted for prostate health either have not been studied adequately or have failed.

LIFESTYLE CHANGES

Heart healthy = prostate healthy! I have said this in medical journals for more than 10 years, and lifestyle studies are proving it as well. Anything that helps your heart will help your prostate. Specifically, researchers have found that tobacco use and higher caloric intake, both risk factors for heart disease, may be risk factors for CP/CPPS as well. And it's not just about diet and not smoking: A clinical study from Florence, Italy, found that men with CP/CPPS who walked vigorously three times a week for 40 minutes (achieving an intensity of 70 to 80 percent of their maximum heart rate) reported an improvement in symptoms, pain, and quality of life. (Sadly, approximately 25 percent of the participants dropped out of the study by 18 weeks, which is one of the serious limitations of lifestyle-change trials.) Exercise releases pain-fighting compounds in the body. In my experience, patients also see improvements in urinary function when they exercise more often (5 to 7 days a week).

Take a bath. Magnesium sulfate baths (a.k.a. sitz baths) can reduce the pain associated with CP/CPPS.

Keep a food diary. For some people, certain foods and beverages can make symptoms worse, so keep track of what you eat for several weeks and note whether there are any changes in your CP symptoms. Surveys suggest spicy foods, coffee, hot peppers, alcohol, tea, and chili can make symptoms worse.

WHAT ELSE DO I NEED TO KNOW?

Acupuncture or percutaneous tibial nerve stimulation (PTNS), which is just a conventionally modified form of acupuncture (Google it, please), should also be a standard of care for CP/CPPS. These techniques have led to some significant improvements in urinary function. In a perfect world, a patient would be offered a prescription drug, supplements, and acupuncture or PTNS for their CP/CPPS!

Colon Polyps and Colon Cancer C

Dr. Moyad Secret Do you know why colon cancer screening will probably never be questioned the same way prostate, thyroid, and even breast cancer screenings have been? Because colon cancer can be screened for and cured (at least the existing premalignant lesions/polyps) at the same time. Imagine receiving a breast, prostate, or thyroid biopsy and then having the doctors cure you or substantially reduce your risk of getting these cancers right then and there? It is my dream that most other cancer screenings will develop a tool or injectable product (drug/supplement) that will do the same thing.

When it comes to colon cancer prevention, there is no greater advice than, "Heart healthy = colon healthy." The latest research on reducing the risk and progression of colon cancer through exercising and achieving a healthy weight along with other heart-healthy changes (diet, quitting smoking, and so on) is outstanding!

Aspirin. In people with a high risk of colon cancer, no supplement can beat it. A recent study showed that in individuals with a high genetic risk of colon cancer, such as Lynch syndrome patients, two aspirin per day (600 milligrams) compared to a placebo reduced the risk of colon cancer after taking it for more than 2 years. There was a 44 percent reduction in the risk of colon cancer in the aspirin group. And those who continued to take aspirin for 2 years or more saw a 63 percent reduction in risk. (Although aspirin comes from willow bark originally, there is no supplement—including white willow bark—that comes close to aspirin's results.) Keep in mind very high doses of aspirin were used.

Even a baby aspirin (81 milligrams) every day or every other day appears to lower the risk of colon cancer in women and men, but you would need to use it for 5 to 10 years minimum to see a potential benefit. Doctors would probably feel more compelled to encourage baby aspirin use in an individual with a strong genetic/family history of gastrointestinal cancer or in someone who was previously treated for colon cancer. However, here comes the catch (because everything comes with a catch): Aspirin can worsen kidney and liver problems, and it increases the risk of ulcers and serious internal bleeding. This risk also increases with age.

Omega-3 fatty acids. There's a large Japanese trial under way looking at 2,700 milligrams of EPA (an omega-3 fatty acid) daily versus a placebo in people at higher risk of colon cancer. Stay tuned! In another study, high-risk individuals who took 2,000 milligrams of fish oil daily (in the form of free fatty acid EPA only) for 6 months had fewer and smaller polyps.

139

Red yeast rice. Red yeast rice, which people often take for high cholesterol, seems to be the dietary supplement with the most potential against cancer: In its largest cholesterol-lowering clinical trial, red yeast rice appeared to significantly lower the risk of dying from several cancers (see the High Cholesterol section, page 234). I am convinced that cholesterol-lowering drugs and supplements have some role in preventing aggressive polyp formation.

Fiber. Getting 20 to 30 grams per day from diet could improve both heart and colon health. If eating that much is difficult, it's easy to add 5 to 10 grams in the form of a fiber powder, like psyllium or inulin.

Calcium and vitamin D. A normal daily intake of calcium and vitamin D might reduce the risk of colon polyps (and possibly even cancer). But calcium rarely needs to be supplemented with a pill today because it's in so many fortified foods.

Vitamin C. New data from the Physicians' Health Study II trial has found that vitamin C supplements could potentially lower colon cancer risk. Stay tuned.

WHAT'S WORTHLESS

Curcumin. This is the most promising supplement for colon cancer prevention according to some "experts," but it hasn't been tested in enough well-done clinical trials, even though it has shown an anti-inflammatory effect in the laboratory.

Folic acid. The Aspirin/Folate Polyp Prevention Study (AFPPS) was perhaps one of the best randomized clinical trials to look at aspirin and also folic acid in people with a history of colon polyps. The US study required that each participant have a complete colonoscopy and removal of all known polyps within 3 months of enrolling in the study. Investigators found that a daily baby aspirin (81 milligrams) reduced the risk of colon polyps, but folic acid (1 milligram per day) did not work better than a placebo and was even associated with a higher risk of having three or more polyps and possibly with an increased risk of other cancers (primarily prostate cancer). This still needs more research, but overall it seems that folic acid supplements do not lower the risk of colon cancer. Plus, people in the United States and Canada already get plenty of folate or folic acid from fortified foods (like breakfast cereals), multivitamins, and vegetables. Taking more just doesn't make sense for most people.

Common Cold and Flu

C

Dr. Moyad Secret Every year in the United States, there are more than 1 billion upper respiratory tract infections and colds. In addition, 5 to 25 percent of Americans get the flu, which results in 200,000 hospitalizations and anywhere from 20,000 to 36,000 deaths, depending on the year. The vast majority of over-the-counter conventional and alternative products have no adequate clinical evidence that they can prevent or treat colds and the flu. That's why I like to say, "Treat a cold and it will only last 7 days, but if you do not treat it, well then you might be sorry because it can last up to a week."

While there are a few supplements that have clinical data suggesting they can prevent or treat colds and the flu, what you really want to look for is a supplement that might be able to prevent or help treat pneumonia (along with conventional medicine) because that is the real killer. It's the most common life-threatening complication of the flu, and young children and the elderly are at the highest risk for it. In the United States, pneumonia is the number one cause of death from an infection and the sixth most common cause of death overall. Therefore, the annual debate about which dietary supplements do and do not prevent colds and the flu is a nonproductive distraction. Being hospitalized or dying from a cold is unheard of, but dying from the flu is common because it's easy to develop a deeper lung infection. One last tip: Don't look for a supplement that "boosts your immune system"; this means nothing, and many companies have gotten in trouble with regulatory agencies over these claims in the past.

WHAT IS IT?

Colds and the flu—considered cytokine diseases—are caused by viruses. When you are otherwise healthy and get sick, your immune system pumps out protein molecules called cytokines, which help battle the virus and lead to many of the symptoms you experience—sneezing, coughing, a runny nose, and puffy eyes. It's the body's immune response to the virus that makes you feel so bad, not the virus itself. In fact, there were so many deaths in the flu pandemic of 1918 (it killed 3 to 5 percent of the global population) because a lot of people had never dealt with such a strong virus and their immune systems *over*reacted! That's why it makes no sense when supplements claim they can "boost" your immune system. It's already boosted! What you really want is higher-quality immune surveillance with a strong memory for any previous infections (imagine a home security system that could track people who have

141

come into your house, recognize them, and then immobilize them if necessary).

Rhinoviruses cause 30 to 80 percent of colds each year, but there are more than 200 other viruses that could be the culprit. Cold viruses take hold and proliferate primarily in the nose (people like me who have big noses can hold a lot of virus!), and they're passed by touch, like when people wipe their noses and then shake hands or grab a bar on a bus or subway that someone else touches a short time later. Flu viruses, on the other hand, can enter through the nose, eyes, and mouth. They get passed around when infected folks cough, sneeze, or talk, which transmits small virus-filled water droplets out of their mouths and noses and into yours. You can also come in contact with flu viruses by touching infected surfaces, such as desks and doorknobs. Some flu viruses can live up to 3 days on surfaces!

If you have symptoms that come on gradually and are primarily above the neck—sneezing, sore throat, watery or itchy eyes—you probably have a cold. If you have symptoms that come on quickly, are severe, and are above and below the neck—fever (a key symptom of the flu), shivering, sweating, achy muscles and limbs—you've probably caught the flu. I like to say "one is a nuisance and the other

---

MOYAD FACT: One cough expels 2,000 to 19,500 virus-filled droplets, according to recent research from Hong Kong.

---

is a knockout." You can differentiate them with testing, but symptoms often overlap.

WHAT WORKS

1. Vitamin C 250 to 1,000 milligrams a day for prevention during periods of intense exercise and stress and especially for treatment along with conventional cold and flu medicines

I can hear it already. You're thinking, *I can't believe Moyad made cheap, old vitamin C number 1!* Well, give me a moment to explain. In the 1920s, American physician Alfred Hess discovered that pneumonia was one of the most common causes of death from untreated scurvy. Later he said that a lack of "antiscorbutic factor" (vitamin C or ascorbic acid) can lead to scurvy and increase the risk of lung infections. In 1934, Polish-born biochemist Casimir Funk (what an awesome name for a researcher or musician), who is credited with inventing the name *vitamin*, noted that an epidemic of pneumonia in Sudan went away when doctors gave vitamin C.

Fast-forward to today, and there is more research suggesting benefits: A meta-analysis of vitamin C research, which was published in the prestigious *Cochrane Database of Systematic Reviews*, concluded that "overall, the results of the five identified trials suggested vitamin C is beneficial in preventing and treating pneumonia." The largest meta-analysis of vitamin C demonstrated that ingesting several hundred milligrams or more per

IS THE FLU SHOT WORTH IT?

Some natural medicine enthusiasts get upset at me for recommending flu shots, and to this I respond, "We'll just have to agree to disagree." Given that between 20,000 and 36,000 people die *each* year from the flu and we have enough data to suggest an inexpensive vaccine can dramatically reduce deaths, I'm going to vote in favor of the vaccine until someone finds something that's proven to be better at saving lives. As more Americans get flu shots, we will see a dramatic drop in the death rate from this disease, which is what happened in 2014, as well as a reduction in cardiovascular disease events, due to inflammation control. I remember a similar concern 25 years ago over the hepatitis B vaccination, but the resulting drop in cases has been historic (it is 95 percent effective in preventing infection). Recent research suggests there has been up to a 90 percent reduction in death from liver cancer and complications from this virus where vaccination has been implemented.

day was associated with a significantly lower risk of pneumonia, and a faster recovery from pneumonia when used *with* conventional medicine. (Remember, pneumonia is often what kills people who have the flu.) No other dietary supplement has this kind of pneumonia data, which involved school kids, Marine recruits, and the elderly. Vitamin C is also safe to use during pregnancy, and this speaks volumes about its safety for children and adults.

After 30-plus clinical trials involving more than 11,000 individuals, we know that taking 1,000 milligrams a day (2,000 milligrams max) of vitamin C lowers the duration of the common cold in kids and adults by up to 20 percent. Individuals who have an increased risk of temporary immune suppression due to stress, intense exercise (which is a type of stress), or extreme environments may have the most to benefit in

terms of vitamin C: Five clinical studies involving approximately 600 soldiers, runners, and skiers under extreme stress (subarctic exercise conditions) showed a more than 50 percent reduction in the risk of getting a cold. (If I'm training for a marathon or long race and am putting in ridiculous amounts of exercise over several months, I'll take 500 to 1,000 milligrams of vitamin C daily.) Researchers have also found that vitamin C helps reduce common cold–induced asthma. There isn't much data in the area of flu prevention or treatment, which is true for all dietary supplements, but preliminary investigations suggest vitamin C may help produce certain compounds, like interferon, that can help in the fight against the flu as long as you're vaccinated.

There has been some concern over the potential for ascorbic acid to increase urinary oxalate levels in individuals at risk for kidney stones, but this is mainly after long-term use of high dosages (1,000 or more milligrams daily), and most people need extra vitamin C for only a week or two when they feel like they're getting a cold or are susceptible to one. Additionally, in my own research I've found that a nonacidic form of vitamin C known as calcium ascorbate (I used Ester-C) has the potential to reduce or have no impact on oxalate levels in individuals without a history of kidney stones. There are only a few very rare circumstances where vitamin C should not be taken, such as with the medical condition hemochromatosis (a genetic defect that leads to too much iron absorption, and vitamin C encourages absorption).

So, how can vitamin C prevent colds in some people, reduce the duration of a cold in others, and help treat pneumonia?

- It may protect against cellular stress caused by infections.

MOYAD FACT: Some animals have extremely large requirements for vitamin C. For example, monkeys and apes consume 10 to 20 times the human Recommended Dietary Allowance. And an adult goat produces its own vitamin C and will make 10,000 to 15,000 milligrams of C per day; if it's under stress, the goat will increase production manyfold. Of course, this doesn't prove that humans need more; it just demonstrates the importance of this vitamin in the animal kingdom. Long ago, we used to be able to make vitamin C from sugars, like glucose, right in the liver (which is how other mammals make it today), but now we've lost that ability because of a simple mutation (and perhaps because we get enough in our diet).

- The concentration of vitamin C in immune cells is much higher than in the blood (10 to 50 times higher, on average) and in most organs of the body, which suggests a greater need for vitamin C for immune cells so they can do what they do.

- It may also help certain immune cells mature and release compounds that help kill bacteria and viruses. Some infections actually impact the metabolism of vitamin C, which reduces amounts in the blood, urine, and immune cells.

- Vitamin C is involved in the chemotaxis of monocytes and macrophages, which means it might provide our immune cells with added energy to help them migrate to the source of infection.

- It regenerates the antioxidant form of vitamin E in the body, which may also help with immunity.

- Vitamin C increases levels of a compound called glutathione, which enhances the immune system.

Still, it is incredible to me how some health care professionals dismiss the research related to vitamin C and the common cold (more than 30 good clinical trials have been completed—probably the most for any dietary supplement).

A lot of folks have told me through the years that Emergen-C, Airborne, and other cold formulas really appear to work, and I always point out that they all have one thing in common—they all have about

1,000 milligrams of vitamin C per tablet or packet! You could just take vitamin C. You might ask, why not just eat the recommended five servings of fruits and vegetables a day? Won't that be enough? No. That will only get you about 200 to 300 milligrams of vitamin C, and only *if* you're lucky to consistently pick the few fruits and veggies with the most C (like papaya, strawberries, oranges, and broccoli). Plus, only 10 to 20 percent of the population eats five servings a day!

2. (tie and moving up fast) *Pelargonium sidoides* 30 drops (1.5 milliliters) three times a day for 10 days for cold treatment

I'm going to break two rules of not recommending 1) a supplement that requires taking a lot of drops or pills and 2) a homeopathic product. The first is primarily a convenience and compliance issue, and as for the second, since there are still detectable levels of active ingredient in this herbal product, I think *Pelargonium sidoides* should be considered a dietary supplement (unlike many other homeopathic remedies, which are very diluted). *P. sidoides* is a species of South African geranium that's been used for centuries in Zulu medicine and has two randomized trials showing it can improve symptoms of acute bronchitis (which is usually caused by a virus). Its consistent history of effectiveness for respiratory symptoms and safety in kids and adults is what spurred me to include it in my top three for cold treatment (not

for prevention). It appears to work by inducing the interferon system and upregulating cytokines in protecting host cells from viral infection.

This liquid herbal product is easy to find (look for Umcka ColdCare and follow the dosage instructions on the box), and the side effects are similar to a placebo. The primary product used in clinical trials comes from Willmar Schwabe Pharmaceuticals in Germany and is also known as EPs 7630 in many studies. It appears to reduce the duration and severity of common cold symptoms within 5 days, but more commonly 10 days. It worked better for nasal congestion and drainage, sneezing, sore and scratchy throat, hoarseness, and headache than for fever, cough, and muscle aches. Weakness, exhaustion, and fatigue were also improved. By day 10, about 79 percent versus 31 percent (placebo group) felt better, and it reduced days missed from work by about 1 to 1½. It could be argued that since most positive *P. sidoides* studies have been funded by the company, we should be skeptical. This is fair, but it does not change the fact that the studies had good methodology, efficacy, and safety.

2. (tie) American ginseng (*Panax quinquefolius*) 200 milligrams twice a day **or Panax ginseng** 100 milligrams a day for prevention during cold and flu season

Research has shown that American ginseng can activate some immune cells (macrophages), may increase cytokine and antibody production, and can even help natural killer cells in the body that go after infections. It's been studied against a placebo in at least five different clinical trials, and it reduced the number of colds by 25 percent (not that impressive, but not that bad) and the duration of colds or acute respiratory infections by as much as 6 days (very impressive). The most common dosage was 200 milligrams twice a day for 8 to 16 weeks (with 4 percent ginsenosides).

In one impressive trial with Panax ginseng (Ginsana), 227 healthy adults who had been vaccinated for the flu took 100 milligrams of a ginseng extract or placebo for 12 weeks. The ginseng group had a 65 percent reduction in colds. Panax ginseng is getting funding for some large future trials, so keep your eye on it. (Preliminary results with larger dosages, up to 3,000 milligrams per day, have shown some benefit for flu prevention.)

Here's the catch with these products when it comes to colds and flu: While the effective active ingredient in ginseng for improving fatigue is something called ginsenosides, some ginseng products that have shown benefits for colds do *not* contain them. So there may be other active ingredients responsible for the benefits that researchers aren't aware of yet. In other words, it's difficult to say exactly which product is the best to choose, whether it's a supplement like COLD-FX or Ginsana (Panax ginseng), which contains 4 percent ginsenosides. I don't endorse one type of ginseng product over another because the research is unclear (they both may work in a similar fashion).

Side effects reported with American ginseng include gastrointestinal upset, headache, anxiety, and insomnia. (The last two are not surprising since it is one of the only dietary supplements proven to reduce fatigue and improve energy levels in some people when taken long term.) So taking it in the late afternoon or evening can increase the odds that you'll have trouble sleeping. But if you're sick and need to keep working, ginseng could play a role in reducing the fatigue and weakness associated with colds or the flu.

Never take ginseng if you're pregnant or breastfeeding because this has not been adequately studied. Similarly, I do *not* believe kids should take it because it hasn't been well studied in this population either. Also, there have been some case reports of drug interactions (warfarin, phenelzine, and alcohol), so, as always, check with a pharmacist or doctor you trust before taking this supplement. Overall, side effects generally have been similar to a placebo in trials.

3. (tie) Brewer's yeast–derived fermentate or beta-glucans from yeast 250 to 500 milligrams a day for prevention and treatment of cold and flu symptoms

Modified yeast products are essentially yeast that has been placed under some sort of laboratory-induced stress to produce more immune-fighting compounds. The product EpiCor has the most human research so far. People who took 500 milligrams per day for 12 weeks had fewer cold and flu symptoms and a shorter duration of symptoms than with a placebo. They also reported less nasal stuffiness, hoarseness, and weakness. (These supplements have also been found to reduce nasal allergy symptoms and improve gut immune antibody levels in separate clinical trials.) Full disclosure: I assisted in the design and research of some of these clinical trials for EpiCor, and our research was given one of the highest awards in the supplement industry. I no longer consult for this company, but I am as convinced of the research today as I was many years ago when these trials were conducted. I am happy with the overall research done on yeast-based products for cold and flu symptoms.

Other components of yeast, such as beta-glucan, have immune surveillance and modifying properties that can increase the strength of the immune response. Yeast-based products, such as EpiCor and Wellmune, are interesting because they contain so many potentially beneficial ingredients that identifying the one that is clearly responsible for a particular outcome is kind of like asking which compound from a multivitamin is the most important.

The safety of these products has been excellent in trials, with side effects similar to or even less than a placebo. There is some concern that people with inflammatory bowel disease should not use yeast products because the immune response they prompt could theoretically cause a flare-up in symptoms, but this is not definitive so talk to your doctor.

People often ask me if just using brewer's or baker's yeast has the same impact. It is safe but does not have near the amount of research, so I like to stick with what worked in the clinical trials. I believe modified forms of these yeasts provide enhanced immune benefits beyond what the original forms deliver. It's certainly safe to experiment and be your own guinea pig.

3. (tie) Zinc (acetate or gluconate)
10 to 15 milligrams every 2 to 3 hours until cold symptoms disappear or 10 to 20 milligrams a day for cold and flu symptoms (*only* for treatment)

Zinc is an essential mineral that's used in hundreds of metabolic pathways in the body. There is no doubt that a deficiency of this mineral can increase the risk of infection. Research has shown zinc can block cold viruses from attaching inside the nose and protect cell membranes from toxins produced by these infectious agents. Yet, there is that side effect thing! The reason zinc comes in tied for third place—and at low dosages—is because it is very toxic in large doses. Even when zinc works, many people quit taking it because they feel the benefits do not outweigh the side effects (bad taste and nausea).

One of the largest reviews of past clinical trials of zinc supplements found that they appear to reduce cold symptoms in adults (by 1 to 2 days more than placebo), but not kids, when taken within 24 hours of symptom onset and that zinc acetate impacted symptoms a little more than the gluconate or

MOYAD FACT: In the past year, more than 60 percent of Americans who were hospitalized or died from the flu were between the ages of 18 and 64. Yet another reason to get vaccinated!

sulfate forms. Subjects took 10 to 15 milligrams every 2 to 3 hours until symptoms began to disappear. Overall, more than half of these clinical trials showed efficacy. The acetate and gluconate forms have the most research in general, but they're also less apt to bind to additives in supplements and other products, which could reduce the amount absorbed by the body.

There is some research showing that normalizing zinc levels (because there's a deficiency) could improve cell-mediated immunity, which is needed when you're fighting the flu and pneumonia.

Do not take zinc to *prevent* colds or the flu; only take it when you're sick. And avoid zinc inhalers and nasal gels; they can reduce your sense of taste or smell, sometimes permanently. Also, take zinc with food to reduce the risk of stomach upset.

HONORABLE MENTIONS

Elderberry has shown promise for the treatment of colds and the flu. In two small studies done more than 20 years ago, up to 4 tablespoons of elderberry extract per day for 3 to 5 days along with conventional treatment cleared up flu symptoms faster than a placebo. (Both studies used the "original formula" Sambucol supplement, with 3.8 percent extract.) While I'm a bit skeptical due to the age of the studies, it appears safe, so I cannot reject it as an option unless some study proves that elderberry extract is clearly ineffective. Throw in a few recent laboratory studies and it still seems that the benefit of these extracts (now there are many) outweighs the risk.

Andrographis paniculata, or Nees extract, is an herbal extract that's also known as Chiretta, King of Bitters, or Kalmegh, that has been used widely in India (one common brand is Kalmcold). The herb has demonstrated some anti-inflammatory and immune-enhancing benefits, which stem from its potential primary active ingredient known as andrographolide. It has been studied over and over for the treatment of colds, but researchers still haven't been able to identify the exact amount needed of the active ingredients. The most common dosage of andrographolide used in most of the clinical trials was 60 milligrams per day for 3 to 7 days. There is no good research on the potential for allergic reactions to this herbal, and the number of reports has been small. In other words, use at your own risk.

Vitamin D might help, but only in cases of extreme deficiency. Let me repeat that: I recommend this for cold and flu prevention and treatment *only* if your blood test is very low—10 ng/mL or less. If you're deficient, raising blood levels higher (20 ng/mL) or back to normal (30 ng/mL) could have a large impact on your risk of getting colds and the flu as well as pneumonia and other serious infections, such as tuberculosis. Known as the sunshine vitamin, D activates cathelicidins, a group of natural antimicrobial peptides made by immune cells and other cells in the body. It also stimulates immune cells to protect the body from infections.

If you have normal or near-normal levels, vitamin D won't help you fight off viruses. The VIDARIS (Vitamin D and Acute Respiratory Infection Study) randomized trial—one of the best and most rigorous ever conducted—looked at whether healthy individuals can benefit from D supplementation. Participants received 200,000 IU of vitamin D_3 (one megadose) at the start of the study, another 200,000 IU dose 1 month later, and 100,000 IU monthly thereafter for a total of 18 months (the recommended daily intake for adults is 600 to 800 IU per day). Compared to a placebo, the D supplementation did not reduce the incidence or severity of an upper respiratory tract infection in healthy adults (332 of them) with near-normal vitamin D levels.

Juice concentrate supplements, concentrated extracts of fruits and vegetables, can be a convenient way for some people to get their five servings a day. Although these supplements don't contain fiber, they can be helpful for some people who can't tolerate the real thing for whatever reason. Recent research shows that people (health care workers) who took these juice concentrate supplements daily saw a potentially significant reduction in cold-symptom days (fewer colds in general and less severe symptoms) over 8 months compared to placebo. This looks interest-ing, and I'm hoping we see more research in this area.

WHAT'S WORTHLESS

Echinacea. This supplement has had some positive research, but it hasn't been consistent. The biggest problem with echinacea is that it hasn't done well in more rigorous studies. On top of that, echinacea is a member of the large Asteraceae family (aster, daisy, sunflower), which can cause serious allergic reactions in certain people and may increase the risk of side effects from some drugs. Given the lack of research and the potential side effects, the risk is higher than the benefit to me.

Garlic. There are no well-done clinical trials that show these supplements aid in the prevention or treatment of colds or the flu. Malodorous belching is the biggest problem with these supplements.

Probiotics. They're being promoted for everything these days, but the research is weak in this area right now. When experts boast that taking probiotics in food or supplements may reduce antibiotic use, well that's groovy, but you don't need antibiotics for the majority of cold and flu cases because they're caused by viruses, not bacteria.

Miscellaneous. Reviews of more than 50 other products showed that there isn't enough data out there to support any other supplements for colds and the flu beyond what is recommended in this section. There is a ton of competition, but you have to look at what has been tested the most;

what has the most consistent impact against colds, the flu, and pneumonia; and what is safe enough to use for kids, cost effective, and easy to find.

WHAT ARE THE OPTIONS FOR KIDS?

Vitamin C (250 to 500 milligrams per day) is safe and may shorten the duration of a cold in kids. (You can also pair it with conventional flu remedies for the flu.) In one of the only recent reviews of past clinical trials with children, researchers found that zinc could reduce the risk of pneumonia, with more of a potential impact on severe pneumonia. Yet the good studies have come from India, Bangladesh, Peru, and South Africa, where there may be large zinc deficiencies, and critics suggest these results would not be the same if the studies had been done in the United States. I believe zinc supplementation is controversial for kids, and I would never recommend a child take more than 10 milligrams a day of elemental zinc from gluconate, sulfate, or acetate for several days. And since there's such a high risk for nausea and bad taste, giving your kids zinc supplements isn't really worth it anyway.

LIFESTYLE CHANGES

Heart healthy = immune healthy. You saw this one coming, right? People are always asking me how they can improve their immune health. Anything that is heart healthy also promotes normal immune function and can reduce the risk of illness. Factors associated with a lower risk of heart disease (low cholesterol; normal blood pressure, blood sugar, and weight; and no tobacco) are all associated with lower rates of illness, including hospitalization from the flu. Exercise in moderation (30 to 45 minutes daily) also improves immune function, and so does adequate sleep. Gee, what a shocker! Even a heart-healthy diet (which is low in calories and high in fiber, omega-3s, fruits, and especially vegetables and incorporates healthy fats) is the best diet for the immune system.

Gargle frequently. Irrigating the back of the throat, where bacteria and viruses can set up shop, can significantly reduce the risk of infection. Gargle with several ounces of water several times a day. Using warm salt water can soothe a sore throat because the salt draws out excess water in throat tissues, reduces inflammation, and clears mucus and other irritants from the back of the throat.

Wash your hands regularly. Antibacterial soaps are a waste of money because they haven't been shown to work better than regular soap and they promote resistance. Wash your hands with regular soap and water, making sure you clean the front and back of your hands and your fingernails each time. Follow this up with a 62 percent (or more) ethyl alcohol hand sanitizer gel.

Flush your nose. Use a metered saline nose spray in each nostril several times a day to loosen potential bacteria

THE BEST RX FOR COLD AND FLU

These simple research-proven strategies can help alleviate your most irritating symptoms.

COUGH AND SORE THROAT First, you probably do not need an antibiotic for your sore throat because most are caused by viruses, not bacteria. But here's a surprise: Honey beat the number-one-selling over-the-counter cough suppressant (dextromethorphan) in a head-to-head study in kids and adults. (Do not use honey for children younger than 2 because it can increase the risk of an infection known as botulism.) I love the science behind this: Nerves that control coughing may interact with parts of the brain that detect sweetness, so the taste of honey may calm the area of the brain that makes you cough. Honey also contains a compound that can be converted into hydrogen peroxide, and it has other antimicrobial compounds that may prevent infection, or at least improve recovery from it. Of course, honey—like all cough meds—is viscous and can coat your throat. Take 2 teaspoons every 4 to 5 hours during the day and 30 minutes before you go to bed. Darker types, such as buckwheat honey, might have more antimicrobial compounds (and they have more clinical research).

CONGESTION AND SORE THROAT Chicken soup eases cold and flu symptoms by loosening nasal secretions, reducing throat soreness, and preventing inflammatory reactions. Hot liquid in general is a demulcent, which means it forms a soothing film over mucous membranes, helping to relieve sore throat or cough symptoms. Spicy soups and other food generate airway secretions that can calm an inflamed throat.

COUGH Vicks VapoRub contains camphor and menthol, and when applied topically to the chest and neck, it can reduce a cough. (Do not use camphor for kids younger than 2.)

and viruses; it can also get rid of allergens that are stuck in there.

Get happy. Research actually shows that upbeat, positive people are less likely to develop a cold, and when they do get sick, they're more likely to report milder symptoms (happy person = happy immune system).

Fight stress. Significant stress and crowds can increase the risk of colds. This is the reason why researchers love to conduct their cold and flu studies in military boot camps, schools, and office environments.

Lose (or clean) your tie. Preliminary research suggests that health care professionals infrequently wash their neckties, which are reservoirs of pathogenic microorganisms. Want to do your family and friends a favor? Skip the tie during cold and flu season. Next comes the stetho-scope, another hotbed of bugs.

WHAT ELSE DO
I NEED TO KNOW?

An antihistamine, like the kind you use for allergies, can help tame sneezing, a runny nose, and watery eyes, and combining it with a decongestant will reduce symptoms even more. However, antihistamines do not work better than a placebo for a cough.

If you think you've caught the flu, get to your doctor within the first 48 hours of having symptoms and see if you qualify for Tamiflu. A recent review of the research, published in the journal *BMJ*, showed concerning side effects, such as nausea, vomiting, and headaches, and potentially less efficacy against the flu compared to previous reviews. Talk to your doctor about this latest controversy.

Complex Regional Pain Syndrome

C

THE JURY'S STILL OUT

Dr. Moyad Secret Complex regional pain syndrome, or CRPS (formerly known as reflex sympathetic dystrophy syndrome), is a very painful condition of the feet, legs, hands, or arms, which usually occurs after some kind of trauma to the area (fracture or surgery). Common symptoms include diffuse pain and edema, a difference in skin temperature, and limited active range of motion. It's also one of the best examples in this book of how generalizing supplements—how they're all bad or all good—is rarely effective. For years I've heard that vitamin C doesn't treat anything; it's worthless and no one needs it. However, there's a clear indication that it can help with prevention, and perhaps even treatment, of CRPS. So throw your vitamin C prejudice out the window!

Vitamin C. Taking 500 milligrams of C (plain ascorbic acid) on the day of a fracture and for 50 days thereafter is one of the best ways to prevent CRPS; it appears to reduce the risk by more than 80 percent. Higher doses of vitamin C (1,500 milligrams per day) have not worked better than 500 milligrams in terms of wrist fractures. Now, whether vitamin C can be helpful in the *treatment* of this condition is still unknown. Although all of the initial research with vitamin C and CRPS was after a wrist fracture, new studies are looking at other sites of the body. A small study of individuals having foot and ankle surgery demonstrated that 1,000 milligrams of vitamin C every morning beginning on the first day after surgery and continuing for 45 days may also reduce CRPS postsurgery. (The researchers in this study now recommend 500 milligrams of vitamin C because 1,000 milligrams could increase oxalate levels in the body and the risk of kidney stones in certain people. Plus, 1,000 milligrams per day doesn't appear to work any better than 500 milligrams anyhow!)

153

Congestive Heart Failure

Dr. Moyad Secret Congestive heart failure (CHF) means your heart, for a variety of reasons, including hypertension and heart disease, can no longer meet your body's oxygen demands. For decades I watched so many people tout the benefits of hawthorn herbal products in conjunction with conventional medicine for CHF. But when there were finally some larger clinical trials, no benefit was seen. In the HERB CHF (Hawthorn Extract Randomized Blinded Chronic Heart Failure) study, investigators found no symptomatic or functional benefit at dosages of 450 milligrams twice daily versus a placebo. (This was a trial led by several University of Michigan researchers.) Hawthorn also increased the risk of noncardiac side effects—such as nausea, diarrhea, vomiting, and loose stools—in this study. And in another well-known study (the SPICE trial from Germany), there was also no overall benefit with hawthorn compared to a placebo. What it comes down to is this: I would be scared to use a supplement for this serious condition unless there was some really, really good evidence to recommend it.

CoQ10. There has been some good preliminary clinical trial data supporting the use of this supplement along with conventional medicine for CHF. It's found in high concentrations in heart tissue and may help improve heart function. An analysis of more than 13 placebo-controlled trials suggested a positive effect: CoQ10 increased left ventricular ejection fraction (the amount of blood being pumped to the rest of the body by the left ventricle) by approximately 4 percent (a significant change) and resulted in a small potential benefit in the New York Heart Association (NYHA) functional classification (a gauge of the severity of heart failure), which suggests it may improve prognosis. Researchers used dosages of 100 to 300 milligrams on average, but higher dosages did not necessarily translate into better benefits. Those with less severe CHF benefited more. The most recent studies have shown less of an impact with CoQ10 compared to older studies, but part of the reason for this is the fact that drug treatments just keep getting better.

The biggest trial yet for CoQ10 is Q-SYMBIO, where more than 400 patients took a daily dose of 2 milligrams of CoQ10 per kilogram of body weight along with conventional treatments. It reduced death from all causes at the 2-year period compared to the placebo. We're waiting on more details from this study, so stay tuned.

Constipation

Dr. Moyad Secret As I've gotten older, I've noticed that at some point—I'm not sure when, exactly—my wild oats have turned into All-Bran. I use this line at conferences for laughs, but let's face it, things don't "move" like they used to as we age. There are a ton of dietary supplements out there for constipation, but they usually only contain inexpensive soluble fiber, which can help, but it can also cause terrible gas, bloating, and stomach pain if you overdo it. *In*soluble fiber is just as important for preventing and treating constipation and rarely causes the gastrointestinal side effects associated with the soluble kind. This is something patients just don't know! Eating more foods with fiber (like most fruits and veggies), especially insoluble fiber, and making some key lifestyle changes can prevent and treat constipation better than any pill in this section.

WHAT IS IT?

Physicians have different definitions for constipation, but one commonly accepted description is having three or fewer bowel movements per week. People who experience it, however, often have their own definition, including straining to go; hard stools; infrequent stools; and bloating, cramping, or other abdominal discomfort immediately before or during a bowel movement. You could say "constipation is in the eye of the beholder." You get the picture.

So why does it happen? The intestines move in a wavelike motion, known as peristalsis, to propel food through your system and out of the body. If the wave slows or the contents are too dry, the stools become hard and difficult to pass. And if constipation becomes chronic, it increases your risk of anal and rectal cracks, breaks, and infections; rectal bleeding; fecal impaction (where stool gets stuck in the intestines, a medical emergency); and hemorrhoids.

Many medications, including more than 100 prescription drugs and some over-the-counter products, can increase the risk of constipation, especially pain medications, such as codeine and hydrocodone, which are notorious for causing severe or chronic constipation. Calcium supplements, anabolic steroids, antihistamines, and antihypertensives also increase the risk of constipation, and the more medications you take, the better your odds of being constipated.

Common (and not so common) causes of constipation include:

- Age
- Lifestyle habits (dehydration, lack of fiber, high-protein diets, too little exercise)
- Irritable bowel syndrome
- Neurological causes (spinal cord injury, Parkinson's disease, multiple sclerosis)
- Obstructive causes (like colon cancer or Crohn's disease)
- Gynecologic issues (hormonal fluctuations, pelvic relaxation, pregnancy, and childbirth)
- Metabolic/hormonal problems (diabetes, low thyroid levels, low magnesium, low potassium, high calcium, high blood sugar)
- Connective tissue disease (scleroderma)
- Psychological problems (depression, eating disorders, stress)

Women are two to three times more susceptible to constipation, mainly due to gynecologic issues and hormonal changes, and—no surprise here—they are also more likely to schedule a doctor visit for it than men. Some experts also believe that living in colder climates increases the risk of constipation, perhaps from being less active and dehydrated in the winter. Having lived in Michigan most of my life and a few years in Florida, I tend to agree with this.

Chronic constipation (lasting more than 3 months out of the year), sudden constipation, or constipation that's accom-panied by rapid weight loss, bleeding, or fever should be brought to your doctor's attention. There are a variety of tests available to determine the underlying issues.

WHAT WORKS

Note: If there are no red flags (fever, weight loss, bleeding) that prompt further testing, the first line of treatment will generally include switching to a high-fiber diet or adding fiber supplements, exercising, and increasing your fluid intake. Keep in mind that relying solely on supplements to have a bowel movement can create numerous complications, including bowel dependence (from stimulant laxatives) and even pneumonia (from lubricant laxatives). In other words, you won't be able to poop without them. Also, chronic use of constipation products can cause serious electrolyte imbalances and dehydration. Finally, women who are pregnant or breastfeeding and children under the age of 16 should only take a laxative for the shortest amount of time and only with a doctor's approval because they have generally not been tested in these populations. It's just not worth taking a chance.

1. Psyllium 10 to 15 grams a day

I like psyllium (ispaghula husk) because it is one of the only fiber supplements that has enough clinical trials behind it suggesting that it can do all of the following:

- Reduce constipation
- Help control blood glucose

- Reduce LDL (bad) cholesterol levels

- Help with weight loss and reduce appetite in some cases

- Reduce blood pressure slightly in some people with high blood pressure

- Increase stool frequency as good as some prescription drugs (lactulose)

- Help with diarrhea in some cases

- Produce less gas and bloating compared to other commercial soluble fiber sources, such as inulin, since it is a mostly soluble viscous fiber

And psyllium is gluten free (less than 20 ppm gluten) and generally low in calories (45 calories per tablespoon).

Other natural fiber supplements (guar gum, locust bean, inulin) just don't have the amount of human evidence that psyllium has. I recommend the powdered form over the pills because you would have to take at least six capsules to equal the equivalent dose of 1 tablespoon of psyllium. Plus, the powders are so much cheaper. Always take it with at least 8 ounces of water (per tablespoon) and at least 2 hours before or after other medications or supplements. It works so well and so quickly that it can prevent your other medicines from being absorbed in the intestines.

Finally, fiber supplements are not as helpful in rare types of constipation where there is some kind of underlying physiological disorder, such as slow transit time through the intestines or pelvic floor dysfunction.

2. Magnesium citrate 400 to 600 milligrams a day

Physicians have been using magnesium drinks (magnesium sulfate or Epsom salts) for years to treat constipation. They work by acting like a sponge to draw or attract water into the colon to make the stool softer. *A word of warning:* Taking more than the dosage recommended here can cause serious side effects, including cardiac and respiratory toxicity. And individuals with kidney problems should stay away from magnesium supplements unless cleared by a doctor to take them. Daily doses of 400 to 600 milligrams of elemental magnesium from magnesium oxide, slow-release magnesium, and chelated magnesium appear to be absorbed almost as well as the citrate form and are just as effective; sometimes they're cheaper than the citrate form, too, so experiment to find what works best for you. Your doctor might allow magnesium citrate for constipation if you're pregnant or breastfeeding, but always check.

Some people experience constipation because they're deficient in magnesium. Acid reflux drugs (especially the proton pump inhibitors), metformin (the number one drug used for type 2 diabetes), high-protein or meat-based diets, daily alcohol consumption, daily exercise, and heavy menstrual periods can increase your risk of being magnesium deficient. It's hard to get enough magnesium in your diet to treat constipation, but high-fiber foods often contain it, so you get a twofer!

3. Senna one to four pills a day

The active ingredient in the senna plant is sennosides (also known as anthraquinone glycosides), which have stimulant laxative properties. This means it works by increasing the activity of the intestines so the muscles contract and keep those stools moving forward. Senna is frequently found in tea or herbal products and often with cascara (a.k.a. sacred bark or California buckthorn), but due to quality control issues, I am more comfortable recommending known commercial senna products, such as Senokot (or a pharmacy generic), that contain sennosides or a standardized senna concentrate. Although this is a "natural" plant-based supplement, you should take it only as needed and for no more than a week. Again, it's easy to become dependent on these stimulant laxatives and then your bowels won't work without them.

WHAT'S WORTHLESS

Probiotics. They're the hot topic these days, but probiotics are not a cure-all by any means. They're being overhyped for all sorts of problems, especially constipation. Let me say this right now: There is *no* probiotic pill that has enough evidence to recommend it for constipation prevention or treatment (there is a probiotic drink called Yakult, however, that can be beneficial; see Lifestyle Changes on the next page). *Bifidobacterium lactis* DN-173 010 (the probiotic strain found in Dannon Activia yogurt) may slightly increase the number of bowel movements. Many people don't notice any change at all, but they're still paying a lot of money. (I feel the same way about *Bifidobacterium lactis* BB-12, a probiotic supplement strain found in various products.) You're much better off just eating more fiber, which does so much more for you than just moving your bowels.

Calcium. *All* calcium dietary supplements—carbonate, citrate, and even antacids with calcium—have a high risk of gastrointestinal side effects, including constipation! I see this all the time, especially now that so many men and women are getting enough calcium from food and also taking calcium supplements. Please check with a dietitian or do your own calculation over 3 days to determine how much calcium you're getting before taking any supplements. If you need to take calcium supplements, try to find a brand that contains some magnesium (50 to 100 milligrams) because it could reduce the risk of constipation.

Iron. Again, one of the most common side effects of iron supplementation is constipation and nausea. If this occurs, talk with your doctor about reducing the dose or changing the type of iron you're taking. One option that is gaining popularity and has been studied many times is "intermittent iron supplementation." You take the supplements once, twice, or three times a week on nonconsecutive days to reduce side effects.

Aloe supplements. The aloe plant contains compounds called anthraquinones, which have a laxative effect when they interact with intestinal bacteria on their way through your system (some of the sugars in aloe may also act as a laxative). But research on these effects is scarce and inconsistent, and aloe supplements rarely work better than fiber or magnesium, in my experience. The other problem is that they can cause severe potassium reductions that could lead to abnormal heart rhythms. It's for this and other reasons that the FDA believes aloe supplements need more research on safety and efficacy before they can be promoted for improving constipation.

WHAT ARE THE OPTIONS FOR KIDS?

Fiber, such as psyllium, is your safest option for kids, based on the research. Studies have found that it helps reduce abdominal pain and increase the frequency and consistency of stools. Probiotics and other supplements have *not* been found to be helpful in kids, and I do not recommend them. One of the better clinical trials tested a probiotic in 159 constipated children. There were no serious side effects, but the commercial probiotic product did not work any better than a placebo.

LIFESTYLE CHANGES

Diversify your diet. Powders and bars are okay sources of fiber, but they're usually soluble fiber and only a few of them match what you can get in high-fiber foods or cereal. Getting the recommended 20 to 30 grams of fiber a day from diet alone is not easy unless you find diverse sources, such as cereals, fruits, veggies, beans, and nuts. Remember, most healthy foods are a mix of soluble and insoluble fiber, which is ideal. Soluble fiber dissolves in water, slows the absorption of some foods, and interacts with bacteria in the intestines, often causing gas. Insoluble fiber absorbs water and helps to rapidly move stool through the colon. It's like having a brake and a gas pedal in a car—one without the other is useless.

Get moving. Individuals who are sedentary have a higher risk of constipation than people who work out regularly. Exercise helps stimulate digestion, but it's also dehydrating, which can make constipation worse. If you work out, as we all should, make sure you drink more fluids (especially water). (*Note:* Excessive exercise, where you're working out for many hours and can become extremely dehydrated, can make constipation worse!)

MOYAD FACT: Tobacco, like caffeine, is a stimulant, which is one reason constipation is a side effect of quitting smoking. Tobacco smoke was actually suggested as a laxative in 1643, and more than a hundred years later, the Royal Humane Society of London recommended the tobacco enema: "It is not only the admission of kindly warmth into the internal parts of the body which proves advantageous, but it is a stimulus to excite irritability and to restore the languid peristaltic motion of the intestines." I'll pass, thanks (no pun intended)!

LAXATIVE CATEGORIES AND HOW THEY WORK	PRODUCTS (ALWAYS ASK ABOUT CHEAPER, GENERIC OPTIONS, TOO)
Fiber supplements/bulk-forming laxatives (they draw water into the intestine to make the stool softer, so they *must* be taken with water)	• Citrucel • Metamucil • Fiber (generic)
Lubricant laxatives (they lubricate the stool and allow it to move through the intestines more easily)	• Mineral oil
Saline laxatives and osmotics (these are poorly absorbed ions that work like a sponge to draw or attract water into the colon to soften the stool)	• Lactulose (Rx only) • Magnesium citrate/salt • Milk of magnesia • Polyethylene glycol (generic MiraLAX) • Phillips' MO • Sorbitol
Stimulant laxatives (they increase the movement or activity of the intestinal muscles to keep stools moving forward)	• Aloe (the laxative drug from the plant has FDA issues) • Correctol • Dulcolax • Bisacodyl (generic Correctol) • Ex-Lax • Senokot • Senna (generic Senokot) • Castor oil
Stool softeners (they moisten the stool and prevent dehydration to make it easier to pass)	• Colace • Dialose • Surfak • Docusate (generic Colace)

Limit processed foods. Whenever you take a fruit or veggie and manipulate or process it, you end up with little to no fiber. Packaged/processed foods in general often provide calories without adding fiber, so opt for fresh, "real" foods.

Watch your protein intake. It's an essential part of your diet, but eating too much—especially if you're cutting out high-fiber foods—can cause constipation.

It's the primary complaint I hear from people on high-protein diets.

Go tiny for more power. While nuts and seeds in general aren't high in fiber, ground flaxseed and chia seeds are great sources that can be added to foods or beverages. (There are some claims that taking 1 to 2 tablespoons of flaxseed oil or olive oil can help lubricate the stool, which may be the case, but there is no fiber in the oils.)

DR. MOYAD'S FAVORITE FIBER SOURCES (THEY CONTAIN BOTH INSOLUBLE AND SOLUBLE FIBER)

FRUITS	GRAMS OF FIBER PER SERVING
Dried plums	6
Apple with skin	3–3.5
Prunes	3
Raspberries	3
Strawberries	3
VEGETABLES	**GRAMS OF FIBER PER SERVING**
Artichoke (cooked)	6
Broccoli	4.5
Brussels sprouts	4.5
Green beans	3
Kale	3
LEGUMES	**GRAMS OF FIBER PER SERVING**
Baked beans	9
Kidney beans	7–8
Navy beans	6
Lima beans	4.5
Lentils	4–5
GRAINS/CEREALS	**GRAMS OF FIBER PER SERVING**
Wheat-bran cereal (All-Bran Buds)	13–15 (per just $\frac{1}{3}$ cup)
Fiber One cereal	13–15
Oatmeal	4
Spaghetti (whole wheat)	4
Whole wheat bread	2–3

Chew gum. It's been shown to stimulate or maintain peristalsis after surgery, so it may also keep the bowels moving when you have a mild case of constipation or are just trying to get them to operate normally again.

Grab a cup of Joe. Caffeine is a stimulant, and in moderation it can keep your colon moving.

Eat *this* bug. The only real probiotic I trust for constipation is *Lactobacillus casei* Shirota. It's sold around the world under the brand name Yakult, but it was created in Japan by fermenting the live *L. casei* Shirota strain with skim milk. In one study, people with chronic constipation who drank 2 to 3 ounces of Yakult daily experienced relief within 2 weeks. This product has also been tested in kids with chronic constipation at even lower dosages and appears to be helpful.

Just chill out. Abdominal massage? Biofeedback? Maybe. If stress is contributing to your chronic constipation problem or if constipation is stressing you out, then light abdominal massage or other tension-busting therapies might help.

WHAT ELSE DO I NEED TO KNOW?

I've created the chart shown on page 160 to give you a quick overview of the different types of laxatives (stimulants, osmotics, lubricants, etc.) and the associated products you'll see on store shelves.

Contrast-Induced Nephropathy

C

Dr. Moyad Secret There's always risk involved with any medical procedure. And when you inject dye or other chemicals into the body during certain imaging procedures, that risk is primarily to the kidneys; this is called contrast-induced nephropathy, or CIN (also known as contrast-induced acute kidney injury, or CI-AKI). Currently, there are many clinical trials going on with supplements for the prevention of CIN. NAC (N-acetylcysteine), which is the same product used to save the liver in the case of an acetaminophen overdose, is being studied, but overall the results have been weak. Vitamin C has some early positive research (nine randomized trials), and it's worth discussing with your doctor for before and after a procedure. Dosages and timing have been all over the place, though. Subjects took anywhere from 500 to 1,000 milligrams either the night before the procedure, the day of the procedure, or the day after the procedure.

Of course, heart healthy = kidney healthy: There's new evidence to suggest that the body and kidneys are better able to tolerate these procedure-induced injuries when the heart is healthy. In fact, new research on statin drugs (the ROSA-cIN trial) suggests they may have some anti-inflammatory and protective effects when used short term for these procedures. For this reason, hopefully someone will test red yeast rice supplements as well, since they work similarly to a low-dose statin (see the High Cholesterol section, page 234).

COPD (Chronic Obstructive Pulmonary Disease) or Chronic Bronchitis and Emphysema

THE JURY'S STILL OUT

Dr. Moyad Secret COPD essentially means the airflow in your lungs has been compromised, making breathing difficult. Emphysema and chronic bronchitis are two primary types of COPD. Tobacco kills, and even though many smokers never get lung cancer, many do get COPD, which is one of the primary reasons smoking is now one of the top five killers of men and women in the United States. It's also the primary reason people should quit using tobacco immediately. Regardless, nonsmokers can also get it. COPD treatment has many goals that supplements could help with, including reducing respiratory tract infections, exacerbation rate (worsening of disease/symptoms), number of days of suffering and length of hospital stay, and lung function decline and improving quality of life.

Pelargonium sidoides. When patients with stages II and III COPD took 30 drops (EPs 7630) three times per day for 24 weeks, they experienced fewer exacerbations, less antibiotic use, greater quality of life and patient satisfaction, and better ability to work. Some minor gastrointestinal side effects were higher than with the placebo. Find it in Umcka ColdCare and follow the directions on the label.

NAC (N-acetylcysteine). NAC may reduce inflammation and oxidative stress (the normal wear and tear that happens to all cells through the course of daily living and exposure to environmental factors, such as sun and loud noises, and toxins, such as lead or smoke) by activating cellular defense mechanisms. Ultimately this lowers sputum/mucous production, reduces mucous viscosity, and improves lung function and breathing. It might even prohibit bacteria from adhering to respiratory tissue. More than 30 clinical trials have demonstrated improvement when taking 600 to 1,800 milligrams of NAC per day for several months to a year. However, newer preliminary data is suggesting 600 milligrams is not effective, based on the large, multisite BRONCUS trial; dosages of 1,200 to 1,800 milligrams per day are more promising. Side effects have been similar to a placebo in most studies, and even if it only slightly reduces exacerbations and not the progression of the disease, it might be worth discussing with your doctor, especially for people who are having trouble tolerating conventional medicines.

Cystic Fibrosis

Dr. Moyad Secret Cystic fibrosis (CF) is one of the most common autosomal recessive genetic disorders in Caucasians of northern European descent. It's characterized by deteriorating lung function and pancreatic abnormalities. People with CF experience thick mucus in the bronchi and numerous infections of the airways, leading to a decline in respiratory function. Approximately 75 percent of CF patients now use complementary medicine to treat symptoms.

NAC (N-acetylcysteine). NAC acts as a precursor to raise glutathione (an antioxidant) levels in different body tissues, meaning it helps the body fight off free radicals and other toxins. It can also help thin out mucus, which is why it's called a mucolytic. Doses of 700 to 3,000 milligrams per day have been preliminarily tested and appear to be safe over several weeks (testing of long-term use hasn't been completed).

Magnesium. In one study, 300 milligrams per day of magnesium (in the form of an amino acid chelate, which may improve utilization of magnesium throughout the body) for 8 weeks improved respiratory muscle strength and possibly reduced disease severity when used with conventional CF treatments. The median weight of kids and adolescents (7 to 19 years old) in the study was 40 kilograms, and 7.5 milligrams of magnesium per kilogram was given.

Whey protein powder. Whey protein is getting a lot of attention for CF right now because it may improve muscle development and function and quality of life (see the Athletic Enhancement section, page 77).

L-arginine and L-citrulline. Theoretically, L-arginine can improve nitric oxide amounts in lung tissue, which helps expand the airways and improve breathing, but in reality it has had mixed results in studies. First of all, much of L-arginine gets degraded by the liver and intestines (see the Erectile Dysfunction section, page 186), so patients need to take 3 grams or more, based on a German university study, to see any potential benefit. However, L-citrulline solves this problem because it bypasses liver metabolism and is converted into L-arginine by the kidneys and then into nitric oxide. Plus, you can use half or less of the L-arginine dosage. More research with L-citrulline needs to be done, though.

Zinc. People with CF who have low zinc levels may reduce the number of days antibiotics are needed with 30 milligrams of zinc per day.

Depression

Dr. Moyad Secret The WHO (World Health Organization) has stated that depression (also known as major depressive disorder) is now the leading cause of disability world-wide and the second largest global disease burden next to heart disease. It can negatively impact all aspects of physical health, and it's so complex that without a comprehensive approach—including medication (*only* if needed), exercise, therapy, dietary supplements, and other lifestyle changes—the chances that treatment will be successful drop dramatically. Many doctors just want to throw some drugs at it. One randomized study from Duke University published in the *Archives of Internal Medicine* (since renamed *JAMA Internal Medicine*) more than 15 years ago showed men and women with major depressive disorder (MDD) had a greater chance of remission when they exercised just three times a week for 30 minutes a session (high-intensity walking or jogging) in addition to taking their prescription meds compared to taking medication alone. Overall, the impact of exercise on MDD was just as good as the drug itself over time (together they are synergistic). Did you hear about this study? Not many people did, although recent research has confirmed it. In another of my favorite unsung studies, men and women with MDD had a greater chance of responding to conventional prescription drugs for depression—after failing to respond to them initially—when a specific dietary supplement was added (hint: the supplement is ranked number one in this section).

Sometimes we fool ourselves in conventional medicine, just like in alternative medicine, and tell ourselves we have all the answers for patients. The truth is that conventional antidepressants have been lifesavers for many people, but in academic center studies as many as 50 percent of individuals do not see their depression get better with drugs. Other studies point to even higher numbers. This serves as a gentle reminder of the desperate need to continue to be open to all kinds of options for treating this very common, debilitating, and life-threatening condition.

WHAT IS IT?

Major depressive disorder is a remarkably heterogeneous condition; two patients with the same diagnosis can have few if any symptoms in common. It's often caused by abnormal changes in neurotransmitters in the brain (dopamine, serotonin, and norepinephrine), and it can also be triggered by age, life events, illness, medication, and even seasons.

Symptoms include feelings of sadness or absence of emotion, decreased interest or pleasure in activities, appetite change with weight loss or gain, decreased or increased sleep, fatigue or loss of energy, feelings of guilt or worthlessness, agitation or feelings of moving in slow motion, trouble concentrating, and recurrent thoughts of death or suicide. While doctors usually look for the presence of at least five of these symptoms, a diagnosis can be made based on just one or two. The major issue is that it disrupts your life.

Subtypes of MDD include atypical depression (where sufferers may not have the classic symptoms, and they don't respond to the classic treatments either), postpartum depression, seasonal affective disorder, melancholic depression, and catatonic depression. Dysthymia, mild depression lasting for at least 2 years, is not considered a type of MDD.

WHAT WORKS

Note: The concept "everything in moderation" is always a good rule, especially when it comes to treating depression. Most antidepressants work by increasing brain neurotransmitters (dopamine, norepinephrine, and serotonin). Get too much serotonin, though, and you can induce "serotonin syndrome," a potentially life-threatening condition that can cause diarrhea and shivering in mild cases and seizures and death in more severe situations. It usually happens when you add a new drug or supplement to your antidepressant regimen. I'm not trying to scare you, although maybe it's good to be a little

scared. Talk with your doctor before taking any supplements if you're already on antidepressants; supplements can work just as well as Western drugs in raising serotonin levels in some individuals, so you have to be careful.

1. SAM-e (S-adenosylmethionine)
800 to 1,600 milligrams once a day or 400 to 800 milligrams twice a day

SAM-e improves the production and use of several brain neurotransmitters, including dopamine and serotonin. Overall, it appears to work similarly to other antidepressants, but there are some differences. A review of approximately 50 studies on the treatment of MDD with SAM-e reported significant benefits with this drug over a placebo. Recent preliminary research funded by the National Institute of Mental Health suggests individuals who haven't responded to conventional SSRI (selective serotonin reuptake inhibitors) medications can see a significant improvement in depression (primarily MDD) when taking 400 milligrams of SAM-e twice daily for 2 weeks, and then transitioning to 800 milligrams twice daily for 4 weeks *with their conventional medications.*

There has been a concern in the past that SAM-e raises blood levels of homocysteine (a controversial marker of heart disease), but recent studies haven't shown this. Your doctor can always follow up with a blood test after you start taking it if you're concerned. Rare side effects include stomach upset, diarrhea, dry mouth, headache, mild insomnia, anorexia, sweating, dizziness, nervousness (especially at high dosages), and feelings of anxiety. Be aware that SAM-e might cause a toxic reaction when used with the cough suppressant dextromethorphan, certain antidepressants, or narcotic pain relievers, and it could worsen Parkinson's symptoms when taken with the drug levodopa.

There are two positive side effects with SAM-e: It doesn't appear to cause sexual dysfunction, which some other antidepressants commonly do, and it may be one of the best supplements out there for osteoarthritis pain (it works as well as over-the-counter pain relievers, with fewer side effects). I have recommended this supplement to patients for almost 2 decades with outstanding success. (It's also being studied specifically for atypical depression.) The primary problem is the price; I've seen bottles going for anywhere from $10 to $100, so you have to shop around. Also, always check the expiration date. SAM-e oxidizes quickly and the date marked on the bottle is the date to follow; it's not one of those pills you can take for a year or two after it expires.

2. St. John's wort (*Hypericum perforatum*) 500 to 1,200 milligrams a day in divided doses

St. John's wort was used in ancient Greece and has been used in Europe for depression since the 1980s. Researchers aren't sure exactly how it works yet, but it seems to block serotonin uptake in the brain and alter levels of multiple brain neurotransmitters, including dopamine, norepinephrine, and GABA (gamma-aminobutyric acid). A review of 29 trials with approximately 5,500 patients found that it may work as well as conventional antidepressants and that participants were 50 to 75 percent less likely to drop out compared to those taking a prescription. The most commonly used dosage in clinical trials was 900 milligrams daily, but doses between 500 to 1,200 milligrams (taken in divided amounts two or three times a day) over 4 to 12 weeks have been effective. The active ingredient in St. John's wort is hypericin, and whatever product you choose should be standardized to contain 0.3 percent hypericin.

Side effects have been low or rare in clinical trials, but they can include insomnia, vivid dreams, anxiety, dizziness, and skin sensitivity. However—and this is a biggie—it has the potential to interact with or reduce the effectiveness of almost half of all available prescription drugs, including birth control pills. And unlike SAM-e, you shouldn't combine St. John's wort with prescription antidepressants, such as SSRIs, tricyclic antidepressants, or MAO (monoamine oxidase) inhibitors. You should also avoid it if you're taking immunosuppressants, antiretrovirals (anti-HIV drugs), blood thinners (like warfarin), and chemotherapy drugs. Still, it's worth talking with your doctor about it; St. John's wort has been inappropriately tagged as the poster child of why supplements cannot be combined with prescription drugs, and this is not entirely fair.

Many alternative medicine experts say St. John's wort works as well as most conventional drug options for depression, but that's not exactly true; many of the positive head-to-head clinical trials with St. John's wort were with older prescription drugs that are no longer used. Still, many doctors recommend it as a monotherapy (by itself) for depression.

3. 5-HTP (5-hydroxytryptophan)
200 to 300 milligrams a day

An extract from the *Griffonia simplicifolia* bean or plant of West Africa, 5-HTP (also called L-5-HTP) is an intermediate metabolite in the conversion of L-tryptophan to serotonin. In other words, it helps increase the production of serotonin in the brain. There have been many positive small clinical studies over the past few decades showing reductions of depression-related symptoms in 33 to 66 percent of participants with 5-HTP supplementation. The dosage usually ranges from 20 to 3,250 milligrams per day, but most of the positive studies that had good safety used 200 to 300 milligrams, with results noticeable in 2 to 4 weeks. Critics would argue that many of the past clinical trials (there have been more than 100 of them) were not adequate enough and that it still has not been proven to be effective or safe, but I disagree. What these critics fail to mention is that even in the few high-quality clinical trials, there were positive results and overall safety was not a serious issue.

You can take 5-HTP with meals, but be aware that higher doses can lead to night-mares and vivid dreams, dizziness, nausea, vomiting, and diarrhea. Most important, don't combine 5-HTP with any other medications that also impact serotonin levels, such as antidepressants, without talking to your doctor because there is an increased risk for serotonin syndrome (although it hasn't been an issue in studies so far). This, like SAM-e, is also being studied specifically for atypical depression.

HONORABLE MENTIONS

Folic acid, B$_{12}$, and L-methylfolate are showing promise. In some people, these B vitamins play a larger role in the production of brain neurotransmitters, so doing a blood test for them would be helpful. In addition, there are individuals who have abnormal changes in the gene that impacts folate, known as the "MTHFR" gene, and your doctor can test for this to determine if you have an increased need for folate or B$_{12}$. A form of folate, L-methylfolate at 15 milligrams a day has recently shown some real promise in initial clinical trials of people with MDD who were not responding or partially responding to selective serotonin reuptake inhibitors (SSRIs), a type of antidepressant, when added to their conventional treatments.

Inositol (a vitamin-like substance present in all body tissues, with the highest concentrations being in the brain and heart) supplementation may modulate serotonin activity, and it's being tested for depression in bipolar disorder. The only issue I have with this supplement is large doses—as high as 12 grams—have been used in some successful preliminary studies, which can be hard to take and isn't very realistic in the real world of patient care.

Rhodiola rosea (look for the extract called SHR-5), a hardy plant that grows in very cold climates, has already accumulated some interesting data in terms of improving mental performance and reducing anxiety, and there are signs that it may help people with mild to moderate depression as well (see the Stress and Anxiety section, page 414). Basic scientific studies suggest it can increase levels of a variety of neurotransmitters—including serotonin, dopamine, and norepinephrine—by blocking enzymes that reduce these compounds. It may also work by affecting opioid levels in the body (natural stress reducers).

Researchers believe they've found the active ingredients—rosavin and salidroside—and the extracts used in many studies have been standardized to 3 percent rosavin and 0.8 percent salidroside. A fairly recent 6-week study of 340 or 680 milligrams per day of SHR-5 compared to placebo found both dosages reduced depressive symptoms without side effects. Try it first at the lowest effective dosage, about 340 milligrams daily, for 4 to 8 weeks. If that doesn't work, you can increase the dose to 680 milligrams for another 4 to 8 weeks. Take it 30 minutes before meals and early in the day because it could cause some insomnia and vivid dreams. Not much is known about drug interactions with this supplement, except that it appears *not* to interact with the blood thinner warfarin or theophylline, a drug used for asthma and COPD.

Overall, the safety of *R. rosea* has been good, but mild and uncommon side effects—such as irritability, allergic reaction, fatigue, insomnia, and restlessness—have been reported in some studies, especially as the dose increases. Some experts have suggested that *R. Rosea* may be most promising in people with a history of a more "lethargic" depression, who require physical and mental energy-boosting.

Omega-3 fatty acids, both plant and fish sources, may slightly reduce depression, and the latest evidence suggests that the compound EPA may be better at preventing and treating depression than DHA (both are omega-3 fatty acids found in fish oil). Regardless, there have been many clinical studies, but they've been too short. The best trials have used 1,000 to 2,000 milligrams daily of the active ingredients in fish oil, which means a higher ratio of EPA to DHA (fish and inexpensive fish oils tend to have more EPA than DHA). Doctors may be more inclined to add omega-3s to current conventional antidepressants instead of other supplements because there's less risk of drug interactions. The reason omega-3s made my list isn't because I believe their impact is profound; it's just that the benefit at these dosages completely outweighs the risk. Good sources of omega-3s from fish include salmon, mackerel, anchovies, sardines, trout, and whitefish; good plant sources include chia seeds, flaxseeds and flaxseed oil, canola oil, and even walnuts.

WHAT'S WORTHLESS

Lemon balm, borage, and mimosa. These have all been tested for depression (individually) in the lab, but we need more human studies to support the lab findings. Results for lemon balm have been weak so far, and manufacturers need to improve the standardization of ingredients in borage so customers know what to look for. Mimosa has no real studies to support it at all.

Saffron. The research on this herbal has mostly been dominated by one group of researchers in one area of the world (Iran), and even though I am half Iranian and damn proud of it, there needs to be some outside research to support it (no different from what is expected from ginseng or maca, which also tend to be grown predominantly in certain areas and heavily researched in those areas as well). In the Appendix in the back of this book, you'll see I take country and supplier bias into account when considering the validity of research on any supplement, so this definitely raises a flag. I'm excited about saffron because it appears to have some potential as a treatment for MDD, but I do not believe it has quite found its niche yet.

Lavender. We need human research to support the laboratory research that's been done with lavender. It's mostly used as aromatherapy for depression, but

results from some of the largest studies haven't been very promising. Still, for aromatherapy purposes it has been proven safe, and if it can help some people, then that works for me.

WHAT ARE THE OPTIONS FOR KIDS?

There is a small amount of data to suggest that 150 to 300 milligrams of St. John's wort taken three times a day may help adolescents (12 to 17 years old) with depression. There is also some positive research on SAM-e, starting at really low doses, such as 200 milligrams. However, the data on any supplement helping children with depression is generally weak. Always work closely with your physician when using these with kids, and remember that socialized exercise (group sports or games) is perhaps the strongest lifestyle change that has had a positive impact on depression in children. Recent research also suggests an improvement in physical strength and muscle mass in children and adolescents may be predictive of a lower risk of suicide. This is a preliminary finding, but I believe it's due to the impact of physical health on mental health.

LIFESTYLE CHANGES

Heart healthy = brain healthy. Almost everything associated with improving heart health can improve brain function. Eating a Mediterranean diet—rich in fish, fruit, vegetables, fiber, and whole grains

171

and low in unhealthy fats and processed foods—is good for your heart and appears to improve mood as well.

Work out! Three large clinical trial reviews found that exercise can enhance the effects of prescription antidepressants and can also reduce the risk of depression when used by itself. In other words, there is no greater lifestyle change you can make to help reduce depression or improve your response to an antidepressant drug. Aim for at least 30 minutes a day of aerobic exercise and consider joining a gym or working out with a group because it increases your socialization, which can help depression as well (plus, most of the studies looked at group or trainer-directed exercise).

Moderate to vigorous exercise appears to result in even more profound mental health benefits. The release of neurotransmitters and endorphins increases with exercise intensity—maybe to take your mind off all the hard work! Weight lifting, yoga, tai chi, Pilates, and other modalities may also provide a mental health boost, but the vast majority of clinical trials involved aerobic exercise. Again, I believe the social factor played a role in the positive effects seen in these studies. And we're going to be seeing a lot more research about this. Personally, every morning I either run with a friend or sprint on a treadmill, and it turns me from groggy and grumpy to happy and healthy within minutes.

Grab a java. A large prospective study (the Nurses' Health Study), which included more than 50,000 women who did not have depressive symptoms at the beginning, found that those who consumed coffee daily had a significant reduction in the risk of depression compared to those who drank a cup or less a week. It was the same for ingesting caffeine in general, and there was no benefit seen for decaffeinated coffee. Caffeine crosses the blood-brain barrier and appears to improve neurotransmitter function in the brain.

Diabetes and Prediabetes*

Note: While this section is focused on type 2 diabetes, many of the options listed here could be discussed with your doctor if you have type 1 diabetes.

Dr. Moyad Secret The number one prescribed drug in the world for prediabetes and type 2 diabetes is now a cheap generic drug originally derived from the French lilac, called metformin. Although it's approved for the treatment of diabetes, it's now arguably also the safest (but not the best) weight loss drug ever invented, and it has been proven to prevent type 2 diabetes. More than 100 clinical trials are currently testing it to potentially prevent and help treat a variety of cancers (breast, colon, and prostate) as well, along with conventional medicine.

Metformin works by reducing the amount of glucose produced by the liver, making muscle tissue more sensitive to insulin, blocking the absorption of some carbohydrates in the intestines, and controlling blood sugar and insulin levels. Plus, it can help those with and without diabetes lose weight. One very important thing to note, however, is that the same large clinical trial that showed metformin can prevent diabetes (the Diabetes Prevention Program study) also showed that comprehensive lifestyle changes (exercising, following a heart-healthy diet, and losing weight) worked *better* than this drug! You will never see that advertised on TV, though, despite the fact that type 2 diabetes is a superepidemic all over the United States, Puerto Rico, and now the world, affecting both adults and kids.

WHAT IS IT?

Insulin is a hormone produced by the pancreas that shuttles blood sugar (glucose) out of the blood and into cells to be burned for energy or turned into fat for storage. Type 1 diabetes—which usually strikes in childhood—occurs when the cells fail to produce insulin. The resulting buildup of glucose in the blood (hyperglycemia) leads to many (often life-threatening) health problems. Type 2 diabetes is usually the result of lifestyle in combination with genetics/family history, and it occurs when the pancreas gets worn out from trying to make more insulin to lower blood sugar levels or the body becomes resistant to it. Type 2 is preventable in some cases, while type 1 is usually caused by a genetic or autoimmune disorder. Having elevated blood sugar levels that aren't high enough to be considered type 2 diabetes is known as prediabetes, and it's a sign that you need to make lifestyle changes immediately.

Symptoms of diabetes include frequent urination, large appetite and thirst (even though you're eating and drinking), vision changes, slow wound healing, numbness or tingling in the hands or feet, and fatigue. Those with type 1 diabetes might experience unexplained weight loss. Chronic diabetes can lead to vision loss (diabetic retinopathy), cardiovascular disease, circulatory and nerve problems (peripheral neuropathy), kidney damage, and infections. And it increases your risk for most health problems, especially heart attack and stroke.

New American Diabetes Association (ADA) guidelines suggest anyone with a body mass index of 25 or more (about 75 percent of Americans and growing), which is a known risk factor for type 2 diabetes, should be tested. More than 80 percent of people with type 2 are overweight or obese, and studies have shown that weight loss—even as little as 10 pounds in those with prediabetes—can reduce the risk of developing full-blown diabetes by more than 50 percent.

Lifestyle changes and inexpensive medications to prevent type 2 diabetes should be your main focus. However, research has shown that the following supplements can help lower or maintain blood sugar levels, and the benefit may outweigh the risk for some people.

MOYAD FACT: Doctors will use a hemoglobin A1c, or HbA1c, blood test to track blood sugar levels over a 3-month period to see how well they are being controlled. A result of 6.5 percent or higher is associated with diabetes. This test is becoming a more accurate gauge for diagnosing diabetes than a fasting blood glucose test, but both are still important.

WHAT WORKS

1. Fiber, especially soluble fiber powder 5 to 15 milligrams a day (10 milligrams on average if taking psyllium)

Anyone concerned about diabetes should get the recommended daily amount of fiber per day (20 to 30 grams) primarily from foods that contain soluble and insoluble fiber. Fiber pills are mostly a waste of money, but fiber powders and some bars can help you reach your target (I don't recommend getting more than 5 to 15 milligrams per day in this form). Fiber slows gastric emptying and delays the absorption of nutrients, so it helps promote insulin sensitivity and control or reduce glucose spikes. It could also help with weight loss, so it's a cornerstone of diabetes prevention and treatment. Many soluble fibers have been researched for controlling blood sugar in prediabetes and diabetes, including psyllium (the most researched), beta-glucan, guar gum, and even glucomannan.

2. Chromium picolinate 600 micrograms a day and biotin 2 milligrams a day

These two in combination can improve insulin sensitivity and help regulate carbohydrate metabolism along with conventional medicines for better glucose and cholesterol control in type 2 diabetes. There have been many fairly well-done clinical trials in this area, and the commercial product Diachrome was one of the first to show positive results when used along with conventional drugs. The research has been impressive, especially in people with higher hemoglobin A1c levels, meaning they're having a hard time controlling or reducing blood sugars. Why more "experts" don't pay attention to this research and implement it is beyond me. Chromium picolinate by itself in doses of 200 to 1,000 micrograms (1 milligram) per day—or a similar dosage of chromium from a brewer's yeast source—could have a mild benefit. Chromium has no impact on prediabetes.

Note: These next two supplements are for a common symptom or consequence of diabetes called diabetic peripheral neuropathy or diabetic neuropathy. It's a result of nerve damage caused by high blood sugar, and it happens in the hands and feet. These aren't for glucose control or treatment.

3. (tie) Alpha-lipoic acid (ALA)

600 milligrams a day for the prevention and treatment of peripheral neuropathy and 1,800 milligrams a day for weight loss (600 milligrams approximately 30 minutes before each meal)

Alpha-lipoic acid (a.k.a. thioctic acid) is used as an IV and oral prescription drug around the world to help prevent and treat some symptoms of diabetic neuropathy, but in other countries, like the United States, it's a dietary supplement. Researchers believe it works like a far less potent version of metformin, activating a path-

way called AMPK that can increase metabolism (see the Weight Loss section, page 448). Many supplement companies advertise that the R-form, or more expensive form of ALA, is absorbed better, which is true, but the lower cost R/S-form has been used in some of the best clinical trials, including for weight loss.

Distal symmetric sensorimotor polyneuropathy (DSPN), a type of peripheral neuropathy, impacts one-third of people with diabetes, and it can reduce quality of life and increase the risk of death. The NATHAN (Neurological Assessment of Thioctic Acid in Diabetic Neuropathy) trial—which was done in 36 centers in Canada, Europe, and the United States—found ALA may slow the progression of DSPN. Researchers discovered that 600 milligrams of ALA daily moderately improved small nerve fiber and muscular function.

In a well-done clinical trial in Korea, researchers compared 1,800 milligrams per day (600 milligrams before each meal) of ALA with a placebo over 5 months. The ALA group had significant weight loss (one-third of the participants had type 2 diabetes). All of the participants (ALA and placebo) also followed a 1,200-calorie-per-day flexible diet plan. The average weight loss in the ALA group was around 4.5 to 5 pounds greater than the placebo group, but approximately 23 percent of the subjects lost 5 percent or more of their body weight (versus 10 percent of the subjects in the placebo group). *Note:* ALA can cause a harmless malodorous urine smell (like asparagus does) and rash and itching, and it can lower glucose substantially in really rare situations.

3. (tie) Capsaicin cream (0.075 percent) applied up to four times a day for diabetic peripheral neuropathy

Capsaicin (the hot active ingredient in hot chile peppers) works by reducing levels of a compound in the body called substance P, which effectively interrupts transmission of pain. When used at a concentration of 0.075 percent up to four times a day, it can provide relief for some individuals who have pain near the surface of the skin (versus deep bone pain), so try it for at least a week or two. However, you should always use gloves and a cotton swab because if you get capsaicin on your fingers and into your eye, the burning sensation can be quite painful (and potentially harmful). When applying to your feet, always put on socks afterward so you don't risk transferring the capsaicin to other surfaces that might somehow come in contact with your (or a loved one's) eye. I love that the American Association of Neuromuscular and Electrodiagnostic Medicine, the American Academy of Neurology, and the American Academy of Physical Medicine and Rehabilitation recommend capsaicin at 0.075 percent for diabetic peripheral neuropathy. Ahhh, another supplement moves into mainstream medicine.

You can ask your doctor about even higher concentrations of capsaicin (up to 8 percent) that are being tested in clinical trials now. It could work better, but it's only available through a prescription in the form of a patch (it's called Qutenza). Currently, the 8 percent capsaicin patch is being used for shingles with good results, but there is good reason to believe it works with other forms of neuropathic pain, depending on the individual. Side effects have been low, but the prescription can cause a rapid change in blood pressure at first. (Never combine capsaicin with anything else that can heat the skin, such as a heating pad, because this combined effect can burn or otherwise damage the skin.)

Oral capsaicin dietary supplements are starting to be researched for a variety of conditions, but I don't think they will garner evidence in the area of peripheral neuropathy anytime soon, plus, as you would imagine, oral capsaicin can be really harsh on the gastrointestinal tract. If you want more capsaicin, order hot peppers on your next veggie burger.

HONORABLE MENTIONS

Berberine can be found in many plants, and it has preliminary data as an antimicrobial agent. It appears to increase insulin receptors and sensitivity and may impact one of the pathways that the drug metformin affects (5'-AMP-activated protein kinase, the body's metabolic master switch). Researchers have used 1,000 to 1,500 milligrams per day with some conventional medicines, such as metformin, to lower blood glucose and potentially improve cholesterol levels in people with type 2 diabetes, but a large, well-done trial is still needed before we get too excited about it.

Cinnamon (*Cinnamomum cassia*) extract contains cinnamaldehyde, the active ingredient in cinnamon, and it can improve insulin sensitivity. Dosages of 120 to 6,000 milligrams per day have been used in at least 10 clinical trials lasting from 4 to 18 weeks, and though it appears to reduce glucose and even some cholesterol levels, it has had minimal impact on the hemoglobin A1c blood test. The biggest problem with many of the trials is that they have had a high risk of bias. The most common cinnamon extract dosage is 1,000 to 2,000 milligrams per day, and it has an excellent safety record. Keep in mind that metformin can lower glucose twice as well as cinnamon, though, and it's inexpensive.

Magnesium—which can be found in squash, pumpkin, watermelon, flaxseed, sesame seeds, sunflower seeds, almonds, cashews, peanuts, and Brazil nuts—may reduce the risk of type 2 diabetes and prediabetes. However, since many of these foods also contain fiber (and vice versa), researchers aren't sure whether it's the fiber or the magnesium that's responsible for the benefits. Still, most of the research on magnesium is for the prevention of diabetes, not treatment. Several studies of magnesium supplements—for example, 365 milligrams per day of magnesium aspartate hydrochloride—improved insulin sensitivity in overweight individuals at risk for type 2 diabetes.

Vitamin D is overhyped for everything, but there's one area that shows promise and needs more intense study. Children who currently have normal D levels and whose mothers had normal D levels when pregnant with them appear to have a lower risk of getting type 1 diabetes. Vitamin D plays a role in immune surveillance and improving immune function, and since type 1 diabetes is really an autoimmune disease, D may have a role in preventing the body from attacking the cells of the pancreas that produce and secrete insulin.

WHAT'S WORTHLESS

L-cysteine, gurmar, and resveratrol. An amino acid, L-cysteine gets a lot of hype as a potential diabetic agent, but in reality, apart from the amount found in whey protein powder, which *can* be beneficial, there is little research to support its use. I feel the same way about *Gymnema sylvestre* (also known as gurmar, which means "sugar destroyer" in Hindi). The clinical studies are weak, and the isolated reports of liver inflammation and problems with standardization or identifying a true active ingredient only make me more skeptical (not just for diabetes, but weight loss, too). When it comes to resveratrol, it's all hype and no substance. We need more consistent clinical data before I recommend spending any money on this supplement made from the skin of grapes.

Ginseng. It can lower blood sugar, especially American ginseng, but the results have been inconsistent, probably because standardization of the active ingredients, called ginsenosides, is all over the place. Panax ginseng has been shown to have weak glucose-lowering effects. Basically, I see no role for ginseng currently in prediabetes or diabetes to reduce glucose or hemoglobin A1c.

High doses of B vitamins. We used to think B vitamins could protect the kidneys, but recent research suggests they can harm kidney function and do not lower the risk of cardiovascular disease. In fact, they may *increase* it. A typical multivitamin contains 400 micrograms of folic acid, 6 micrograms of B_{12}, and 2 milligrams of B_6. In the latest megadose studies, individuals were taking 2,500 micrograms of folic acid, 1,000 micrograms of B_{12}, and 25 milligrams of B_6! So be careful and avoid B-complex multis, too, because people with diabetes have a high risk of kidney problems.

LIFESTYLE CHANGES

Heart healthy = blood sugar healthy! The leading killer of people with diabetes is cardiovascular disease (CVD). More than 80 percent of individuals with type 2 diabetes are overweight or obese, and doctors now treat patients with diabetes similarly to patients who have already had a heart attack. In other words, they try to aggressively reduce CVD risk factors, which has worked brilliantly. It's one reason many people with diabetes now can live as long as people without the disease.

Add flaxseed. Getting 10 to 30 grams of flaxseed powder in your diet daily—sprinkle it on oatmeal, bake with it, and more—provides a good, cheap source of fiber. Chia seed powder is another great source (it has as much fiber as flaxseed).

Get more caffeine. It appears to improve insulin sensitivity and is being studied as a way to reduce the risk of type 2 diabetes and improve liver function. Moderate daily amounts—what you'd find in one to two 8-ounce cups of coffee—have the most research, but even smaller amounts—like what you'd find in many teas—may also be beneficial. In the largest review of clinical studies looking at caffeine and diabetes to date, the reduction in risk was significant and appeared to be even greater in those who didn't smoke and were not overweight. Coffee and caffeine both have anti-inflammatory properties that can improve metabolism enough to reduce the chances of becoming insulin resistant. I think they could even help keep type 2 diabetes from getting worse.

Diverticulitis

THE JURY'S STILL OUT

Dr. Moyad Secret If I had a beer for every person who has come up to me at a lecture and told me he was treated for diverticulitis—an intestinal condition that causes pain, bloating, nausea, and possibly fever—and wished he knew how to prevent it from happening again, I would have at least five cases of free beer by now! The secret is fiber and conventional medicine! Fiber is one of the only supplements that can potentially reduce the risk of another attack. There's also research suggesting that combining fiber with some drugs (such as rifaximin) might reduce the risk of another attack better than taking either fiber or the drug alone. And since it can lower the risk of heart disease, fiber should always be a part of your diet anyway. Heart healthy = gut healthy, folks! (You had to know that was coming.)

MOYAD FACT: Hospital admissions for diverticulitis have increased by 26 percent and elective operations by almost 30 percent over the last 10 years.

Diverticu*losis* occurs when small "pockets" form in the wall of the bowel, usually in the last part of the colon (sigmoid), right before the rectum. I call it small pouch syndrome of the colon, or SPSC, because I like to come up with ridiculous names like this when I'm writing. Many folks find out they have this condition as they get older and have procedures like colonoscopies and CT scans, but it usually doesn't cause any symptoms; rarely people experience bleeding, bloating, cramps, and changed bowel habits.

Only about 10 to 20 percent of these pockets of diverticulosis ever turn into diverticulitis, which happens when the area becomes infected and inflamed. Some people call it left-sided appendicitis because the pain happens in the lower left abdomen (and appendicitis is in the lower right); there's usually fever present too. Doctors typically prescribe a combination of antibiotics (like ciprofloxacin and metronidazole) and a liquid diet to soothe the bowel. But some people get these attacks over and over again, to the point where the colon is damaged enough to warrant surgery before it tears or perforates, leading to a life-threatening infection. The goal here is to prevent an attack so you never have to worry about surgery. (Ask your doctor about the latest preventive drugs, such as mesalamine or rifaximin, if you're at risk of another attack.)

Fiber. Getting 20 to 30 grams a day from food is key, and adding a fiber powder supplement to help you get there is a good idea. Get 5 to 10 grams of your daily total from psyllium or inulin, or even from another over-the-counter product like methyl-cellulose, which has been tested in some diverticulitis patients.

Probiotics. These may help because the damaged microenviron-ment of the colon, including abnormal gut bacteria, can increase chronic inflammation and make the disease worse. Some probiotic studies reported less abdominal pain, bloat-ing, and fever but no significant reduction in recurrence rates. More research is needed to uncover whether they work better than a placebo.

MOYAD FACT: For a long time researchers thought nuts, seeds, peas, skins of raw vegetables, corn, popcorn—basically small food items—could become trapped in the intestinal pouches caused by diverticulosis and turn the condition into diverticuli-tis, but recent research (with more than 47,000 health care professionals) has discredited this the-ory. Now, researchers believe diverticulitis is caused by chronic inflammation from diverse sources, lead-ing to a small break in the tissue and then infection. And those same foods that patients were told to avoid are now encouraged because many of them are healthy and good sources of fiber.

Dry Eye

Dr. Moyad Secret This may show my age, but when I think of tears, I immediately think of Barbara Walters interviewing the celebrity du jour and inevitably making that person cry. But lack of tears, or just dry eyes in general, is actually the number one reason for eye doctor visits (maybe doctors should keep videos of Barbara Walters interviews in their offices). It's common—about 50 percent of the population will experience dry eyes (also called xerophthalmia)—and often easily treated. But I think that physicians prescribe Restasis, a medicine that increases tear production, way too often (it's a good drug, but it's also pricey—maybe because of all the advertising they buy!). You should try a low-cost dietary supplement first; it's safer, cheaper, and often just as effective. In addition, the active ingredient in Restasis is cyclosporine, which is an immunosuppressant. They are very safe drugs, but people often get hooked on them, and I get nervous about taking anything that's an immunosuppressant long term, even if it's been deemed safe.

WHAT IS IT?

The surface of the eye is protected by tears, and tears themselves consist of three layers: an outer lipid layer (fatty or oily), a middle water layer, and an inner mucous layer—who knew? If your body manufactures insufficient tears or if they're faulty (maybe they only have one layer instead of three or they produce less of the watery layer), the whole tear mechanism can become dysfunctional and the eye becomes dry and irritated. Symptoms include itchiness, a gritty feeling, stinging or burning, blurry vision, increased mucus, redness, sensitivity to light, trouble wearing contact lenses, and even bouts of excessive tearing. Chronic dry eye can lead to infections and in some cases loss of vision.

But it's not just tears and their funky structure that are to blame here. To keep your eyes properly lubricated, you need meibum (rhymes with sebum, which is an oily, waxy secretion on your skin), an oily substance that keeps tears from evaporating too quickly. There are about 30 to 40 small meibum glands on the rim of each eyelid, and if those glands become clogged or irritated, it can cause dryness. (Meibomian gland dysfunction is another name for dry eye.) Turns out, these little glands start going haywire as we age, sometimes due to hormonal fluctuations.

Environment (airplanes, excessive

heat or air conditioning, low humidity, smoke, and pollution) is a big trigger, as well as computer use, contact lenses, and aging. I find this interesting because the risk of dry skin increases with aging, too, which suggests a common phenomenon occurring with the glands of the eye and skin. LASIK, a common vision-correction surgery, can also cause dry eye. With the exception of aging and eye surgery, the rest of these triggers generally cause temporary or less severe dry eye.

WHAT WORKS

Note: The goal with supplementation is to reduce inflammation and thin out some of the tear secretions (thick tears do not drain well and can plug up the drainage area on the side of the eye). The options I recommend here are quickly gaining converts in the conventional medical world, but, unfortunately, they aren't being touted in any television commercials like some of the pharmaceutical products.

1. Omega-3 fatty acids and omega-6 fatty acids dosage varies by type

Warning: Be on the lookout for expensive dry eye supplements that are really just simple, low-cost omega-3 or omega-6 products!

Omega-3s: You can take flaxseed oil as a softgel, but you would need to down six or seven to get the 3,300 milligrams per day of alpha-linolenic acid, or ALA, that has shown anti-inflammatory benefits for the eyes in studies. It's much easier to just take 1 or 2 tablespoons daily of flaxseed oil (my favorite is Omega Swirl from Barlean's). Alternatively, you could take 800 to 1,500 milligrams (one or two pills) of the active ingredients in marine or fish oil (EPA and DHA omega-3 fatty acids); Omega Swirl also has an incredible-tasting fish oil option. Many studies have found potential benefits at a variety of dosages, and even the American Optometric Association recommends omega-3s for dry eye now.

Omega-6s: We're often told that omega-6 fatty acids are bad for us because they *create* inflammation, but this is a gross generalization. They're not all bad. Some omega-6 compounds have *anti-*inflammatory effects, which is why they are potentially effective for the treatment of dry eye. Taking 57 to 224 milligrams of linoleic acid (LA) or 30 to 300 milligrams of gamma-linolenic acid (GLA) has been found to reduce symptoms of dry eye in studies. The human study that impressed me the most—and that also relates to my experience with patients who have dry eye from diverse causes, including contact lenses—used 300 milligrams of GLA from evening primrose oil (you can also use borage or black currant oil) or just two or three softgels per day (my favorite here is Barlean's evening primrose oil because it is so concentrated and easy to take).

I recommend combining omega-3 and omega-6 supplements only if your dry eye condition does not improve in 3 months of taking either type on its own. The benefit in combining them is that they fight inflammation in different ways, so it's possible for someone who's not responding to omega-3 supplements to get a better response from omega-6s and vice versa. Both reduce inflammation and pain, but in some individuals one works better than the other or the combination works better than either one alone. By combining them, you're essentially covering all your bases. Regardless, many sources of omega-3s (like flaxseed) also contain some omega-6s and vice versa, but larger doses are often needed to really see a benefit. If you want to combine them, try taking either 750 to 1,000 milligrams of fish oil or 1,000 milligrams of flaxseed oil *plus* up to 100 milligrams of GLA or 150 milligrams of LA.

2. Vitamin A eye drops apply 4 drops a day of a 0.05 percent retinyl palmitate formula

This antioxidant and anti-inflammatory vitamin has specific benefits for the eye. Vitamin A deficiency is a common cause of dry eye in Third World countries, but not as much in the Western world. Still, make sure you're getting it in your multivitamin (most have at least half if not the full 5,000 IU recommended daily intake). Or, if you like to eat fruits and vegetables (especially those deep green and orange veggies), chances are you're getting plenty. There was a large Korean study that used vitamin A drops (the product studied is sold under the brand name VIVA) four times daily and found that they improved blurred vision and tear film about as well as the cyclosporine. Both the vitamin A drops and cyclosporine significantly improved the symptoms of dry eye within 2 to 3 months.

3. Sea buckthorn oil (*Hippophae rhamnoides*) 2,000 milligrams a day in divided doses

This product contains omega-3s (ALA) and omega-6s (LA) as well as several antioxidants that are important for proper eye function, such as vitamin E and carotenoids. The dosage used in studies is 2,000 milligrams a day (two capsules twice daily with meals). Over 3 months, subjects saw improved tear film and reduced redness and burning. (If you're trolling for information on sea buckthorn oil online, you may read about something called an omega-7 fatty acid, but nobody really knows if these omega-7s do anything, so don't buy it because the extra fatty acid impresses you.)

WHAT'S WORTHLESS

There aren't many supplements out there being billed as dry eye treatments, besides the ones I've just mentioned, but there are a few that can *cause* dry eye, including niacin, echinacea, and kava. Some herbal products have also been associated with dry mouth, which could lead to dry eye (*Rhodiola rosea* and St. John's wort). This is because the toxicity that affects salivary glands can also impact the glands or cells that produce tears.

LIFESTYLE CHANGES

Reel in your dinner. Studies have shown that diets higher in omega-3 fatty acids from fish and plants may reduce the risk of dry eye (in other words, we're talking about prevention here). Diets high in omega-6s (plant oils, nuts, and seeds) don't seem to have the same benefit, but there have only been a few studies looking at this so far. Interestingly, consuming certain fish, such as tuna, several times a week was associated with one of the lowest risks of dry eye. You are not going to like this, but I have had several people recommend eating a few pieces of anchovy in oil daily for 2 weeks. I told patients about it and it worked! Of course, if you don't like anchovies then it works too because you'll be crying about having to eat them.

Exercise your eyes. Blinking produces meibum (the ever so tiny eye muscles squeeze the glands around the eyes). If you're working at a computer for a long time, take several full blinks, where you forcefully squeeze your eyelids shut then open them, every 15 to 20 minutes. Moving your eyeballs from side to side and up and down (think of it as eye yoga) helps activate these glands, too. Finally, massaging your upper and lower eyelids with a cotton swab (small circles around each eyelid) also helps the glands produce more fluid.

Wear glasses. Sunglasses protect your peepers from the sun, naturally, but also wind that can cause tears to evaporate quickly, leading to inflammation. Eyeglasses also discourage the evaporation of tears. (It's always good to give your eyes a break from contacts, which can aggravate dry eyes, every few days.)

Use a humidifier. Dry air can make your eyes feel worse, so use a humidifier in rooms where you spend the most time.

Baby your peepers. Use a hot compress to loosen and release hardened oil in clogged meibomian glands. Twice a day, wash your face and then soak a cloth in warm water and use it as a compress over your closed eyelids for 30 seconds. Next, clean the lower lids with a dry, tightly wrapped cotton swab. This will help remove lid debris that could be disrupting the tear film. It also stimulates your own reflex tears.

Check your meds. There are a ton of prescription medications that can potentially cause dry eye, so talk to your doctor if you're experiencing irritation. The list includes beta-blockers, antidepressants, anticonvulsants, anti-Parkinsonians, antihistamines, decongestants, antipsychotics, pain medications, antithyroid drugs, cancer drugs, antiemetics, acid reflux medications, blood pressure meds, urinary incontinence drugs, antivirals, antimalarials, respiratory medications—you get the idea.

Epilepsy/Seizures

Dr. Moyad Secret Ketogenic (90 percent fat) and modified Atkins (70 percent fat) diets have a long history of being effective in the treatment of epilepsy, especially for patients who don't respond well to drugs (called refractory epilepsy) or are not good candidates for surgery. Some clinicians actually believe, as I do, that these diets should be offered as a potential first-line therapy (the first thing doctors try for some patients). Results have been equivalent to drug treatments, but compliance is an issue due to the high fat intake (modified Atkins is less extreme and has better compliance). Still, there is no dietary supplement that can come close to beating a ketogenic diet for seizure reduction.

Erectile Dysfunction

Dr. Moyad Secret Treating erectile dysfunction (a.k.a. ED; I always wonder how guys named Ed feel about this acronym) is challenging on several fronts. First, the ED supplement category is the most recalled or penalized area of dietary supplements in FDA history; this is due to lack of testing and good quality control. I tried to shake up the industry a few years ago and force quality-control testing, but to no avail. (Some of the world's most legitimate, nonbiased quality-control testing agencies did not want to test well-researched ED supplements because they were too worried about how it would appear!) It's completely insane and shameful, and I am *still* crazy upset about this. Unfortunately, most people just assume that ED supplements don't work or are dangerous. Another challenge is that the stereotype of ED drugs—let's call it the "Hugh Hefner phenomenon"—clouds the fact that ED is a legitimate medical condition. If more physicians treated it as such, I believe couples would have access to better, higher-quality dietary supplement options. Finally, the current cost of prescription ED drugs is ridiculously high at $10 to $25 a pill, which makes it the most overpriced drug and the most egregious case of drug price gouging that I have ever come across in my career! The average per pill cost of a prescription ED drug is 20 to 40 times that of an effective supplement, plus these drugs often come with numerous minor toxicities and some serious ones. As a result, according to research done by the pharmaceutical companies themselves, only one-third to one-half of first-time users refill their prescriptions!

WHAT IS IT?

ED is the inability to achieve or maintain an erection sufficient for intercourse or for other sexual activity. Any heart-unhealthy condition (high bad cholesterol, excess weight, low good cholesterol, inactivity) can contribute to ED, but there are also many other potential causes, including hormonal, neurological, psychological, vascular/cardiovascular, extrinsic (a medication or surgical procedure), disease-related (liver disease, kidney problems, etc.), structural (such as fractures or curvature of the penis), or any combination of these.

ED is very complex and does not just include issues related to erectile function; it also encompasses orgasm and sex drive (libido). Some dietary supplements help more with erectile function while others help more with libido, but ED prescription drugs *only* address erectile function.

So is ED in the big head or the little

(continued on page 189)

THE PENIS AS A BAROMETER OF OVERALL HEALTH

Here are some common habits, disorders, and diseases that can impact a man's sexual health.

- Alcohol in excess
- Anxiety and other emotions in excess (guilt, low self-esteem, fear, grief)
- Blood disorders (e.g., anemia)
- Cardiovascular disease
- Depression
- High blood glucose (those with diabetes are at very high risk for ED and heart disease)
- High blood pressure
- High cholesterol (especially higher LDL or triglycerides)
- Hormonal abnormalities (prolactin, testosterone, thyroid)
- Kidney disease
- Lack of exercise
- Lack of sleep and obstructive sleep apnea
- Low amount of "good" cholesterol (HDL)
- Medication use (some prescriptions and over-the-counter medicines)
- Neurologic diseases, such as multiple sclerosis and Parkinson's
- Penile abnormalities (Peyronie's disease)
- Peripheral vascular/artery disease (also called PAD)
- Prostate problems (cancer treatment, enlargement, infection, inflammation)
- Smoking (and smokeless tobacco, too; sorry, cowboys)
- Stress
- Substance abuse
- Trauma or surgery to the pelvis or spine
- Weight gain

THE DRUG-ED LINK

Approximately 25 percent of ED cases can be linked to prescription and over-the-counter (OTC) medications! *Some* medicines (not all of them) in the following categories can cause problems.

- Acid reflux drugs (prescription or OTC, especially H2 blockers, such as cimetidine and ranitidine)

- Antianxiety meds

- Anticholinergics

- Anticonvulsants

- Antidepressants (30 to 70 percent of men and women who take these drugs experience sexual problems, which leads to poor compliance rates)*

- Antihistamines, including those that prevent motion sickness

- Antipsychotics

- Blood pressure medications

- Cardiac drugs

- Cholesterol-lowering drugs in excess (so that cholesterol drops too low)

- Diuretics

- Hair loss pills (finasteride)

- Marijuana (it has carcinogens, so it can kill, which also does not help anyone's sex life)

- Pain medications (OTC and prescription)

- Prostate enlargement pills

- Steroids (especially anabolic steroids)

*Harvard researchers have found that the dietary supplement SAM-e (see the Depression section, page 166) may enhance the mood-boosting effects of SSRIs (selective serotonin reuptake inhibitors, the most commonly prescribed antidepressant class), and it can be used by itself in some cases. So far, researchers haven't found any noticeable negative impact on sexual health with SAM-e; it may even promote sexual health by stimulating an area of the brain that promotes sexual function.

head? Just a decade or two ago, experts thought that most cases of ED were caused by psychogenic/psychological factors, but now we know that this is false (only 20 percent of cases are psychogenic). The remaining 80 percent are due to an organic cause (some kind of underlying physical medical condition) or a mix of organic and psychological factors. The question to work out with your doctor before deciding on a dietary supplement—or any intervention—is whether your ED is mild, moderate, severe, or very severe. This is important because I believe that men with mild to moderate ED have the most to gain from dietary supplements. Men with moderate to very severe ED generally don't respond as well to supplements and need more aggressive conventional medicines, devices, or procedures.

WHAT WORKS?

Note: Always get your doctor's approval before combining these supplements with other ED drugs. Also, unlike Viagra, which is taken "on demand," most supplements need to be used daily to see an impact.

1. (tie) L-citrulline (free form) 1,500 to 6,000 milligrams a day maximum

Citrulline is derived from the Latin word for watermelon (*Citrullus vulgaris*). It's primarily found in watermelon rind, but it's virtually impossible to get sufficient amounts through diet, unless you like to eat watermelon rind all day long (perhaps after reading this section you might!). It increases nitric oxide levels, which boosts bloodflow to the penis, improving erectile function, especially hardness. Research continues to show that it's hardness—not size—that matters to partners when it comes to sexual satisfaction. Keep in mind that L-citrulline improves erections but rarely impacts libido and the most tested dose is 1,500 milligrams a day.

Nitric oxide may have antiplatelet effects, which means it acts as a blood thinner, so be careful when combining this with other blood-thinning drugs, like warfarin. It also may cause a slight reduction in blood pressure in some individuals, so check with your doctor about combining this medicine with prescription ED drugs that can significantly drop blood pressure. (You need to have adequate kidney function for this product to work well because the kidneys facilitate the conversion of L-citrulline into nitric oxide by way of L-arginine.)

Although there hasn't been any research yet looking into combining L-citrulline with prescription ED medicine in general, it seems promising; ED drugs work best when there is a sufficient amount of nitric oxide available, and Viagra works by helping nitric oxide stick around and function better.

There doesn't seem to be a "best" way to take this supplement, so you can decide whether to down it with or without food or in divided doses during the day. The higher doses can get pricey, so you'll want

INCREASE PENIS SIZE NATURALLY!

As a man gains weight, the excess abdominal tissue begins to pull or retract the penis in toward the abdomen, exposing less of the length of the penis. However, every 10 to 15 pounds of weight loss can add an extra half-inch of exposed penis length! Lose 30 pounds and "say hello to my big friend!"

to do some comparison shopping to find the best deal. And make sure to give it 1 to 4 weeks to see a difference. Finally, make sure you look for L-citrulline by itself (free form) and not the malate form, which is used for exercise enhancement but has no data yet for ED.

1. (tie) Panax ginseng (or, ideally, Korean red ginseng) 1,800 to 3,000 milligrams a day in divided doses, depending on ginsenoside content

This famous herb improves libido, but it also improves erectile function. Ginsenosides (also known as ginseng saponins or glycosylated steroidal saponins), which are unique to the *Panax* species, are the primary active ingredients in ginseng, and more than 30 different ginsenosides have been isolated from the root of *Panax ginseng*. They appear to improve the enzyme reaction that converts L-arginine to nitric oxide in the body, which allows for adequate bloodflow into the penis.

A study published in the *Korean Journal of Urology* provides some of the best clinical research to date for this supplement: A multicenter, randomized, double-blind, placebo-controlled study of 69 men

used a highly concentrated ginsenoside but low-dose overall ginseng product (800 milligrams per day). After 8 weeks, every single sexual health parameter was significantly improved by Korean ginseng compared with a placebo, including erectile function (primary endpoint), sexual desire, orgasmic function, intercourse satisfaction, and overall satisfaction. Furthermore, every single question on the medically validated ED questionnaire (which tracks patients' subjective assessments of their problems) was improved. Additionally, there were no significant differences in adverse events reported for ginseng compared with a placebo. The results of this trial should strengthen the clinical evidence for ginseng and the evidence that concentrated ginsenosides are the active or effective ingredients in ginseng when it comes to treating ED.

Here is the catch! This clinical trial used a specialized formulation that was a 50-50 combination of an almost 100 percent concentrated ginsenoside product and a standard extract of more than 8 percent ginsenosides. And it's not easy to get this kind of product from Korea or China without paying a *lot* of money for it. This is the Holy Grail of ginseng! Now all that

GET PRESCRIPTION ED PILLS TO WORK BETTER

The secret is exercise! A clinical trial from Padova, Italy, published in the very prestigious *Journal of Sexual Medicine,* demonstrated that men taking drugs for erectile dysfunction (ED) who also exercised for 3 or more hours per week over 3 months increased their sex drive and most other areas of their sexual health. This improvement was *significantly* better than a group of men who only took the drugs. This is exactly what I have observed with patients. If I were a marketing person for an ED pharmaceutical company, I'd be cross promoting with a fitness company. (How about giving away a treadmill with every Viagra prescription because that would certainly justify the high price of these drugs!) Seriously though, what this study clearly shows is that exercise makes ED drugs work so much better *and* it increases sex drive, something the pills have never been able to do in clinical trials.

consumers need is a ginseng supplement like this at a reasonable price. Here's the dosage that I recommend: 1,800 to 3,000 milligrams per day for a ginsenoside content of 4 to 8.5 percent. For a ginsenoside content of 16 percent or higher, take 600 to 1,500 milligrams per day. Divide whatever amount you opt for into two or three daily doses with or without food and take it for at least 4 weeks .

Some laboratory studies have suggested that ginseng may increase testosterone, but I disagree because this has not been observed in clinical trials, and I have not seen this in any patients. A fascinating mechanism of action of ginseng that I *have* witnessed is its effect on the brain, and we all know how important your noggin' is when it comes to sex. By binding to areas that can promote relaxation, improve mood, and impact dopamine receptors, it may stimulate sex drive. (The doctors I've been able to convince to try ginseng have called it the "happy pill," regardless of whether it affected their erections.)

Ginseng also improves energy levels, which can impact libido and erectile function. That stimulant effect *may* increase blood pressure (it has not been seen in the clinical studies), so anyone with high blood pressure should be vigilant. Conversely, it's also being studied to help *lower* blood pressure—go figure! Regardless, it's important to be aware of this potential side effect. Also, there have been rare drug interactions with an older drug class known as MAO (monoamine oxidase) inhibitors (a type of antidepressant), and the research is controversial on whether it interacts with the blood thinner warfarin. Personally, I would not take this product if I were on warfarin, even if the overall research suggests it is probably safe.

One last word of warning: There are serious quality control and contamination issues with Panax ginseng, so once you've found a company whose products you're interested in, make sure it has verified the ginsenoside content and checked its supplement for heavy metal contaminants.

1. (tie) L-arginine aspartate
2,800 milligrams a day and
Pycnogenol 80 milligrams a day

L-arginine is the intermediary step between L-citrulline and nitric oxide, which increases bloodflow and possibly erectile function. The kidneys convert L-citrulline to L-arginine, which is then converted to nitric oxide. But you'd really need to take megadoses of L-arginine as a dietary supplement to see an impact on erectile function. That's because the liver and intestines remove huge quantities of L-arginine when the supplement is taken and very little ends up being converted to nitric oxide (your organs take a more hands-off approach, if you will, with L-citrulline, allowing more to be converted to nitric oxide). But the news isn't all bad. Multiple studies have shown that the combination of L-arginine aspartate and Pycnogenol can improve erectile function. The drawback is you have to take several pills a day and it's not cheap, but there is always the option of trying fewer pills at first (this is true of any supplement). One of the best-selling products is called Prelox; another is EDOX. In fact, Prelox is one of the only dietary supplements for ED that was studied in a 6-month clinical trial against a placebo! The results (increased orgasmic function, sexual desire, intercourse, and overall satisfaction) were not dramatic, but it's still one of the best-researched options on the market.

Just like with L-citrulline, you need to be careful about combining any supplement that increases nitric oxide levels with prescription ED drugs because both can cause a drop in blood pressure, so I would not combine them without your doctor's approval.

HONORABLE MENTIONS

Note: These supplements look interesting and have some initial research, but I think they still need a bit more to convince me that they work better than my top three.

Tongkat ali (*Eurycoma longifolia*) comes from a plant or a common shrub found along the slopes of hilly areas in the Malaysian rainforest, and there is preliminary human data showing that 200 milligrams per day might improve various aspects of male health, including sex drive, testosterone, and sperm quality and quantity. The product that has the most research—and the only one with real clinical data—is the standardized water-soluble extract of *Eurycoma longifolia* root called Physta (from Biotropics Malaysia). Another study with Physta (300 milligrams per day for 12 weeks) showed improvement in erectile function and libido.

Maca (*Lepidium meyenii*) had early promising research, but it seems to have dropped off. I have always called maca the pride of Peru! It's a plant that grows only at higher elevations in the central Peruvian Andes. There have been multiple clinical studies with maca, and about half have shown an improvement in sexual desire for men and sexual function for women. It has not been standardized in studies, so all I can tell you is that 1,500 milligrams worked as well as 3,000 milligrams in a study completed more than 10 years ago in Peru. It has *not* been found to raise testosterone or estrogen, which means it probably works by some unidentified central (brain) activating mechanism, *if* it truly works. I definitely think it does something to slightly improve libido and sexual function, and it appears to be safe as maca is used widely in Peruvian culture. There is no research on whether it should be taken with or without food, and no serious drug interactions have been reported, but, again, it only has several preliminary clinical trials.

Horny goat weed (*Epimedium sagittatum*) is a tacky name, but the research on this supplement is increasing. Unfortunately, quality control is a major problem. There is a compound in this herb known as icariin that has been shown in laboratory studies to have a similar mechanism of action as prescription ED drugs (making nitric oxide stick around longer), but I don't believe it's anywhere near as effective. The other problem is that there still hasn't been a good clinical study completed, but this will happen soon.

WHAT'S WORTHLESS

Note: The list of worthless or dangerous male enhancement supplements is so long that I decided to shorten it a little, but it illustrates why this category is so suspect. It's no surprise that the FDA has removed at least 100 over-the-counter male enhancement products from the market over the past decade.

Yohimbe. Yohimbine HCL is the active ingredient found in the bark of a West African tree. Many supplement manufacturers sell yohimbe, the bark that supposedly contains yohimbine HCL, but the products, in many cases, have little to no—or variable—quantities of yohimbine HCL in them. In other words, when you buy the supplement yohimbe, you may or may not be getting any active ingredient. All of the positive data regarding yohimbine HCL came from studies that evaluated the active ingredient in drug form, not as a supplement. Yohimbine HCL works and can be tried in rare cases (Viagra and other drugs work 10 times better). I say *in rare cases* because it's dangerous. Most dietary supplements that claim to contain yohimbine HCL have serious quality-control problems and are just as dangerous. Side effects for both the drug and supplements include headache, sweating, nausea, dizziness, nervousness, tremors, sleeplessness, antidiuresis (can't pee), and elevated blood pressure and heart rate. It should not be used by anyone who is taking antidepressants or other mood-altering drugs or who has kidney disease or specific cardiovascular, neurological, or

193

psychological issues. In short, I would never take this supplement or the drug!

DHEA (dehydroepiandrosterone). This is the only official prohormone (a compound that gets converted in the body into a hormone, such as testosterone or estrogen) that's allowed to be sold in supplement form. (Other prohormone supplements were banned by the FDA many years ago because of safety concerns.) The thing about DHEA is that it can increase estrogen levels in men as much as it increases testosterone when taken at higher doses (100 milligrams or more). (Those athletes who were taking DHEA for athletic performance enhancement many years ago were probably getting more in touch with their feminine side!) The prescription drug testosterone does everything DHEA can do—and more— and it's safer and smarter. There's a saying I trot out at lectures: "If you want to go to the Super Bowl, don't try and sneak in the back door, just buy a ticket." In other words, you're better off just taking testosterone. Studies have also shown that DHEA can lower your good (HDL) cholesterol, which is not heart healthy (what's good for the heart is good for the penis!).

Tribulus terrestris. Don't mess around with this herbal DHEA copycat. Just get a prescription of testosterone. Manufacturers claim it increases testosterone, but human studies have failed to demonstrate that.

Fenugreek. Again, human studies have failed to demonstrate that this herb/spice supplement increases testosterone

consistently, contrary to manufacturers' claims. In fact, in one study it actually significantly *reduced* levels of free testosterone! Some experts are pushing it as an ideal substitute for testosterone replacement therapy for men, but the studies are so weak. Now, if you buy fenugreek seeds (*not* concentrated pills) and just use them once in a while in your diet, they may slightly lower cholesterol because they have fiber in them.

L-carnitine. This compound helps with energy production in the body, and it may also play a role in repairing injuries. There has been a lot of research with it in regard to reducing fatigue and improving sexual function, but most of the studies are in the area of male fertility. However, although it has a good safety record, it's very expensive and the required dose is huge. In one older clinical trial, it took 4,000 milligrams (that's several pills a day) to get a questionable improvement in sexual response. L-carnitine, in my personal experience, rarely improves ED beyond what a placebo or lifestyle changes can accomplish.

Ginkgo biloba. The majority of the research on ginkgo and ED was done with individuals who were also on prescription antidepressants, which are a known cause of sexual dysfunction for many people. In one of the better studies, researchers saw no difference between ginkgo versus a placebo, and side effects included increased risk of bleeding and potentially increased blood sugar levels.

Zinc. Zinc is commonly advertised for male sexual health because there are claims it can improve testosterone levels (sorry, this is only true in super-rare cases of profound zinc deficiencies). Some bone-headed experts recommend megadoses of zinc for ED (80 to 100 milligrams daily), but the evidence has demonstrated that such large amounts may lead to prostate-related problems, including benign prostatic hyperplasia and cancer. It also may increase the risk of hospitalization for urinary tract infections and kidney stones. In fact, in one of the largest studies of zinc supplements in medicine (a Harvard study), researchers found a significantly higher risk of advanced prostate cancer in men consuming large amounts of zinc supplements. In Canada and some other countries, there are now restrictions on dosages of over-the-counter zinc pills. In other words, this supplement does nothing for sexual health.

LIFESTYLE CHANGES

Heart healthy = penis healthy! Any time the risk of heart disease is reduced through lifestyle changes penis health is improved. In the official ED treatment guidelines for European doctors, published in the medical journal *European Urology*, lifestyle changes were considered the top evidence-based treatment for ED (they can be used along with conventional medicine or by themselves). When will this finally be recognized in the United States?

Cardiovascular disease is the number one killer of men and women and, of course, the number one cause of sexual dysfunction and reduced erections in men. Erectile or sexual dysfunction can be an indicator of a future life-threatening disease, especially in younger men. After all, the same type of cells that line coronary blood vessels also line the penile artery. The artery itself is just 1 to 2 millimeters in diameter, about the same as a coffee stirrer; the blood vessels that supply the heart (coronary arteries) are 3 to 5 millimeters in diameter, similar to a regular straw, and the blood vessels that supply the brain (carotid arteries) are 4 to 6 millimeters in diameter, which is the size of two straws combined. Most research suggests that the penis runs into trouble before the heart does because the "pipes" that lead to it are smaller and more vulnerable to damage. If a man has erectile issues early in life, there are many doctors who will refer that patient to a cardiologist, and I could not agree more. You will never look at a coffee stirrer the same way again, and you shouldn't because it's a vivid reminder of how easy it is to harm your sex life. Men, take care of the one and only coffee stirrer you've got!

Drink in moderation. Alcohol in excess is a sedative, which also makes a man's penis soft and weak. However, a small amount (one to two drinks, maximum) of alcohol increases the release of nitric oxide in the blood vessels, which slightly improves bloodflow to the penis.

Female Sexual Dysfunction

Dr. Moyad Secret So far in my lifetime, every drug that researchers thought would improve female sexual function has been rejected by the FDA. Why can't we find a Viagra equivalent for women? For starters, the situation for women is a little more complicated than for men. The female sexual response usually involves neurovascular, hormonal, and psychological factors (it's similar for men, but a major improvement is seen when enhancing just the neurovascular component with them). Simply increasing bloodflow to the clitoris or vagina—the way Viagra does for the penis—does not improve desire, arousal, orgasm, or other aspects of female sexual dysfunction. And what works for menopausal women may not work for premenopausal women and vice versa (this is also a critical difference compared to men), making the picture even more complicated. Let's just say that female sexual dysfunction, or FSD, is a medical specialty that should have embraced lifestyle changes and dietary supplementation long ago because there are so few other options. (Of course, that means doctors will have to start asking their patients about it as well, which they're not doing consistently now.)

WHAT IS IT?

Between 25 and 63 percent of women have some form of female sexual dysfunction, which involves problems with one or more of the following:

- Desire/libido (most common complaint)
- Arousal (second most common complaint)
- Orgasm
- Pain (known as dyspareunia, usually due to lack of lubrication, vaginal atrophy, or thinning of the vaginal lining)
- Lubrication
- Overall sexual satisfaction

FSD can be chronic or it can occur periodically or even situationally, and the underlying cause—physical, psychological, or both (see "Potential Causes of Sexual Dysfunction" on page 200 for a list of these)—can be hard to pinpoint. Here are some eye-opening FSD facts.

- Fewer than 30 percent of women experience orgasm on a regular basis with a partner.
- At least 30 percent of women report having some issues with sexual desire, arousal, or orgasm.
- About 30 to 50 percent of women report having sexual complaints, but the actual number of women who are

bothered enough to seek medical treatment is lower (research statistics conflict here a bit). That's an important difference. Many experts and some professional medical organizations believe that unless a woman has "personal distress" about her sexual dysfunction, it should not necessarily be recognized as a problem that needs to be treated. Although this makes some sense, I believe part of the problem is that women, regardless of age, are not given the opportunity to have an open discussion about their sex lives—and any complaints or problems—with health care professionals. The typical checkup is so rushed that it's just not conducive to a frank, thoughtful discussion.

WHAT WORKS

Note: When talking with your doctor, it is critical to ask whether a suggested supplement or product is for premenopausal or postmenopausal women. As you will see, the research often differs by age group.

FOR PRE- AND POSTMENOPAUSAL WOMEN

1. Lubricant (oil-, silicone-, or water-based) as needed

Vaginal dryness or inadequate lubrication is a *major* issue for women of all ages and their partners, and it's a relatively easy fix. (Granted, these aren't technically "supplements." I'm taking some liberties here because lubricants work better than supplements for many people, and lots of them contain supplement ingredients.) A few more stats: Fifteen percent of women between 18 and 64 report always or usually experiencing dryness during sexual activity. Lack of lubrication occurs "very often" in about 10 percent of women over the age of 50, and even younger women report problems with adequate lubrication. Finally, as many as 24 to 48 percent of women have reported experiencing pain during intercourse, and lack of lubrication is a major cause (some studies are suggesting that dyspareunia is more common in younger women). Overall, research continues to show that lubricant use is associated with higher sexual pleasure and satisfaction for both individual and partnered sex. A Johnson & Johnson study showed it increased sexual well-being for healthy women (they felt more satisfied). Some studies suggest that lubricants work as well as locally (vaginally) applied estrogen to improve dryness in menopausal or postmenopausal women.

An over-the-counter massage oil for women known as Zestra—a blend of borage seed oil, evening primrose oil, angelica root extract, and coleus extract—has had some success in clinical trials. A study (with women ages 21 to 65) published in the *Journal of Sex & Marital Therapy* found that Zestra increased sensitivity and warmth and may improve female

COMMON REASONS FOR LUBRICANT USE

In a study published in the *Journal of Sexual Medicine,* women reported the following reasons for relying on a lubricant (from most to least common).

- Enhance sexual experience (stimulation and arousal) for myself

- Aid with insertion (lubricants also reduce the risk of vaginal or anal tearing)

- Vaginal dryness

- Enhance sexual experience for my partner

- Prevent or reduce pain

- I enjoy taste/smell or my partner enjoys taste/smell

desire, arousal, and overall sexual pleasure when applied to the clitoris, labia, and vaginal opening. Borage and evening primrose oil contain large amounts of gamma-linolenic acid (GLA, an omega-6 fatty acid), which, after it's metabolized through the skin, could increase blood-flow and enhance nerve communication. The only side effect reported (by 10 to 15 percent of participants) was mild genital burning that lasted anywhere from 5 to 30 minutes. I would have liked Zestra to be tested against other over-the-counter products or even against a placebo in a very large study, but beggars cannot be choosers; this is an area of medicine that is woefully lacking in research. There are other massage oils out there, so don't be afraid to try them out and see which one works best. The "don't be afraid" part is key! One of the most-cited reasons for not using lubricant is being too embarrassed to purchase it.

One final note: I recommend looking for a product that contains a thickening or gelling agent, such as hydroxyethylcellulose, which improves the consistency of the lubricant, and a pH-balancing agent, such as citric acid, which wards off infection and maintains good bacteria. If you prefer more natural ingredients, look for a lubricant with organic compounds instead of silicone; they may help protect against infections (Some like beeswax have antimicrobial properties, but don't use them to avoid sexually transmitted diseases!). Many of the best lubricant brands have multiple options to pick from, including Yes and Kama Sutra (my favorites), K-Y, and Astroglide.

LUBRICANT CAVEATS

Lubricants come with different issues. Here's a basic guide to lubes.

- Oil-based products—such as petroleum jelly, olive oil, mineral oil, coconut butter, and vitamin E—should not be used with condoms because they can penetrate the latex. They can also alter the vaginal environment (which could lead to infections). They are safe with toys though.

- Silicone lubricants are not absorbed well by the skin (so they stay "wet" for longer), but they must be cleaned off with soap and water. They are condom-safe but not very hygienic with sex toys. They can also alter the vaginal environment.

- Water-based lubricants can dry out quickly, but they're safe with latex contraceptives—such as condoms, diaphragms, and sponges—and with sex toys. They're less likely to alter vaginal bacteria, unless they contain glycerin.

FOR PRE- AND SOME POSTMENOPAUSAL WOMEN

2. Combination product (L-arginine and Panax ginseng) and/or L-citrulline *dosage varies by form*

L-arginine by itself (3,000 to 6,000 milligrams per day) has shown real promise for FSD because it can increase nitric oxide levels in the body, which improves blood-flow to the sexual organs. A related compound, L-citrulline, which I talk about extensively in the Erectile Dysfunction section (page 186), does an even better job of increasing nitric oxide and it's metabolized more effectively by the body, so I usually recommend it over L-arginine. In fact, L-citrulline (the free form versus the malate form) is one of the supplements I recom-

mend the most for female and male sexual health. Research has shown that 1,500 to 6,000 milligrams per day can increase nitric oxide levels in the body within 1 week. Most of the benefit appears to be in premenopausal women, but some postmenopausal women could also benefit.

There have been mainly two placebo-controlled studies of a combination dietary supplement known as ArginMax, which contains Panax ginseng and L-arginine, along with several other ingredients. The results showed improved arousal, desire, orgasm, sexual frequency, clitoral sensation, and sexual function scores, *but* these effects were mostly observed in premenopausal and perimenopausal women. Postmenopausal women reported improved sexual desire, but that was it. A recent

199

POTENTIAL CAUSES OF SEXUAL DYSFUNCTION

- Alcohol or drug use

- Cardiovascular disease and risk factors (e.g., high cholesterol or blood pressure)

- Childbirth and pregnancy (e.g., difficult vaginal delivery)

- Contraceptives

- Diabetes

- Diet

- Hormonal issues
  (e.g., reduction in estrogen or testosterone)

- Inactivity (lack of exercise)

- Medications (over-the-counter and prescription)

- Mental health (depression, anxiety, bipolar disorder)

- Neurological issues , such multiple sclerosis and Parkinson's

- Sleep problems

- Surgeries

- Thyroid disease

- Tobacco use

- Weight gain

clinical study published in the *Journal of Sex & Marital Therapy* showed a benefit within 4 weeks. This supplement does not appear to have estrogenic enhancement properties, so it could be an appropriate option for women with breast cancer or who don't want to use hormone replacement therapy. A study of this product in breast cancer patients (whose sexual health can be so greatly impacted by cancer treatment) found that it helped, but the impact was not statistically significant; still, the fact that it helped some of these women is a testament to the product. You could take L-citrulline by itself, with the ArginMax (500 to 1,500 milligrams of

L-citrulline, in this case), or with ginseng only. In other words, there are plenty of options here to experiment with. (Ginseng by itself has not worked for premenopausal FSD.)

These supplements need to be used for at least 4 weeks before judging if they work. It does not appear to matter if they're taken with or without food, and there has been no good research in the area of drug interactions or the effect on pregnancy, so check with your doctor. (I'd like to see testing of lubricants containing these two amino acids. I think they could improve bloodflow to the vagina and may even improve arousal and lubrication.)

FOR PRIMARILY POSTMENOPAUSAL WOMEN

3. Panax ginseng up to 3,000 milligrams a day in divided doses

Ginsenosides are the active ingredient in ginseng, and they work in multiple ways. One way is that they improve the conversion of L-arginine to nitric oxide in the body, allowing for adequate bloodflow to the genitals. Another fascinating mechanism of action is their effect on the brain. They bind to areas that can promote relaxation, improve mood, and impact dopamine, all of which may stimulate sex drive. Ginseng also improves energy levels. The future of research in the area of ginseng and FSD involves isolating specific active ginsenosides and testing higher dosages. For example, Panax ginseng contains high amounts of a ginsenoside known as Rg1, which has shown some ability to improve bloodflow, arousal, and libido in the laboratory (for women and men), but it needs to be tested more by itself.

A small, randomized trial published in the *Journal of Sexual Medicine* found that taking 3 grams of Panax ginseng (participants took a form called Korean red ginseng) daily for 8 weeks resulted in a significant improvement in arousal in postmenopausal women. The product contained about 8 percent ginsenosides. The reason I believe this trial should get more attention is 1) the Korean-based research team is one of the best in the business and 2) Panax ginseng has a long history of improving male erectile dysfunction and sex drive. You can also look for a product with 16 percent ginsenosides and just take half the dosage. (Always check the percentage of ginsenosides when browsing products at the store so you're comparing apples to apples.)

Pharmacological reviews have found that the potential for drug-ginseng interactions is low; the concern over this supplement interacting with medications, such as blood thinners and antihypertensives, is mostly based on isolated case reports. I recommend taking it with a meal to avoid stomach upset.

WHAT'S WORTHLESS

General supplements for "women's issues," including depression, PMS, menopause, and more. While FSD can

DEPRESSION AND FEMALE SEXUAL DYSFUNCTION

There is a type of female sexual dysfunction that is caused by medications, especially SSRIs (selective serotonin reuptake inhibitors). These antidepressants are lifesavers in many cases, but the high rate of sexual dysfunction—and the difficulty in treating it—makes some people consider stopping their medications. You should always talk with your doctor if you're experiencing sexual side effects because there are some promising supplement options out there. A small published pilot study from Massachusetts General Hospital found that 3,000 milligrams per day of maca (from the Peruvian plant *Lepidium meyenii*) may increase sex drive in women taking SSRIs. Maca contains compounds that appear to improve male and female sexual function, especially sex drive. Another option is the dietary supplement SAM-e (see the Depression section, page 166). Research from Harvard has shown that it may enhance the antidepressant effects of SSRIs and may override some of their negative sexual impact. It can even be used by itself in some people in place of antidepressants. So far, researchers haven't found any noticeable negative impact on sexual health with SAM-e; it may even stimulate an area of the brain that promotes sexual function.

be caused by or associated with some of these problems, the supplements or drugs that help treat them won't necessarily improve FSD. And they could make it worse! For example, it's well known that prescription antidepressants (drugs like venlafaxine or paroxetine) can reduce hot flashes in postmenopausal women, but they *increase* the risk of sexual dysfunction. Calcium supplements can reduce PMS but have absolutely no ability to improve sexual function beyond the fact that women with less severe PMS might be able to be more sexually active. So until a PMS supplement, like vitex (which has serious quality control issues in the United States), shows some consistent impact on

FSD, I cannot recommend them like other doctors do. I think the idea that what works for one thing must work for the other is a bit demeaning to women and the field of FSD research—so this is one bandwagon I won't be jumping on!

Ginkgo biloba. I'm going to skip this bandwagon as well. The studies for ginkgo and FSD have been very weak and controversial. I realize that the dietary supplement ArginMax (see #2) has ginkgo in it, but I don't believe it's the active ingredient because gingko has shown minimal to no activity in past studies of sexual dysfunction.

Yam-based products. These sound good because they can contain precursors

THE BIG PICTURE

When trying to diagnose the cause of female sexual dysfunction (FSD), it's not unusual for doctors to test for hormone imbalances or other markers of underlying problems. They may look at levels of prolactin, thyroid hormone, adrenal hormones, estrogen, and testosterone, as well as cholesterol, hs-CRP (high-sensitivity C-reactive protein), glucose, and more. But lab results rarely give the complete picture; a number that's too high or too low doesn't always explain the cause of the problem. To truly understand the mechanisms at work in your personal situation, your doctor should examine the test results, perform a thorough medical history, evaluate your current physical and mental health, and review your answers to her questions as well as those on an FSD questionnaire (you can find several online; one of my favorites is the FSFI or Female Sexual Function Index). If that doesn't happen, it may be time to find a doctor who's willing to look at the complete picture.

or compounds that resemble human hormones that impact sexual health—such as DHEA (dehydroepiandrosterone), estrogen, or testosterone—but the body isn't able to convert them into the actual hormones. The research with these products is very weak as a result.

Plant estrogens (a.k.a. phytoestrogens), such as soy, flaxseed, and red clover. Having low estrogen can result in a dramatic reduction in bloodflow to the clitoris, vagina, and even the urethra, and it can cause the tissue in these areas to thin. The problem with calling these products "plant estrogens" is that they are so weak. Most clinical trials with these compounds do not show any changes in estrogen.

Yohimbe. If you are excited to take yohimbe, please look at the Erectile Dysfunction section, page 186, to see why many of the yohimbe products are a scam and why they are not safe in general.

LIFESTYLE CHANGES

Heart healthy = sexually healthy! The following heart-healthy habits can improve or prevent some forms of FSD.

- Exercise for at least 30 minutes or more every other day; try to break a sweat.

- Lose weight or maintain a healthy weight.

- Reduce your overall caloric intake by 100 to 200 calories per day if you need to drop pounds.

- Increase your intake of high-quality protein from lean, grass-fed beef; fish; eggs; or even whey, soy, and brown rice protein powders.

DHEA AND FEMALE SEXUAL DYSFUNCTION

DHEA (dehydroepiandrosterone) is a natural prohormone (and the only legal prohormone supplement) that gets converted into estrogen or testosterone in the body (you don't get to choose which one), both of which can improve sexual health. As a result, some women take DHEA in hopes it will improve female sexual dysfunction (FSD). However, you should only take it after your doctor has determined that you have low levels of DHEA (through a blood test for DHEA and DHEA-S) *and* has ruled out other potential causes of FSD. Low DHEA doesn't necessarily cause FSD, but there is one rare situation, something called androgen insufficiency, where it can, and this is where dietary supplementation can be helpful. In women without an insufficiency, DHEA (at a daily dose of 25 to 50 milligrams and higher) hasn't consistently worked better than a placebo. However, pre- and postmenopausal women with androgen insufficiency have seen an improvement in desire, arousal, orgasm, and satisfaction in some past studies.

There is some renewed excitement in the potential for a vaginally inserted DHEA product that improves vaginal thinning or atrophy in postmenopausal women with low estrogen, and it may also improve other aspects of sexual function. It could be available soon in prescription form, so ask your doctor about it.

Anytime a supplement or drug has the potential to increase testosterone levels in women, the potential side effects have to be discussed with your doctor. Acne, deepening voice, clitoral enlargement, and a reduction in "good" cholesterol are just a few of the potential side effects of getting too much DHEA or prescription testosterone in women.

One last note: There are so many supplements that claim to have DHEA-like effects, including yam products and the herb *Tribulus terrestris,* but the research hasn't proven these claims, so I recommend avoiding them. Plus, they tend to be more expensive than a simple low-cost DHEA supplement, so if you really want to try DHEA, just opt for the supplement.

- Increase your intake of monounsaturated fats and omega-3s from plants (do this with flaxseed, chia seeds, or heart-healthy cooking oils, such as canola, olive, and safflower).

- Get 20 to 30 grams per day of fiber.

- Eat at least two servings of fatty, omega-3-rich fish daily.

Fibromyalgia

Dr. Moyad Secret Fibromyalgia is a chronic pain syndrome that also involves fatigue, sleep problems, and other complaints. Since there is really no single drug, including traditional pain medication, that is effective, more supplement and lifestyle research is needed. I suggest taking the guinea pig approach: Find a doctor who's willing to monitor you while you try a different supplement every 3 to 6 months to see what works. In many clinical guidelines, aerobic exercise, low-intensity strength training, and cognitive behavioral therapy (individualized to each person's situation, of course) are recommended. I'd add acupuncture, hypnosis/guided imagery, and tai chi to the guinea pig approach list, as well. (See these sections for more information on treatment of specific symptoms: Low Energy and Chronic Fatigue, page 293; Insomnia and Jet Lag, page 266; and Depression, page 166.)

Capsaicin cream. In one study, subjects applied topical capsaicin (0.075 percent) to 18 different tender points three times a day for 6 weeks and reported some moderate improvement. Research suggests fibromyalgia patients have higher levels of a compound called substance P, which is a neuromodulator; the higher the amount, the greater the perception of pain. Topical capsaicin (derived from hot chile peppers) reduces neuropathic pain in people with diabetes by reducing or depleting levels of substance P. Even though it's had mixed results in studies, the overall effects appear to improve as the strength of the capsaicin increases (you can get higher doses in patch form via a prescription).

Vitamin D. There is some controversial preliminary evidence from recent randomized trials that suggests normalizing blood levels of vitamin D (to 30 to 40 ng/mL) can reduce muscle pain. Although a larger study is needed, it is already known that muscle tissue contains receptors for vitamin D, so it makes sense that having a lack of D could lead to pain. Always get a blood test to evaluate your levels before you start taking high doses, though. Also, keep in mind that healthier lifestyle behaviors, from exercise to weight loss and improved diet, could increase blood levels of vitamin D as well.

Melatonin. In numerous studies, taking 3 to 6 milligrams of melatonin, usually at bedtime, reduced pain, depressive symptoms, and fatigue and improved sleep in people with fibromyalgia. Some studies have even combined it with prescription medications to achieve better results.

Acetyl-L-carnitine. In a preliminary clinical trial with fibromyalgia patients, taking 500 milligrams of acetyl-L-carnitine twice a day for 2 weeks and then 1,500 milligrams per day for 8 weeks reduced depressive symptoms. Acetyl-L-carnitine moves fatty acids further into cells to produce energy and possibly help regulate neurotransmitter function (a neurotransmitter imbalance may lead to increased musculoskeletal pain). This is interesting, but it's from an older study.

Creatine. In one study with fibromyalgia patients, using 20 grams daily for 5 days (divided into four equal doses) and then 5 grams a day for 15 weeks resulted in improved muscle function compared to a placebo. This could be critical in helping those with the condition maintain regular exercise.

Miscellaneous. Almost everything else that has been suggested for fibromyalgia comes from cases series (which are more observational versus trials that test an intervention of some sort). For example, high doses of vitamin B_1 (600 to 1,800 milligrams per day) were reported to dramatically help with pain. The researchers theorized that fibromyalgia may lead to a problem with how the body uses B_1. Higher doses of the vitamin could overcome this issue (it sounds good, but this is why it all goes back to trial and error and being a guinea pig while working with your doctor). Similarly, 100 milligrams of CoQ10 per day may reduce fatigue in juvenile fibromyalgia patients; these patients often have lower levels of CoQ10, and this nutrient is crucial for proper energy production. D-ribose is a naturally occurring carbohydrate that is sold as an energy-boosting dietary supplement. It received a lot of attention about a decade ago in a study using 5 grams three times a day for fibromyalgia and/or chronic fatigue patients, but there has been very little evidence since then.

Gout

G

Dr. Moyad Secret Yes, gout is still around, but it's not just prime rib–downing, beer-swilling guys who get it. Women can develop it, too; in fact, it's more common than rheumatoid arthritis in females! But what's really surprising is that it's really easy to *cause* gout with dietary supplements. I spend more time telling patients with gout what *not* to take as opposed to what to take to prevent this disease. Many doctors are surprised by what actually works and what's worthless.

WHAT IS IT?

Hippocrates called gout "the unwalkable disease" for obvious reasons. It's an inflammatory condition of the joints that can be very painful. The culprit: increased blood levels of uric acid, which crystallizes and gets deposited in the joints. Elevated uric acid can be caused by diet (you're at risk if your daily menu is heavy in meat, seafood, or alcohol, especially beer), genes, and reduced elimination by the kidneys (for some reason you're not peeing enough out). Some medications, including diuretics and low-dose aspirin, can increase levels as well.

The risk of gout increases as we get older because our bodies are no longer as efficient at getting rid of uric acid and because our lifestyle choices, unfortunately, often lead to weight gain. And this leads me to the true reason gout is on the rise worldwide: because conditions like obesity, hypertension, metabolic syndrome, and type 2 diabetes—the epidemics of our time—increase uric acid levels.

Classic gout attacks cause sudden onset of pain, redness, and swelling and tenderness in one or more joints, especially the big toe (people say it feels like the big toe is on fire). Repeated episodes over the years can lead to clumps of uric acid called tophi in or around the joints as well as deformities in and around the affected joints. Besides pain and deformities, gout needs to be controlled and prevented because it is also a potential risk factor for chronic kidney disease, hypertension, and cardiovascular disease.

All that said, as a researcher and physician, I believe uric acid is one of the most fascinating compounds in the human body because it has antioxidant properties. For example, uric acid is found in the brain, where it may protect cells from oxidative stress. A higher level of uric acid is associated with a lower risk of the progression of Parkinson's disease, and whether uric acid can slow the progression of multiple sclerosis is being studied. In other words, in the short term and in "normal" amounts, uric acid can potentially protect tissues from damage. But if it's abnormally elevated over a long period of time, it can increase the risk of gout and other problems, like uric acid kidney stones. So, uric acid has both a positive and negative role in the body depending on the levels.

WHAT WORKS

Note: I can count on one hand the number of well-done studies in the area of gout prevention. Most of the dietary supplement research on it never got out of the laboratory and into clinical trials where these supplements could be tested in humans (or they simply failed to work). So I'm only going to recommend one supplement that might lower uric acid.

1. Vitamin C 500 milligrams a day

In one clinical trial, people taking vitamin C (500 milligrams) reduced their uric acid levels by an average of 0.5 mg/dL; there was no change in the placebo group. The same dose reduced uric acid by as much as 1.5 mg/dL on average in individuals who had abnormally high uric acid levels to start with (>7.0 mg/dL). Good old cheap vitamin C appears to work by increasing the rate at which the kidneys filter uric acid into the urine and by preventing its reabsorption as it moves through the kidneys. Some studies suggest that higher daily doses—1,000 to 1,500 milligrams—may be more effective, but I believe they're also risky because large doses of vitamin C can increase the chances of getting kidney stones. Per usual, I recommend starting at the lowest effective dosage for 2 to 3 months and working your way up if needed. If you've had kidney stones before, stick to the 500-milligram dose.

If regular vitamin C upsets your stomach, buffered or pH-neutral vitamin C (calcium ascorbate) might have fewer side effects, but its impact on uric acid levels is not as well known. Talk to your doctor if you want to give vitamin C a try.

HONORABLE MENTION

Cherry extract supplements are being studied by researchers to reduce the risk of gout attacks, with positive results (there's strong data suggesting that eating cherries and drinking cherry juice can help as well.) The extract products I reviewed have much larger quantities of anthocyanins (anti-inflammatory compounds that may reduce gout attacks) and virtually none of the calories that the juice provides. When buying cherry extract, always look for an anthocyanin content of 100 milligrams per 500-milligram pill, or at least 20 percent.

But there may be another compound at work here: Bing cherries contain an unusually large amount of dehydroascorbic acid, a form of vitamin C that's absorbed more quickly by the body than regular ascorbic acid. It's also able to get to places that "normal" vitamin C can't. For example, vitamin C itself cannot enter the brain via the blood due to the blood-brain barrier, but your noggin' still has large concentrations of vitamin C. How is this possible? Dehydroascorbic acid *can* pass through the blood-brain barrier, and the moment it crosses over, it gets changed back into ascorbic acid to help support brain functions! Kind of awesome (something my kid would say) and kind of groovy (something my father would say when he was my age) and kind of awesome-groovy-amazing (something I would say)! I have seen gout attacks reduced in plenty of individuals taking cherry extract supplements with prescription gout medication.

Studies have shown that eating 20 to 24 bing cherries daily (that's about two servings and 90 to 100 calories) reduces the risk of an attack by almost 50 percent, but the supplements might work just as well (and without as many calories!). I recommend taking small amounts of liquid cherry extract (a couple of teaspoons a day) or 200 to 500 milligrams of cherry extract supplement (in pill form) with at least 20 percent anthocyanins in addition to your gout medication.

One word of warning here regarding fruit juices and health claims: Juice companies are funding research all over the place, whether it's pomegranate juice for prostate cancer, cranberry juice for urinary tract infections, or cherry juice for gout. The FDA has sent warning letters to approximately 30 companies that manufacture, market, or distribute products made from cherries for making unproven claims about their ability to prevent or treat diseases, such as gout, arthritis, lupus, and fibromyalgia. Cherry juice may help, but I worry about the calories and sugar content. Opt for raw cherries or supplements. Also, watching your calorie intake can help you lose weight, which could correct your uric acid issue by itself, eliminating the need for gout-related pharmaceuticals and supplements altogether.

WHAT'S WORTHLESS

Note: These supplements should be on everyone's list of what to avoid if you have gout or have suffered a gout attack, yet I rarely see them mentioned by other experts. That's probably because they're not career supplement geeks like me! I always have other doctors asking me to figure out what's causing gout attacks in their patients. When I review the list of the supplements these men and women are taking, one or more of the following is inevitably on the list.

Inosine (inosine monophosphate). This compound is involved in energy production in the body, so people frequently take it to improve athletic performance, energy, and general vitality. However, individuals with gout should not take this supplement because it can dramatically raise uric acid levels and increase the risk of kidney stones.

TOP 5 VITAMIN C SOURCES WORLDWIDE

It takes more than the recommended five servings of fruits and vegetables daily to get enough vitamin C to prevent gout. For example, you could eat five oranges a day and still not reach the 500-milligram supplement dose I recommend. I did track down some exceptions here, but good luck finding them!

FOOD/BEVERAGE	AMOUNT PER SERVING (MG PER 100-MG OR 3.5-OZ SERVING)
Kakadu plum (native to Australia)	3,150
Camu camu (a berry native to the Amazon Rainforest)	2,800
Rose hip (found throughout the world)	2,000
Acerola (a cherrylike fruit native to the West Indies and northern South America and cultivated in India)	1,600
Amla (known as Indian gooseberry)	720

In some cases, though, raising uric acid levels can be a good thing: Inosine is currently being studied in the treatment of relapsing-remitting multiple sclerosis and Parkinson's disease because patients with these disorders often have lower-than-normal uric acid levels, which may lead to increased inflammation. Individuals with more uric acid (also known as urate) appear in some cases to have a slower progression of their disease. (See the Multiple Sclerosis section, page 331, and the Parkinson's Disease section, page 359.)

Niacin (vitamin B$_3$). For some reason, many experts believe that only the prescription drug niacin can increase the risk of gout, but supplements are equally guilty. It's a small increase, but check with your doctor regardless. Niacin (in both forms) is under a lot of scrutiny right now anyway because it may not be as beneficial in reducing heart disease as researchers once thought.

Ribose (a.k.a. D-ribose). Ribose (it usually comes in powder form) is a naturally occurring carbohydrate or simple sugar (monosaccharide) that is best known for being part of the structure of RNA, which is found in every cell and tells the body which proteins to form for various bodily functions. Ribose is also a component of ATP—the energy "currency" that your cells run on. It's a popular energy-booster, and researchers are looking at

D-ribose's role in enhancing exercise performance and increasing energy levels in people with chronic fatigue and similar disorders. A few clinical trials found small increases in uric acid levels with supplementation of 5 to 10 grams per day of D-ribose. Although the bump wasn't statistically significant—research-speak for being big enough to make any claims about—and the levels returned to normal after 14 days on average, I believe it is clinically significant for individuals who need to keep an eye on their uric acid levels, so I would avoid it if you have gout or a high risk for it.

White willow bark. This supplement is considered a "natural" version of aspirin because the active ingredient in it acts like aspirin. But aspirin can raise uric acid levels, and so can white willow bark. If your doctor tells you that you should be taking a low-dose aspirin daily, opt for a cheap, proven, over-the-counter brand and not the dietary supplements; they're not standardized and you just don't know how much of the active ingredient you're getting.

LIFESTYLE CHANGES

Adjust your diet. People with gout should avoid foods high in purines, compounds that are converted to uric acid during digestion. This usually means cutting out meat, poultry, seafood, alcohol, and high-fat foods in general. Most people have a hard time doing this, so I suggest practicing moderation. Vegetables, nuts, legumes, whole grains, and fruits (*not* fruit juices or large servings of fruit) may help prevent gout, and dairy products may help encourage excretion of uric acid in the urine. You can still eat protein, just don't make it the focus of every meal. If you're unsure what to eat, speak with a nutritionist to create a healthy eating plan.

Lose weight. Being overweight doubles your risk of having a gout attack; obesity triples your risk. The less you weigh, the better your kidneys will be able to process and excrete uric acid. Increased muscle mass and healthy cholesterol levels are also associated with lower gout incidence.

Amp up. Coffee and caffeine intake may reduce uric acid. Yeah!!!

Limit your consumption of sugary drinks and fructose. Soft drinks and fructose-rich fruit and especially fruit juices (in particular, apple, grape, and orange juice) can increase uric acid levels. Always make sure you read the label and look for phrases like "low-calorie," "zero sugar," or "almost zero sugar." Agave syrup is high in fructose (up to 90 percent in some cases), but sweeteners like brown sugar, brown rice syrup, and honey are lower. Regardless, you should still try to limit your intake. While the increased sugar does lead to uric acid production in the body, the extra calories and weight gain that these sugary drinks can cause is of bigger concern. One could argue that the popularity and increased intake of high-fructose corn syrup is probably partly to blame for the dramatic increase in gout that is being seen around the world.

WHAT ELSE DO
I NEED TO KNOW?

Once you have a gout attack, you're at higher risk for experiencing another one (especially if you don't alter the lifestyle habits that contributed to it), just like with kidney stones. As a result, doctors generally handle it in two ways: They treat the attack and then manage the condition long term. During an attack, the goal is to reduce inflammation and pain, usually with medication. Afterward, the goal is to better control any diseases associated with gout, such as diabetes, hypertension, high cholesterol, and cardiovascular disease. Your doctor may prescribe medication to keep your uric acid levels low.

Gout should not be occurring in kids. If it does, it's time to see a specialist. Doctors never used to see type 2 diabetes in kids, and now it's a freakin' epidemic. So, I assume we will be seeing a lot of gout in kids soon.

Graves' Disease
(Hyperthyroidism)

G

Dr. Moyad Secret Graves' disease is an autoimmune disorder where the thyroid basically works overtime (hyperthyroid), leading to insomnia, weight loss, palpitations, increased appetite, diarrhea, skin warmth, and tremors. When it comes to thyroid disorders, you have to be very careful about what supplements you take. Thyroid replacement drugs come in millionths of a gram (micrograms), so a slight increase or decrease in dose can have profound positive or negative effects. And if a supplement interacts with this very precise dosing, it could cause serious problems.

Selenium. At the time of publishing this book, investigators in the GRAves' Disease Selenium Supplementation (GRASS) trial were testing selenium at 200 micrograms per day to see if it can help with treatment. The thyroid has the highest concentration of selenium per gram of tissue of any organ, and the mineral helps contribute to normal thyroid function in many ways. Selenium has shown some promise in helping people with Graves' disease achieve normal thyroid levels more quickly. A recent European clinical trial, called EUGOGO (the European Group on Graves' Orbitopathy), found a potential benefit with using 200 micrograms of selenium (as sodium selenite) for people with Graves' disease who have mild orbitopathy (bulging of the eyes); it appeared to improve quality of life and eye lesions and slow the progression of eye bulging compared to a placebo over 1 year of treatment. The problem? There is no data from this trial indicating whether the subjects were deficient in selenium at the beginning of the trial. Regardless, this is worth discussing with your doctor and blood levels have to be monitored.

WHAT'S WORTHLESS

Kelp. These supplements contain iodine and are popular for the treatment of thyroid abnormalities. However, some of these kelp pills provide from 500 to 1,000 micrograms or more of iodine per day (the Recommended Dietary Allowance is only 150 micrograms per day). And these excessive amounts of iodine can throw off thyroid function (too little or too much iodine will disrupt thyroid function). The risk here is clearly greater than the benefit, so I never recommend them.

Gray Hair

THE JURY'S STILL OUT

Dr. Moyad Secret There is no secret! Researchers at the University of Bradford in England found gray hair has lower-than-normal levels of the enzyme catalase. Hair cells produce hydrogen peroxide, which lightens hair, and catalase breaks down hydrogen peroxide into water and oxygen. As we age, production of catalase decreases, so hydrogen peroxide builds up. As a result, there has been an explosion of catalase supplements for gray hair, which I have not seen work so far (it's easily digested in the stomach before it can even reach cells to have any impact). So, I do not believe there is a single supplement that works to reverse gray hair. It's primarily genetics—and in rare instances vitiligo, hypothyroidism, vitamin B_{12} deficiency, chemotherapy drugs, and chronic, ongoing stress—that cause graying of hair. (Treating hypothyroidism and taking vitamin B_{12} might help you in these cases.) Obviously, coloring your hair is a temporary solution for the nuisance.

Hair Loss

Dr. Moyad Secret Surprise! The only cure for male pattern baldness is removing a man's testicles at an early age (i.e., castration). Without male hormones (testosterone and a more potent form of testosterone known as dihydrotestosterone, commonly abbreviated as DHT), genetic characteristics affecting the scalp, such as hair loss, can't be fully expressed (turned on). Of course, when a man's testosterone level drastically plummets (whether from a surgical procedure, drug, or just over time), his risk of experiencing all those things women can go through when they hit menopause (such as rapid bone loss, fatigue, hot flashes, loss of sex drive, and weight gain) almost *immediately* increases. So, I imagine most men would rather lose their hair than go through "manopause."

A more realistic option for men experiencing hair loss is to take a prescription drug or supplement, which works primarily by reducing DHT to almost zero or altering testosterone metabolism (drugs can do this, but supplements haven't been as successful with this strategy). However, side effects include reduced sex drive and fertility and an increased risk of erectile dysfunction and possibly even depression. So, the pros need to be weighed against the substantial cons here. It's incredibly ironic that the supplements and prescriptions used by men to keep their hair, which is a cosmetic or superficial feature of manhood, can do so much potential damage (in the short and long term) to real, or physiologic, manhood!

WHAT IS IT?

Androgenetic alopecia is also known as male pattern baldness (women can experience a version of it as well, commonly known as female androgenetic alopecia or female pattern hair loss). *Pattern* refers to the way hair falls out, which tends to be different in men versus women: Men tend to lose hair at the front "corners" of the scalp (called bitemporal recession) and at the crown (back of the head). Women tend to lose it on the central portion of the scalp, sparing the frontal hairline. Up to 70 per-cent of men and 40 percent of women experience this kind of hair loss, and it typically comes down to hormones and genetics (there's usually a family history). In men, hormones turn on the genetic switch that triggers hair loss. In women, it can be due to either hormones, genetics, or a combination of issues. (Other causes of hair loss, such as thyroid dysfunction or infections, are a separate category, which I'm not going to discuss.)

Alopecia areata is a different type of hair loss; in this case, hair falls out in

MOYAD FACT: After bone marrow, hair is the second fastest-growing tissue of the body. In fact, the reason some cancer chemotherapy drugs cause hair loss is because they inhibit or block these rapidly dividing cells.

patches, and the condition remits and relapses. It's really classified as "inflammatory hair loss of unknown origin," and it can be due to a family history, an autoimmune disorder, or emotional stress. By reducing some of this inflammation, hair growth can be stimulated. The reason I am mentioning this condition is that some companies will test a product on these individuals and then show a photo of how they got better, but this condition can resolve on its own (in other words, caveat emptor!). In this section, I'll primarily discuss androgenetic alopecia, which will not improve without treatment.

Two drugs have been approved in my lifetime for androgenetic alopecia. The first is topical minoxidil (also FDA approved for women), which is applied daily to the scalp; it's available over the counter now and as a generic. Finasteride (Propecia) is the other drug, available only through a prescription (it's not FDA approved for women but some do use it). This drug works by blocking the enzyme 5-alpha-reductase, which helps convert testosterone into its turbocharged form, DHT. This hyped-up testosterone is what triggers hair loss. So if you cut off or reduce the supply of the hormone responsible for hair loss, you keep more hair!

When started as early as possible in the hair-loss process, minoxidil and finasteride (which can be used together) can be effective at stopping it, but they usually won't help dramatically regrow hair or fill in a bald spot; at best, some fine, thin hair might spring up. Another drug, dutasteride, can also help with male and female pattern hair loss, but it is much more expensive than finasteride and is *not* FDA approved for this condition. (It's approved for noncancerous prostate enlargement, so a lot of folks get it off-label from doctors.)

The role of androgens (a male hormone) in hair loss is not as well known in women as it is in men, and the majority of women impacted by hair loss have normal blood levels of androgens. In women, genetics are the primary cause, but higher testosterone levels can exacerbate the condition.

WHAT WORKS

1. Saw palmetto 320 to 960 milligrams a day for treatment of minimal hair loss as soon as it begins to happen

This is only number one because something has to come first, but it does *not* mean that this is the best supplement for hair loss. Almost all (99.9 percent) of the supplements that have ever been promoted for hair loss do not work; the ones that might have an effect would essentially have to work in the same way finasteride does—by altering hormones. If they did that, the unavoidable side effects that I mentioned earlier would grab the attention of attorneys and the FDA, and these products would be gone in less than a year.

There are some small studies of saw palmetto or multiple fatty acid components of saw palmetto showing it may minimally help hair growth in the same way finasteride does, but it's far less potent. In other words, instead of reducing DHT by 80 to 90 percent or more, like conventional drugs do, saw palmetto might reduce it by 25 percent, if that. And remember, these were just small studies.

Many saw palmetto supplements contain the following fatty acids (in approximation).

- 30 percent lauric acid

- 28 percent oleic acid (the same mono-unsaturated fat in olive oil)

- 12 percent myristic acid

- 10 percent palmitic acid

- 5 percent linoleic acid (an omega-6 fatty acid) and some stearic acid

Researchers have concluded that all of these fatty acids have the ability to partially block the enzyme 5-alpha-reductase that contributes to hair loss. Some research teams suggest it is the lauric acid and myristic acid (both commonly found in coconut oil) that mostly block this enzyme, as well as oleic acid in small amounts.

Several herbal supplements or ingredients for prostate enlargement—including pygeum, beta-sitosterol, and zinc (see the Benign Prostatic Hyperplasia section, page 98)—have shown the potential to block 5-alpha-reductase, but not nearly as well as saw palmetto. One oft-cited but small clinical trial is a 5-month study of 26 men with androgenetic alopecia who took either a placebo or 200 milligrams of saw palmetto extract combined with 50 milligrams of beta-sitosterol daily. Sixty percent of the men taking the supplement saw improvements versus 11 percent with the placebo.

A recent small study of 100 men taking either 320 milligrams of saw palmetto or 1 milligram of finasteride daily for 2 years showed finasteride was more effective. More than half of the participants with severe hair loss reported improvements with finasteride, and it helped keep and grow hair (fine and thin) in the front and back of the scalp. Saw palmetto apparently benefited some men who had baldness in the back of the head only (there was no placebo). So, what can I say? Trying 320 milligrams of saw palmetto (up to 960 milligrams per day) is probably safer than taking finasteride, but whether it works much better than a placebo is unknown. (Look for saw palmetto with at least 85 percent total fatty acids and 0.3 percent sterols; it can be taken with or without other supplements for prostate enlargement, such as pygeum and beta-sitosterol.) I recommend trying it for 3 to 6 months to see if there's a difference. Keep in mind that none of these male prostate supplements, such as saw palmetto or beta-sitosterol, have been tested in women. (Finasteride is only approved for men, but a lot of dermatologists use it for women and it clearly helps a minority of them, so it's worth talking to your doctor about trying saw palmetto.)

2. FOR WOMEN ONLY: Iron dosage varies depending on blood test results

In some women (premenopausal), iron can help hair thinning and loss. Doctors often test for iron deficiency in women who complain of hair loss, especially if they are still menstruating, are vegetarian, or have a history of anemia. There's no guarantee obviously, and iron supplements should never be taken unless a deficiency is diagnosed with a blood test. Some women report improvements in the quality or quantity of their hair with iron, but others don't.

The doctor may also test thyroid function because abnormal thyroid levels can cause hair loss, and some will also check testosterone and other hormone levels (DHEA-S and prolactin) to see if there's an excess of testosterone or another hormone issue that might explain the hair loss.

WHAT'S WORTHLESS

Selenium (megadoses). Recently in the United States, there was an incident where more than 200 people took a liquid selenium supplement that, unknown to them, contained 200 *times* the dose reported on the label. More than 70 percent of these people reported hair loss, and 18 percent reported *complete* loss of scalp hair.

B vitamins. Numerous companies promote a variety of B-complex supple-ments for "healthy hair." However, I cannot emphasize enough that you should *not* use B vitamins in excess amounts (beyond what is found in a multivitamin) for genetic hair loss because they have no evidence. Biotin is another popular hair and nail supplement, but it will not grow hair or reduce the risk of hair loss from androgenetic alopecia (see the Brittle Nail Syndrome section, page 119). As I alluded to above, these vitamins are often tested with patients who have rare causes of hair loss, like alopecia areata or extreme Third World deficiencies, and you can't apply those results to regular pattern hair loss.

Vitamin D. There is some minimal, weak research on vitamin D supplements to prevent hair loss (either by itself or with a prescription drug), but these studies mostly come from the laboratory and show that vitamin D is necessary to put hair follicles in the growth stage, to prevent hair from toxicity, or just for normal hair growth cycles. There is very little chance that vitamin D impacts hair growth though, except in rare cases of an extreme deficiency. Obese women, however, can have lower levels of vitamin D (the vitamin gets stored in fat cells instead of in the blood) and abnormal changes in hormone levels, including testosterone, which could be the real reason behind the hair loss.

Vitamins A, E, and C. There is no human research to suggest that these vitamins help with hair loss or making hair healthier, unless there is a rare deficiency.

Estrogen-boosting or testosterone-

suppressive (finasteride-mimicking) compounds. Estrogen production may prevent testosterone from impacting receptors that could accelerate hair loss; it simply decreases testosterone use. For this reason, in rare cases some women are given antiandrogen drugs or contraceptive pills to increase estrogen levels. It's a good rationale, but they just don't work for most men and women for hair loss. Some herbs you might see promoted for this purpose are black cohosh, chasteberry, dong quai, false unicorn, flaxseed or soy extracts, and red clover.

Testosterone-enhancing supplements. There aren't many of these that actually work, but dietary supplements that claim to increase testosterone can only make hair loss worse if you're a man; the extra testosterone can get converted to DHT, which turns on the genetic hair-loss switch.

LIFESTYLE CHANGES

Heart healthy = hair healthy? I wish! However, there is some research to suggest that men who have early hair loss (or premature graying, like me) could have an increased risk of heart disease.

Evaluate your lifestyle. All of the following could cause some hair loss, either temporarily or long term.

- Medications (prescriptions and supplements)
- Crash dieting and eating disorders
- Emotional disorders
- Chronic illness
- Excessive daily exercise for long periods of time, such as training for ultra-endurance races

Wash away the bald. Shampoos to make the hair appear more dense and full can have some minor to moderate impact. I like to put them in the "why not try it" category for both men and women. Shampoos containing ingredients such as ketoconazole (2 percent) or pyrithione zinc (1 percent) have been used for years, and they're basically extra-strength anti-dandruff shampoos that may also impact hormone levels in a small way. These shampoos do have the potential to increase hair density and size, and they can increase the number of hair follicles that go into the growth stage. Rotate them with your regular shampoo.

Let there be light. Laser light therapy combs (like something out of *Star Wars*) are selling well in various countries around the world. You run the bulky comblike device through your hair several times a week for 10 to 15 minutes, and you can also use it as a sword to fight the dark side (just kidding). Sounds crazy—and it very well may be—but there is some *minimal* research to suggest these products may increase bloodflow to the scalp and promote slight hair growth for men and women. In one study, participants used a comb with a wavelength of 655 nanometers

(HairMax LaserComb) for 15 minutes three times a week (on nonconcurrent days) for 6 months. About 64 percent of the subjects reported no growth (compared to 58 percent with a placebo comb), 25 percent saw minimal growth, 10 percent had moderate growth, and 1 percent hit the jackpot with dense growth. Overall, it did a little better than a placebo comb. So I'm not sure if these results are clinically significant (I'm skeptical overall), even though some of the results were statistically significant.

Consider waving the white flag. My primary recommendation for many men is to just shave their heads and not worry about it. Of course, I realize that with all the pressure today to look younger, this is not an easy decision. Unfortunately, drug manufacturers have made this condition seem like it's a disease when, in reality, it's mostly just a natural genetic expression, like eye color. Still, men with hair loss can save time and tons of money by opting for a close shave, and it may improve their sex lives because they won't be messing up their hormones with pills. Going bald is proof that you have a decent amount of testosterone flowing in your body. Giving in and shaving what remains of your hair also seems to be associated with the most long-term satisfaction, in my experience.

WHAT ELSE DO I NEED TO KNOW?

There are still only two FDA-approved drugs for hair loss (topical minoxidil and finasteride), which gives you an idea how hard it is to come up with any drug or supplement in this billion-dollar industry. Other antiandrogen drugs—such as oral contraceptives, cyproterone, and spironolactone—might help some women with hair loss.

The prescription drug Latisse (bimatoprost ophthalmic solution, 0.03 percent) is FDA-approved to make eyelashes grow longer, fuller, or darker. It was originally used to treat ocular hypertension and glaucoma, and a notable side effect was increased eyelash growth. In some small clinical studies of men and women with pattern baldness, it seemed to be beneficial. Stay tuned! What I like is that it grows hair via a new and different mechanism that does not apparently impact hormones; it has more of a localized effect—a little similar to minoxidil.

The only permanent solution for hair loss for men and women is hair transplants, but keep in mind that once you get one, you're probably a customer for life! You will have to use minoxidil or finasteride to keep the rest of your hair from falling out. So, to say this option is costly long term is stating the obvious.

Hashimoto's Thyroiditis
(Hypothyroidism)

H

Dr Moyad Secret Again, as I said for Graves' disease (hyperthyroidism), when it comes to thyroid disorders, you have to be very careful about supplements. Thyroid replacement drugs come in millionths of a gram (micrograms), so a slight increase or decrease in dose can have profound positive or negative effects. If a supplement interacts with this very precise dosing, it could cause serious problems.

Hashimoto's is an autoimmune thyroid disorder, and new research suggests it may now be the most common autoimmune disease in the United States. Symptoms include anxiety, depression, dry skin, puffy eyes, muscle cramps and fatigue, constipation, slow thinking, poor memory, and coldness—all due to low levels of thyroid hormone.

Selenium. New evidence suggests selenium (200 micrograms of selenomethionine), which plays a role in immune and thyroid function, can reduce thyroid antibody levels and the dosage of thyroid hormone replacement (synthetic T4, a.k.a. levothyroxine) needed. It's also possible that 200 micrograms of sodium selenite could improve well-being/mood, so either form of selenium looks interesting. The average time subjects took this supplement was 7.5 months. Side effects appeared to be minimal and similar to a placebo, but selenium can potentially increase the risk of diabetes and skin cancer recurrence at these higher dosages in people who are at higher risk for these diseases. Finally, there's a new clinical trial in Denmark called CATALYST, which will evaluate using 200 micrograms of selenium-enriched yeast versus placebo in patients with chronic autoimmune thyroiditis. This is a big deal, so ask your doctor about the latest study results.

Headache
(Cluster Type)

THE JURY'S STILL OUT

Dr. Moyad Secret This is a nerve disorder that involves extremely severe, stabbing or burning headaches that occur in cyclical patterns (or "clusters"). The pain lasts for 15 to 180 minutes on average and is typically centered behind one eye or one temple (the most common complaint is that it feels like a "red-hot poker"). Additional symptoms include runny nose, tearing, drooping eyelids, and facial swelling on the same side as the headache. Oxygen therapy, where you inhale oxygen from a tank via face mask for 10 minutes, really helps many sufferers (about 75 percent), but conventional medicines have most of the evidence.

There is no supplement to treat cluster headaches, but there is some preliminary research regarding prevention that includes taking 10 milligrams of immediate-release melatonin at bedtime (lower doses have not been as successful). Melatonin levels may be lower in the evening in people with cluster headaches, and supplementing may reduce the release of compounds that can encourage cluster headache pain and other symptoms and may play an overall anti-inflammatory role in the brain. This is worth a try for several weeks, especially if you can't tolerate conventional medications. Keep in mind that melatonin in high doses can cause daytime fatigue in some users, so always evaluate your own benefit-to-risk ratio. Low-dose (2 milligrams) controlled-release melatonin was not effective in a past study.

Here's something else that might work: Applying 0.025 percent capsaicin cream inside the nose a few times a day for 7 days on the same side of the face as the cluster headaches might desensitize nerve cells by reducing substance P, a compound that can increase pain perception. Researchers indicated it might reduce future episodic attacks. As you might expect, it's not a popular treatment because the cream can burn, but if nothing else works, it might be worth trying.

Headache
(Tension Type)

Dr. Moyad Secret Tension headaches—which are characterized by a pressing ache that pulsates across the forehead, at the temples, or at the back of the head—can be triggered by fatigue, stress, poor posture, jaw clenching, and smoking. My favorite remedy for these headaches is to first try stress reduction. Whether it's yoga, meditation, or massage, I've found that profound stress reduction works better than any supplement in most individuals (see the Stress and Anxiety section, page 414). Otherwise, over-the-counter pain relievers have been very effective.

5-HTP (5-hydroxytryptophan). The thinking is that if you increase levels of 5-HTP, a precursor of serotonin, you increase levels of serotonin, which improves mood and may activate intrinsic pain-relieving systems in the body. There is positive preliminary data (at 300 milligrams per day) that it can reduce the use of pain medication in people with chronic tension-type headaches. The only problem is that there has not been a follow-up study.

Magnesium. This mineral has some data to support its use for tension headaches, probably due to its ability to relax muscles. There's no consensus on dosage, but there has been evidence that 300 to 600 milligrams per day of magnesium citrate or another form of this mineral may also help prevent migraines and help relieve pain in adults (diarrhea is a potential side effect, though). This supplement is showing some early positive results in kids and adolescents as well.

MOYAD TIP: Rub peppermint oil on your temples and forehead to reduce headache pain.

Hearing Loss

Dr. Moyad Secret Hearing loss from age, noise, and even drugs is caused by oxidative stress. That's why researchers are really excited to test supplements (many low-cost supplements are antioxidants, which have the potential to absorb or prevent oxidative stress). However, it would take years of testing to prove that a supplement might work to treat hearing loss because of the slow nature of the condition. And, of course, it takes time in studies to prove that a supplement (or drug) can actually prevent a condition. Regardless, there's just not enough funding to do such a long trial of dietary supplements unless a researcher is willing to champion this cause (hint, hint!).

Much like the wear and tear on your joints that causes osteoarthritis, intense exposure to sound causes wear and tear on the hair cells in your inner ear that pick up sound wave vibrations and convert them to nerve impulses. These impulses travel to the brain via the auditory nerve and are then interpreted as sound. Listening to your favorite singer with the volume turned up full blast can cause permanent damage. Turning the volume down and using earplugs around loud noises (like at a rock concert or a University of Michigan football game) are easy ways to prevent damage. When it comes to supplements for hearing loss, I always look for ones that have been tested in a setting with lots of noise, like in military studies.

Heart healthy = ear healthy? Maybe. There are some preliminary studies suggesting that higher levels of blood glucose could impair hearing and that obesity at a young age may predict a higher rate of hearing loss in older age. This is because fat tissue produces hormones and other compounds (such as cytokines) that increase system-wide inflammation and can damage organs.

Alpha-lipoic acid (ALA) and NAC (N-acetylcysteine). In animal models, ALA has been shown to protect against both age-related hearing loss and chemotherapy-induced hearing loss. It is a cofactor in cellular enzymes and a free-radical scavenger that could increase levels of protective compounds in the ear (such as vitamins E and C and glutathione). A preliminary study in humans showed a 10-day course of 600 milligrams of ALA daily could protect the inner ear from trauma; it improved both subjective and objective hearing measures. Although ALA can dramatically increase levels of the antioxidant glutathione in the body, the supplement NAC is even better at it. There is some preliminary research using 1,200 milligrams per day with steel workers and 2,700 milligrams per day with military personnel showing it can prevent ear trauma due to noise. Both ALA and NAC supplements have a history of protecting nerves and other cells in the body: ALA protects nerves from damage in people with diabetes, for example, and NAC protects organs, like the liver, and tissues from acetaminophen overdose. So, these supplements could be preventing reactive oxygen species—a.k.a. oxidative stress, the normal wear and tear that happens to all cells through the course of daily living (aging) and exposure to environmental factors (sun, smoke) and toxins (lead, mercury)—due to noise exposure. ALA can cause a malodorous urine smell (similar to what happens when some people eat asparagus) because of the high concentration of sulfur compounds. Also, rarely, ALA can cause rash and itching and a significant drop in glucose levels (very rarely).

Vitamin B$_{12}$. In one study, Army personnel who had a vitamin B$_{12}$ deficiency showed a greater rate of noise-induced hearing loss than those with normal B$_{12}$ levels. High doses of vitamin B$_{12}$ (1 milligram daily for 7 days and then 5 milligrams on the eighth day) appeared to protect the ear from noise damage better than a placebo. It may help by reducing the excitatory impact of high levels of noise stimulation.

Magnesium. While it hasn't been repeated, a small study of magnesium supplements showed a minor questionable benefit at 122 milligrams per day in protecting nerve and hair cells compared to a placebo. More studies are ongoing with magnesium supplements to determine if this mineral could improve hearing loss.

Miscellaneous. Researchers have theorized that other antioxidants—from CoQ10 to vitamin E—can prevent hearing loss, but good studies are lacking.

Hemorrhoids

Dr. Moyad Secret You can treat hemorrhoids with creams, ointments, wipes, and even medical procedures—with good success—but one of the best ways to treat and potentially prevent this condition, especially in its early stages, is to eat more fiber. Low fiber intake can lead to hard stools that raise colon pressure and can damage existing veins and cause hemorrhoids. Soft, smooth stools do not raise pressure in the colon. Some of the best hemorrhoid drugs in the world are also used to prevent and treat varicose veins (they're both related to abnormal vein structure), and in the United States these drugs are called dietary supplements (see the Varicose Veins and Chronic Venous Insufficiency section, page 442)! (Again, the difference between a drug and a supplement is perception, not reality.)

WHAT IS IT?

Simply put, hemorrhoids are a pain in the butt (pun intended). They are clumps of dilated blood vessels that bulge from the lining of the rectum; when they protrude, or prolapse, outside of the anus, they can become very painful. If there is extreme pain, bleeding, incontinence, or ulceration, you might have to consider surgery, but usually that's not necessary.

This will drive some doctors crazy, but I like to think of hemorrhoids as varicose veins of the anal and rectal area because they share some (not all) features with varicose veins. Having one does not predispose you to having the other. However, there is little question that the drugs—and especially supplements—that are promising for treating varicose veins are also excellent for hemorrhoids. These supplements have the ability to increase drainage of fluid and improve the structure and function of the veins.

No supplements or drugs can cure hemorrhoids, but they can treat and reduce the recurrence. Lifestyle changes can reduce the risk of hemorrhoids, but no one can say for sure that they will reduce the chances of hemorrhoids becoming worse.

WHAT WORKS

Note: Attacking hemorrhoids from multiple angles—with supplements, fiber, topical treatments, and wipes—will provide faster pain relief. Also, every dietary supplement that has shown benefits with hemorrhoids also comes with a small number of reported cases of gastrointestinal side effects (nausea, heartburn, and diarrhea). Overall, the supplements in this section primarily have evidence against grade 1 and 2 hemorrhoids, which are less serious and do not require a medical procedure. Check with your doctor because new research suggests these supplements may also improve recovery from a hemorrhoidectomy (surgery to remove hemorrhoids) or other hemorrhoid procedures, such as rubber band ligation.

1. Fiber at least 20 to 30 grams a day (with no more than 5 to 15 grams coming from a fiber supplement)

Pretty much everyone with hemorrhoids should get more fiber, either through diet or supplements, to help reduce symptoms. Notice I say "reduce symptoms"; researchers aren't 100 percent sure if fiber prevents hemorrhoids (I think it does). Fiber promotes soft, bulky stools that can be passed without straining, which is critical for reducing pain, bleeding, and healing time. It's also important to increase your water intake to make the fiber work more effectively (by drawing water into the stool to soften it) and to reduce side effects from it. In studies, supplements with psyllium, sterculia, or unprocessed bran decreased bleeding, pain, itching, and prolapse; most have found that 10 to 20 grams a day of extra fiber can make a difference.

Some studies reported a higher rate of bloating with fiber supplements, which is

MOYAD FACT: People often ask me why blood from their hemorrhoids is bright red versus dark red or blue. Even though your veins look bluish and carry deoxygenated blood, your blood is *always* red (deoxygenated blood is just darker). The blood you see is bright red because hemorrhoidal tissue has veins that connect with arteries, which carry oxygenated blood.

why it's better to increase the fiber you're getting from diet versus pills or powders. I recommend trying to get 5 to 15 grams from a high-fiber breakfast cereal or bar that includes soluble and insoluble fiber as well as another 5 to 15 maximum from a fiber powder, like psyllium (eating a combination of soluble and insoluble fiber delivers the most benefits for heart and gastrointestinal health and helps prevent future straining and constipation).

2. Diosmin 1,000 to 3,000 milligrams a day in divided doses for 1 week for current hemorrhoids; 1,000 milligrams a day in divided doses for 2 to 3 months or longer to reduce symptoms of chronic or recurrent hemorrhoids

The most commonly tested drugs or supplements for hemorrhoids are preparations that include micronized purified flavonoid fractions (MPFF). This jargony-sounding name essentially means they contain a particular combination of plant compounds called flavonoids. *Micronized* means that the particles were reduced in size to less than 2 micrometers (that's

227

really tiny) to improve solubility and absorption. There are other MPFF products out there, but diosmin is the one to look for when it comes to hemorrhoids. Daflon is the best known diosmin-containing product. A semisynthetic prescription drug in France and Europe, it typically contains 450 milligrams of diosmin and 50 milligrams of other flavonoids (a 90:10 ratio). Although it's a drug in Europe, in the United States it's a dietary supplement.

There is evidence that diosmin helps in many ways, including by preventing endothelial damage, reducing the inflammatory response seen in the microcirculation, and improving venous tone and lymph drainage. It can help reduce hemorrhoids and other venous problems, such as varicose veins. In fact, no other product has received more human research in the area of hemorrhoids and chronic venous insufficiency (CVI). A review of more than 10 randomized trials and 1,500 patients suggests that these flavonoid products (diosmin or Daflon) reduce the risk of bleeding by 67 percent, continuous pain by 65 percent, itching by 35 percent, and recurrence rate by almost 50 percent. That's impressive!

At the same time, however, there is no good research on potential drug interactions or potential side effects when using diosmin, but some clinical trials have reported a higher rate of gastrointestinal problems. I would be careful about combining it with aspirin or other blood thinners only because it can cause a reduction in red blood cell clumping and blood viscosity, which means it may increase blood thinning.

In studies, the most common dosages of diosmin used were 2,000 to 3,000 milligrams per day after meals for the first 3 to 4 days of experiencing hemorrhoids, followed by 2,000 milligrams per day on days 4 through 7. This dosage improved pain, bleeding, itching, and anal discharge. Other studies have used 1,800 milligrams of diosmin for 4 days (600 milligrams three times a day) and 1,200 milligrams for 4 more days (400 milligrams three times a day). There is also research showing that taking 2,000 milligrams a day over 60 to 80 days may reduce symptoms of chronic or recurrent hemorrhoids.

Some studies have followed subjects taking 1,000 milligrams of diosmin daily for a year, and this minimal long-term data is one reason I love this supplement. One study looked at pregnant women with hemorrhoids for 8 weeks before delivery and 4 weeks afterward. The researchers used 3,000 milligrams of diosmin daily for 4 days and then 2,000 milligrams daily for 3 days (known as a loading dose); the maintenance dose after that was 1,000 milligrams daily. About half of the women reported a benefit within a few days, and the researchers noted there was no impact on pregnancy, fetal development, birth weight, feeding, or infant growth. Now, this does not prove it's completely safe during pregnancy, but I think it's absolutely worth discussing with your doctor since hemorrhoids are common in pregnancy.

3. Pycnogenol 100 to 150 milligrams a day in divided doses for 1 week with or without 0.5 percent Pycnogenol cream to treat active hemorrhoids

A standardized extract from the bark of the French maritime pine, Pycnogenol contains polyphenols, especially proanthocyanidins (PCOs), which appear to be the active ingredient with protective properties. You should always look for a Pycnogenol supplement with at least 80 to 95 percent PCOs. Unfortunately, these PCOs are not cheap, but other sources of these active compounds include peanut skin and grape seed extract. (The latter is a fairly well-known supplement, but it doesn't have adequate research in the area of hemorrhoids.)

There have not been many studies with Pycnogenol and hemorrhoids, but the best one used a Pycnogenol supplement and topical cream (0.5 percent Pycnogenol) within 48 hours of the onset of hemorrhoids for 1 week. Subjects took 300 milligrams of the dietary supplement for 4 days and then 150 milligrams for 3 days (in three daily divided doses). When the cream was used with the supplement, symptom relief (especially pain) was significantly faster. Pycnogenol is often given with a 10-milligram fiber supplement, such as psyllium, but a high-fiber cereal is another option. The preliminary data for Pycnogenol and varicose veins is pretty impressive, and it has a good safety record, so despite few clinical trials directly with hemorrhoids, I'm comfortable recommending it. The one con: It's pricey.

HONORABLE MENTIONS

Horse chestnut seed extract (*Aesculus hippocastanum*) has been shown to reduce leg pain, swelling, and itching and ankle and calf swelling as well as the use of compression stockings in people with CVI, and many of the supplements that work well for varicose veins of the legs also work for hemorrhoids, as mentioned earlier. However, there has been very little published human research in the area of hemorrhoids, and I have no idea why.

The active compound in horse chestnut is escin (also called complex active triterpenoid saponins or just aescin), which has been shown to block the destruction of structural components in vein walls. However, in half the studies, up to one-third of subjects reported gastrointestinal upset and dizziness; in others, there were mild to minimal side effects reported. But, again, these were studies looking at leg veins, not hemorrhoids.

A human study that was conducted several decades ago gave subjects with hemorrhoids capsules containing 40 milligrams of escin three times a day for 2 months. The researchers saw improvements in as little as 6 days, and the escin group reported greater reductions in hemorrhoid symptoms compared to the placebo group, including less swelling and bleeding. Yet, where are all the other human studies?

This is a big mystery, kind of like the Loch Ness Monster and Bigfoot. So, it is with great reluctance that I give this supplement a basic free pass based on my experience with patients who've used it and its effectiveness in treating other vein problems. But take this with a grain of NaCl (a.k.a. salt—nerd joke). This should be the last supplement that you use on this list, along with the next one.

Rutosides (O-beta-hydroxyethyl-rutosides, a.k.a. rutin or oxerutin), types of flavonoids, appear to protect blood vessel walls from damage in multiple ways, including by discouraging cells from adhering to the walls so that they can continue to function normally. One of the most commonly tested rutoside products has been Venoruton (from Novartis in Switzerland, a prescription drug in Europe), but a potential equivalent can be found over the counter in other countries if you cannot get it from Europe. Look for products containing rutin, which is close in molecular structure to the rutosides that have been used in studies; I believe it works about as well as they do, plus it's cheaper! (Rutin is also found in asparagus and buckwheat and in the rinds of limes, lemons, grapefruits, oranges, and apples, for example.) In studies, dosages of rutosides for CVI have been 2,000 to 4,000 milligrams per day, and some research for hemorrhoids has used from 1,000 to 4,000 milligrams of rutosides per day.

The side effects of these supplements are rare and include gastrointestinal problems, allergic reaction to the products, headache, and hot flashes. Again, I'd look for this only if fiber, diosmin, and Pycnogenol aren't working, which should hardly ever be the case.

WHAT'S WORTHLESS

Witch hazel. There's some good laboratory research showing that witch hazel can reduce inflammation when it is used topically, and it may even block enzymes that contribute to the breakdown of blood vessels and increase the risk of venous problems. The bark and leaves of the plant have astringent qualities (shrink or constrict body tissues), which make it a popular ingredient in many different products, including hemorrhoid cream. But in terms of human studies, there is minimal research supporting its efficacy as a topical for hemorrhoids and nothing to suggest it has any efficacy as a dietary supplement or pill for hemorrhoids. I don't mind it in my hemorrhoid cream because it contains several ingredients that work, but I wouldn't take it as a supplement, especially since there's also a lack of good safety research. Witch hazel is like saw palmetto for prostate enlargement; they've both worked their way into our culture, but essentially on a free pass! No thanks!

Butcher's broom. This herbal has anti-inflammatory properties and the potential to improve mild vein abnormalities of the leg thanks to one of its active ingredients, ruscogenin (a saponin glycoside). Laboratory studies have suggested that butcher's broom has a slight benefit against CVI as a supplement or topical agent because it may block the enzyme elastase, which is part of the enzyme system involved in breaking down blood vessel components. Now here is the problem: The exact quantity of ruscogenins that are effective is not known. Plus, numerous older clinical trials done with butcher's broom were terrible, and the research in the area of hemorrhoids is weak to nonexistent. Now let's talk about side effects. Study subjects have reported dermatitis or an allergic reaction in rare instances, and in one small trial a few participants had to drop out because of swelling, nausea, and other gastrointestinal side effects. Butcher's broom can also contain the compound tyramine, which should never be combined with certain prescription medicines, such as MAO (monoamine oxidase) inhibitor antidepressants. So, as you can see, I have many concerns about this herbal. I'm not saying it's worthless; it's just not worth it, especially for hemorrhoids.

Buckwheat or buckwheat herbal tea. Buckwheat contains rutins, and an older study of people with venous problems who used this for 3 months showed an impact on lower leg swelling that was better than a placebo. However, the average leg volume or size did not actually significantly change in the buckwheat group. And the placebo group claimed a variety of benefits. In other words, this study by itself does not impress me enough to recommend buckwheat supplements or tea for vein problems, especially hemorrhoids. I am happy about the rutin content, and it

may indeed be found to be beneficial in the long term, but other clinical trials with buckwheat are lacking. Plus, it's a common food allergen in several countries around the world, such as Japan, Korea, and Finland. The one condition I wholeheartedly recommend buckwheat (in honey) for right now, though, is cough reduction (see the Common Cold and Flu section, page 141).

LIFESTYLE CHANGES

Heart healthy = vein healthy (= butt healthy)! Keep your blood pressure, cholesterol, and glucose normal; eat a healthy diet with fiber (see the next tip); and maintain a healthy weight. You get it (or you *should* get it!) by now.

Check your diet. Plant-based diets reduce the risk of hemorrhoids and constipation, whereas high-protein or low-calorie (below 1,200 calories a day) diets can *increase* the risk. If you're a fan of high protein and low carbs, make sure the one type of carb you eat a lot of is fiber! (If you have to strain during a bowel movement—or it takes you a long time to go—then you need more.) A high-fiber cereal contains more than 10 grams of mostly insoluble fiber per serving, which means it will not create a lot of gas and bloating. (Soluble fiber promotes heart and colon health, and insoluble fiber helps soften the stool.) Oatmeal is okay with about 3 to 6 grams of fiber per serving, half of which is soluble. If you take one-third of a cup of a leading high-fiber cereal, put some flaxseed powder on it, and add a few ounces of milk, that's about 15 grams of fiber, most of it insoluble.

Take a soak. Sitting in a warm bath with Epsom salts (magnesium sulfate) and then applying a water-based ointment like K-Y jelly can make you feel better than many of the specialized hemorrhoid ointments from the store will. While sitz baths do not have much human research and don't appear to improve recovery from hemorrhoids, I recommend them because they reduce stress and relieve tension when dealing with hemorrhoids, and they just feel good.

Drop pounds. The less you weigh, the less pressure you put on the veins of your rectum and legs. If you're exercising to manage your weight, stay hydrated. Pregnancy can exacerbate hemorrhoids, which tend to spontaneously improve after birth.

Find a cushy seat. Sit in a comfortable, padded chair or use a doughnut cushion. Cotton (or some other breathable fabric) underwear tends to be less irritating, too. I'm convinced seat warmers, which all the cars in Michigan have thanks to the harsh winters, can make hemorrhoids worse. I can't back up this statement with research, but I have my own personal clinical trial of one ("Moyad") that says it's true.

Opt for acetaminophen. Aspirin, ibuprofen, and other NSAIDs (like naproxen) can thin the blood and make bleeding worse. Acetaminophen (Tylenol) is a better choice. Also, avoid alcohol if you have hemorrhoids because it is dehydrating, can thin the blood, and could delay recovery time.

Hepatitis C and B and Alcoholic Liver Disease

THE JURY'S STILL OUT

Dr. Moyad Secret Hepatitis just means inflammation of the liver, which can be caused by different viruses (usually contracted via the mouth, such as through contaminated food, or the blood), while alcoholic liver disease is liver inflammation and injury due to excessive alcohol intake. Whether or not I had these conditions, I would never take a supplement to "clean my liver" (such as artichoke leaf extract). Trying to "detox" the liver makes no sense anyway because every time you take a pill, your liver just works harder to metabolize it. Plus, a recent report, which I agree with, showed that many cases of reported liver toxicity and failure are due to contaminated dietary supplements! And multiple hepatitis studies have demonstrated a worsening of the condition with dietary supplements taken simply for "antiaging" benefits. So the smartest thing you can do for your liver is to avoid taking any unnecessary pills.

For some people, losing weight can take a large burden off an unhealthy liver; it can potentially improve liver enzymes and slow progression of the disease. If you have hepatitis or alcoholic liver disease, ask your doctor how much physical activity you need and what caloric changes you need to make. And remember, heart healthy = liver healthy!

Finally, the greatest development in liver disease, especially hepatitis C, is happening right now. Conventional drugs can now put the condition into remission for years, if not for life. This is one of the greatest medical success stories since the discovery of drugs that can put HIV in remission!

Milk thistle. Some studies have shown milk thistle (*Silybum marianum*) seeds might benefit people with liver problems or liver damage, but others haven't. One of the best trials conducted on milk thistle (also called silymarin) and liver damage found that patients who had failed with interferon had minimal to no response on high-dose (2,100 milligrams per day) silymarin. However, more than 18 randomized trials (for hepatitis and alcoholic liver disease) suggest this supplement warrants a discussion with your medical team at earlier stages of the disease process. I believe it could provide some benefit for those who have more mild and recent liver injury.

Soy protein. Taking 32 grams per day for 12 weeks decreased the liver enzyme ALT in hepatitis C patients better than a placebo. ALT reflects liver health, and abnormally high levels suggest liver injury is occuring. Experts believe soy protein may improve liver function and reduce inflammation.

High Cholesterol

Dr. Moyad Secret So many people are told that if their good cholesterol number is outstanding (HDL of 60 or higher), it mitigates the fact that their LDL (bad cholesterol) is high. My answer to this is "Do you know why there are no support groups for women and men who have suffered from sudden cardiac death?" In the United States 200,000 people die each year from sudden cardiac death. I'm not trying to be shocking here, just honest. Cardiovascular disease (CVD) has been the top killer of men and women for the last 100-plus years, and LDL is the most dangerous type of cholesterol. Yet people are just supposed to ignore their bad LDL levels? Approximately 150,000 people ages 65 or *younger* died last year from cardiovascular disease, and more women are dying of it now compared to men. Many major clinical trials have proven that a high HDL level is not enough to counteract high LDLs. All of your cholesterol numbers need to be normal or low (except HDL, of course, which should be high). And a favorable cholesterol ratio (total cholesterol divided by your HDL) doesn't warrant accepting an abnormal LDL either. Do you want to go up against the number one killer in the United States without maximizing your odds? The price for being wrong about HDL versus LDL is too great and too permanent, so I'm going to err on the side of living! Okay, now I'll get off my soapbox.

WHAT IS IT?

High or unhealthy cholesterol can be manifested in high levels of LDL (bad cholesterol), high levels of triglycerides (this is a measure of fat in the blood), or *low* HDL (good cholesterol). They're all risk factors for cardiovascular disease, either by themselves or in combination. In Dr. Moyad's world, LDLs of 100 mg/dL or higher are too high, triglycerides of 100 mg/dL or higher are too high, and HDLs of less than 40 mg/dL in men and less than 50 in women are too low!

Cholesterol lays the foundation for our hormonal house, if you will. We need it to make estrogen, testosterone, and even vita-min D (which acts like a hormone). It's also a key component of cells. But too much of it starts to clog the pipes. LDLs are stickier inside those pipes than triglycerides, which makes them more dangerous (HDLs remove blockages in the blood and send cholesterol back to the liver).

Poor diet, obesity, tobacco, genetics, a lack of exercise, and certain medical conditions (such as diabetes and many auto-immune diseases) increase the risk of cholesterol problems and CVD. While there are usually no symptoms of CVD until you have a cardiovascular event (usually a heart attack or stroke), there are some subtle tip-offs that something abnormal may be going on, such as sexual dysfunction, especially in younger men and women. Lowering your cholesterol keeps all of your pipes clean, including your sexual pipes, and it also reduces the risk of high blood pressure and blood clots.

Simple cholesterol testing is a wonderful way to see where you stand. However, since half of first-time heart attack patients have normal cholesterol, another blood test that every person reading this section should ask their doctors about is the hs-CRP or high-sensitivity C-reactive protein blood test (it is also known as cardiac CRP or cardiac hs-CRP). It's a measure of inflammation in your body, including in your arteries, which can lead to clots and heart attacks. An hs-CRP of below 1 mg/L is ideal, 1 to 2 mg/L is moderate, and above 2 is too high! (If you have a bad case of arthritis or the flu, the test can be artificially high. If you're on immunosuppressive medications, such as steroids, it might not be a good idea to get this test either because it could be artificially low.)

Of course, there are many cholesterol-lowering medications, called statins, on the market, but they come with potential side effects, so you want to do everything possible to take the lowest dose available (see "What Else Do I Need to Know?" on page 243). I believe long-term use of statins at high doses can slightly increase the risk of all kinds of problems, from type 2 diabetes to memory loss and even sexual problems. But moderate or lower statin doses—combined with lifestyle changes, especially diet and exercise—are unparalleled in helping prevent disease (including brain, eye, and

heart disease and certain cancers). Not to mention, 10 to 20 percent of people cannot tolerate statins, so they need other options, such as dietary supplements. (See the Statin-Induced Myalgia section, page 408.)

WHAT WORKS TO LOWER LDL

Note: I chose these options for lowering cholesterol because they're generally safe and have been shown to be clinically effective. They all work in different ways to lower LDL cholesterol, so some of them can be combined (talk with your doctor first).

1. Red yeast rice 600 to 3,600 milligrams a day in divided doses (usually 1,200 to 2,400 milligrams total)

This extract is a traditional Chinese herbal medicine that was first mentioned in AD 800 as a way to improve blood circulation. It's produced by the fermentation of a fungal strain called *Monascus purpureus* (red yeast) over moist and sterile rice. Red yeast rice (RYR) has a vibrant and distinct red color, flavor, and aroma, so it's also used as a flavoring agent in a number of Chinese dishes and for brewing red rice wine. In the late 1970s, Dr. Akira Endo (one of my research heroes) discovered that a *Monascus* yeast strain naturally produced a substance that inhibits cholesterol synthesis in the liver, and he named it monacolin K. Researchers were later able to isolate the compound, which has the same structure as lovastatin, the first prescription statin.

So RYR was the first true statin used in medical history! In fact, three of the original statins prescribed in the United States were derived from fungi (lovastatin, pravastatin, and simvastatin). RYR contains at least 10 different compounds known as monacolins, and some of them have the ability to block the same enzyme in the liver that prescription statins do. Of all the monacolins that have been isolated so far, monacolin K is the most potent, and it's the one that is primarily responsible for RYR's ability to lower LDL cholesterol.

There have been more than 100 clinical trials with RYR, and many cardiologists now routinely recommend it for people who cannot tolerate statins. A meta-analysis of 9,625 patients in 93 randomized trials involving three different commercial variants of RYR found a mean reduction in total cholesterol (-35mg/dL), LDLs (-28 mg/dL), and triglycerides (-36 mg/dL) and an increase in HDLs (+6 mg/dL). The largest, randomized, placebo-controlled clinical trial, the China Coronary Secondary Prevention Study, evaluated a RYR product called Xuezhikang. Participants included 4,870 people (3,986 men, 884 women) with a history of heart attack. They took 600 milligrams of RYR twice daily (1,200 milligrams total with a monacolin K content of 2.5 to 3.2 milligrams per capsule) or a placebo and were followed for 4.5 years. Levels of LDL dropped by 18 percent on average, triglycerides went down 15 percent, and HDL increased by 4 percent.

Ideally, you want to find a RYR product that has at least 2.5 milligrams of monacolin K in each 600-milligram capsule. RYR works as well as the lowest doses of low-cost statins, but you have to take more pills to get to that potency. For example, you usually take one statin pill per day (1 to 10 milligrams). However, it can take anywhere from one to six RYR pills (assuming each is 600 milligrams) to achieve a similar result.

But here's the frustrating thing about RYR: Dietary supplement companies are actually legally prohibited from standardizing the amount of monacolin K in their products (meaning the amount of active ingredient is not guaranteed)! Because RYR works too much like prescription statins, supplement companies can get in trouble for selling an over-the-counter product that acts too much like a drug. This is one of the dumbest penalties against dietary supplement companies that I have ever witnessed. Either the supplement should be banned entirely from the United States or companies should be able to standardize the monacolin K amount in red yeast rice!

Because companies can't reveal the amount of active ingredient in their products, you may have to test different brands to see which ones have enough to make a difference. However, many RYR companies in the United States and even globally tend to make products that contain enough monacolin K to reduce LDL. The other issue is that some products might contain a potentially harmful by-

RED YEAST RICE BY THE NUMBERS

This chart summarizes the various cardiovascular disease risk reduction benefits seen with red yeast rice (RYR) in the China Coronary Secondary Prevention Study. All were greater than a placebo, and all were statistically significant, except for fatal heart attack and stroke, which still suggested a benefit for RYR. (Even the risk of dying from cancer was reduced.) No serious side effects were observed during this trial. In fact, the total number of side effects and the number of participants who quit treatment were similar between RYR and the placebo.

MEASUREMENT	RISK REDUCTION WITH RYR COMPARED TO A PLACEBO
Nonfatal heart attack	-62%
Coronary disease death	-31%
Fatal heart attack	-33%
Fatal stroke	-9%
Revascularization	-36%
Cardiovascular disease death overall	-30%
Cancer death	-56%
Total deaths	-33%

product of yeast fermentation known as citrinin (it can damage the kidneys and other organs). Check with the company to make sure there is no citrinin in the product; companies *are* allowed to test for this and report it to the consumer (gee, thanks!). So, this all means you have to put in some effort to find a good RYR product. The potential benefits are worth your time, though.

Note: Do not take RYR if you have liver or kidney impairment or allergies to yeast or fungus. Take it with or after meals for better absorption, but don't take it with pectin or oat bran; these high-fiber products specifically reduce absorption.

Finally, grapefruit juice can interact with RYR just like it can with the cholesterol drug lovastatin (as well as at least two other cholesterol-lowering drugs), so don't drink it while you're taking RYR.

2. Soluble fiber (especially psyllium, but also glucomannan, inulin, pectin, guar gum, oat beta-glucan, and barley beta-glucan)
dosage varies

Soluble (viscous) fiber lowers LDL cholesterol in multiple ways. When it reaches the small intestine, fiber can prevent bile salts from being reabsorbed, which essentially prompts the liver to break down more cholesterol to make more bile salts. (The liver makes bile salts from cholesterol, and the gallbladder releases them into the intestines during digestion to break up fat.) Fiber also keeps sugar from being rapidly absorbed. As a result, less insulin gets released (insulin stimulates the liver to increase cholesterol production, so less of it means less cholesterol). Finally, soluble fiber is a prebiotic, so it feeds good bugs in the gut, which leads to less cholesterol (and bile acid) absorption.

Soluble fiber supplements, primarily psyllium powder, have been studied the most in clinical trials, and at 10 to 15 grams per day (divided into two daily doses), they can lower LDL as much as a low-dose cholesterol drug. Consuming 10 grams of psyllium daily on average lowers LDL by about 7 percent, and in some people slightly higher doses (up to 15 grams) can reduce LDL by 15 to 20 percent. If you're frequently constipated or have poor blood sugar control, then you'll doubly appreciate fiber. Still, it's rarely necessary to take more than 10 grams a day, and higher doses increase the risk of side effects, such as bloating and gas.

In my opinion, inexpensive dietary fibers in powder form (2 to 3 tablespoons in water equals 5 to 10 grams of soluble fiber) are actually easier to take than fiber pills, where in many cases it takes six capsules to get 3 grams of fiber, meaning you'd have to take 12 to 18 capsules *per day* just to match 2 to 3 tablespoons of the powder. Another choice is to try a food product that has 10 to 15 grams of fiber (insoluble and soluble), such as bran cereals, to see if you get the same result.

Other soluble fibers—including guar gum and pectin supplements (10 to 15 grams per day), concentrated oat and barley beta-glucan (5 grams daily), and glucomannan (3,000 to 4,000 milligrams per day)—can also lower LDLs. Do not expect any change in HDLs with fiber, and only expect a drop in triglycerides and inflammatory markers, such as hs-CRP, if you also lose weight on your fiber program. You can expect to see results with daily soluble fiber supplementation in as little as 2 to 4 weeks!

3. Phytosterols (plant sterols and stanols) 2,000 milligrams a day

Phytosterols block the uptake of cholesterol from food and bile sources in the intestinal tract. They reduce LDLs, but don't really impact HDLs and triglycerides. This blockage of cholesterol absorption is followed by an upregulation of LDL receptors in the liver, meaning the liver removes more LDL from the blood, which can also reduce inflammation (so you could say they provide an LDL "twofer").

Phytosterol supplements are really just less potent copycats of the drug ezetimibe (Zetia), which can reduce LDLs by approximately 20 percent (at a 10-milligram dose). At 2,000 milligrams per day, phytosterols have been shown to reduce LDLs by an average of 10 to 11 percent. This has prompted many food manufacturers to add them to their products, including yogurt, margarine, orange juice, mayonnaise, olive oil, and milk. You can get the 2,000-milligram dose by taking one or two caplets twice daily with a glass of water right before your two largest meals (to help block cholesterol absorption). *Note:* Phytosterols may reduce the absorption of some fat-soluble vitamins, so you need to take a multivitamin daily as well.

HONORABLE MENTION

Pantethine (a derivative of vitamin B$_5$) is metabolized by the body from pantothenic acid (vitamin B$_5$). It can block an enzyme in the liver that's used to make cholesterol, and it can also slightly thin the blood. In one study, Japanese researchers gave participants 600 milligrams of pantethine per day (in three divided doses) over 16 weeks and found that it lowered LDLs by 15 percent and triglycerides by 14 percent and increased HDLs by 17 percent. However, the same impressive results haven't been seen in American studies yet (with 600 to 900 milligrams per day); this is partly because participants in the US studies had good cholesterol levels to begin with (LDL was already in the low 100s) and were on aggressive cholesterol-lowering diets. About 1 to 2 percent of participants complained of GI issues, such as stomach upset. Overall, this vitamin derivative has a good safety record and appears to cause a small drop in LDL cholesterol (4 percent in the American studies), but I want to see more studies that it reduces the risk of

heart attack and stroke before recommending it over any of my top three!

WHAT WORKS TO LOWER TRIGLYCERIDES OR INCREASE HDL

Note: Red yeast rice and fiber, mentioned earlier, can also lower triglycerides.

1. Fish oil 1,000 to 4,000 milligrams a day

Fish oil (or the active ingredients EPA and DHA) is FDA-approved to lower high triglycerides (500 or higher) at dosages of 1,000 to 4,000 milligrams per day. However, one of the biggest mistakes I see some doctors and other people make is recommending fish oil for reducing LDL. Not only has fish oil not been proven to lower LDL—the primary "bad" cholesterol—but it *increases* it as you increase the dosage! Some experts discount this increase because they think it might change the LDL particle size in a way that could be healthy, but this has not been proven. Lowering LDLs is still the most powerful way to reduce the risk of cardiovascular disease. And researchers have yet to prove that lowering high triglycerides with fish oil actually reduces cardiovascular events like heart attack and stroke. In the meantime, fish oil (in the Risk and Prevention study) failed to lower cardiovascular events in people at higher risk of CVD.

Most fish oil supplements come from anchovies, sardines, or other very tiny fish that have relatively short life spans compared to larger fish. This means they tend to have little to no mercury, heavy metals, and other pollutants and are very concentrated sources of EPA and DHA—the primary omega-3 fatty acids that have been studied to lower triglycerides (plant-based omega-3s lower triglycerides inconsistently). In short, fish oil supplements tend to have good quality control, and the over-the-counter products appear to work just as well as the prescription ones, so save your money!

If you hate the fishy aftertaste and stomach upset that occur with some fish oil supplements, buy enteric-coated pills.

WHAT'S WORTHLESS

Fish oil to lower LDL. Let me repeat, if you're trying to lower LDL, high doses of fish oil can increase it, so talk with your doctor about your specific cholesterol-lowering strategy.

Vitamin D. It's trendy to be vitamin D-deficient these days, but correcting this deficiency does *not* change cholesterol levels. So, how is it that research suggests higher blood levels of D may be associated with a lower risk of cardiovascular disease? Vitamin D blood levels may simply be a marker of healthy behavior. A lean man or woman with low cholesterol who consumes fish and exercises regularly is more likely to have a higher blood level of vitamin D compared to a physically inactive, overweight or obese man or woman with high cholesterol and other heart-unhealthy factors. That doesn't mean that taking D will help you lose weight or improve your lipid profile. At medical meetings, I like to remind health care professionals that it's more important to raise vitamin D levels naturally through weight loss, exercise, and diet (yes, these things can increase vitamin D!) *before* starting a massive supplementation effort. I think if someone has *super*low vitamin D blood levels (in the single digits, like 1 to 9 ng/mL), which is rare, supplementing might slightly improve heart health by reducing blood pressure. There is a clinical trial going on in the United States (known as VITAL) to determine if vitamin D or fish oil really improves heart health (it was under way as this book was being published). I believe the results will show that vitamin D supplements by themselves have minimal to no cardiovascular benefits, but I hope I'm wrong.

No-flush niacin (inositol hexaniacinate) or even regular niacin. Niacin (both supplements and the prescription form) may help lower triglycerides but not LDLs, and it comes with significant side effects, including facial flushing, liver toxicity, and stomach upset or ulcers. The latest evidence shows that it might not be as clinically effective as once thought for reducing heart attack and stroke. What's more, adding niacin to your regimen to lower your statin dose is very dangerous and can increase liver toxicity. Then there's no-flush niacin (inositol hexaniacinate), which does not cause the telltale facial flushing that regular niacin does, but it doesn't work for reducing triglycerides or LDL. No flush = no work! Also, sustained or slow-release over-the-counter niacin can cause liver damage. To sum it up, current research is casting doubt on the benefits of taking niacin in any form.

Guggulipid or guggul. The herbal extract guggulipid has been used for years in Asia as a cholesterol-lowering agent, and its popularity seems to be increasing in the United States. One of the best clinical trials of this supplement, published in the *Journal of the American Medical Association* way back in 2003, tested two different doses of standardized guggul extract (guggulipid, containing 2.5 percent guggulsterones; I swear to you I am not making up these words) and found that they did not work as well as a placebo at reducing cholesterol in healthy adults with high cholesterol who ate a typical Western diet. It was generally well tolerated, but six patients in the supplement group developed a hypersensitivity rash versus none in the placebo group. I say skip it.

Policosanol. Policosanol is a natural compound that comes primarily from sugar cane wax, but it's also in beeswax, rice bran, and wheat germ. It's sold in more than 40 countries as a cholesterol-lowering agent, but almost all of the research supporting the benefits of policosanol came from a single research center in Cuba. After multiple clinical trials in the United States and Europe, it appears to work about as well as a placebo, which is exactly my experience with this supplement.

Garlic. You can find garlic supplements in a variety of forms, including dehydrated powder, aged extract, steam-distilled oil, ether-extracted essential oil, and oil macerate. Regardless of the type, they just don't work well enough to recommend them. In a research review of 29 clinical trials, garlic had no impact on LDL or HDL and lowered triglycerides only a small amount. Another review of studies showed no impact on any type of cholesterol.

Finally, higher doses of garlic or supplements increase the risk of bad breath, body odor, and gastrointestinal side effects. It also has the potential to interact with blood-thinning drugs, like warfarin. It's not worth it.

Green tea catechins (extract of green tea). A review of 14 randomized trials with more than 1,130 participants that was published in the *American Journal of Clinical Nutrition* demonstrated that green tea beverages or extracts lower LDL by one to two points. In another study, published in the *Journal of the American College of Nutrition* (both highly reputable journals, by the way), doses of 145 to 3,000 milligrams per day over 3 to 24 weeks reduced LDL by only five points on average! This shows you how weak this supplement is and how little it impacts LDL. The really large dosages potentially needed compared to the availability of other more effective options make it a dog (I mean a bad dog—stay away).

B$_6$, B$_{12}$, and folic acid. This one's a little tricky: These B vitamins have been shown to lower blood levels of a compound known as homocysteine, which has been associated with an increased risk of heart disease. However, studies *haven't* found that reducing homocysteine levels results in a reduced risk of heart disease. This is just another example of how altering something that's potentially harmful in the body doesn't mean squat until you can actually demonstrate that it reduces the risk of disease or dying. Regardless, what has been proven is that these supplements do not change any cholesterol levels.

Artichoke leaf extract. This plant was supposed to impact one part of the cholesterol pathway, but the results have been weak and the dosage needed is high. Don't waste your money.

WHAT ARE THE OPTIONS FOR KIDS?

A unique study of children (ages 8 to 16) who were genetically predisposed to having high cholesterol found that a RYR supplement reduced LDL by 25 percent. There were no adverse events in terms of liver or muscle enzyme abnormalities over the 8-week treatment period, so speak with your doctor if you know your child has a risk factor for high cholesterol.

LIFESTYLE CHANGES

Move more, and more often. Exercising regularly while on a statin or another cholesterol-lowering product can reduce the risk of dying from all causes by another 70 percent! Yet exercise acts like one of those drugs that only stays in the body for a short time, so you have to keep doing it. If you exercise daily or every other day, your HDLs will rise, but if you take many days or even a week off, they'll drop.

Watch your diet. A low-fat (especially saturated fat) or, more importantly, a reduced-calorie diet can reduce LDLs as much as a low-dose prescription drug. And a low-carbohydrate diet can reduce triglycerides and LDLs as much as a low-dose prescription drug. Basically, it's very easy to get a 5 to 10 percent reduction in cholesterol by following a Mediterranean diet or similar plan. It's not unusual to see people who've shaved 50 to 100 points from their triglyceride levels or reduced or eliminated their statin pills after losing several inches from their waists through exercise and a low-carb diet.

Add protein. Research has shown that eating 25 grams a day of soy protein might reduce LDLs by 1 to 5 percent (up to 8 to 10 points), but I believe getting concentrated protein from a variety of sources (whey, egg white, pea, or brown rice) can also do this. Increasing your protein consumption and reducing your carbohydrates can lower LDL and perhaps even triglycerides.

Drink moderately. I'm not advocating

STATIN DOSAGE FOR SIGNIFICANT LDL IMPACT

DRUG	DOSAGE (MG/DAY)	LDL REDUCTION (%)
Atorvastatin (generic)	10	39
Fluvastatin (generic)	40–80	25–35
Lovastatin (generic)	40	31
Pitavastatin (Livalo)	2	35–40
Pravastatin (generic)	40	34
Rosuvastatin (Crestor)	5	39–45
Simvastatin (generic)	20–40	35–41

starting to drink if you don't do it currently, but alcohol in moderation (one drink a day for women and one or two for men) can slightly increase good cholesterol; it also works like a mini-aspirin to thin the blood. However, many people have trouble with the moderation part. A new report from the Centers for Disease Control and Prevention suggests that men in the United States now drink as many as 150 calories of alcohol per day, on average, and women down as many as 50 to 75 calories on average. The weight gain from alcohol can raise triglyceride levels (in addition to leading to other health problems), so keep it in check.

WHAT ELSE DO I NEED TO KNOW?

Statins have been the target of recent scrutiny, but don't buy into the negativity. Statins and other cholesterol-lowering drugs have been responsible for huge reductions in the number of cardiovascular procedures, such as bypass surgery and angioplasties, in my lifetime. They have saved billions of dollars in health care costs, and now they are even cheaper than most supplements. Above is a table of currently available statins and the minimum dose needed to reduce LDL cholesterol by at least 30 to 40 percent.

Researchers have found multiple benefits from cholesterol-lowering drugs, probably because they reduce some inflammatory markers and growth factors that can lead to or exacerbate other diseases or conditions. Cholesterol-lowering drugs and supplements are currently being studied for Alzheimer's, autoimmune diseases (including multiple sclerosis), colon cancer, erectile and female sexual dysfunction, eye diseases, and prostate cancer.

HIV/AIDS

THE JURY'S STILL OUT

Dr. Moyad Secret HIV/AIDS, a disease of the immune system caused by a virus (usually blood-borne), really requires its own book because there are just so many issues involved. I address many HIV/AIDS-related problems in other sections, including depression (page 166), nausea and vomiting (page 333), peripheral neuropathy (page 364), and osteoporosis (page 352). Regardless, I believe the "less is more" theory applies here with supplements because conventional drug treatment for this disease—specifically, highly active antiretroviral therapy (HAART)—is one of the greatest medical achievements of my generation. In fact, researchers are just beginning to learn that megadoses of a variety of supplements could reduce the efficacy of some conventional medicines, including HAART, or increase their side effects.

Multivitamins. In Third World countries, multivitamins can help prevent immune suppression and might reduce disease progression in HIV, and I think the benefit exceeds the risk in other countries as well (though it hasn't been tested). Nutritional deficiencies are not uncommon in HIV/AIDS, so it's worth discussing with your doctor or a dietitian. (Always get nutritional testing before supplementing with higher doses of nutrients, though. An older study of megadoses of vitamin A showed a higher rate of toxicity in HIV-infected pregnant women.)

Protein powder. Whether you're trying to gain or lose weight (conventional HIV treatments can cause weight gain), protein powder supplementation can help. A well-done study from the University of Southern California Keck School of Medicine found that although taking 40 grams of whey protein powder daily did not have an appreciable impact on weight, it appeared to significantly improve CD4 cell counts (an important marker of immune status) in HIV patients. I believe taking higher dosages (more than 40 grams) could improve the odds of normalizing weight and improving muscle mass, but this comes with a higher risk of gastrointestinal side effects, too. Divide your dose during the day and use a whey protein isolate that has almost no lactose.

Resistance training. A trial from the University of California San Francisco found that resistance training had the most profound effect on increasing muscle size, strength, and function.

Hot Flashes

Dr. Moyad Secret The real reason researchers cannot find more effective drugs and supplements for hot flashes is due to the placebo effect, which has run as high as 33 to 50 percent in many clinical trials! This means a pill has to really kick gluteus maximus to get FDA approved or sold as an effective supplement, and this just isn't going to happen anytime soon. The placebo response in men with hot flashes (yes, men can also get them in rare cases, such as during prostate cancer treatment when testosterone drops) is just as high.

Hot flashes are the second most common complaint among women going through menopause, and as many as 75 percent experience them. There are two theories about the cause of hot flashes. One is that they're due to roller-coaster levels of estrogen and an increase in norepinephrine, a stress hormone; high levels of a metabolite of norepinephrine known as 3-MHPG are found in the brain after a hot flash. Another theory is that during menopause the body's internal thermostat no longer functions normally, so very small changes cause hot flashes.

When the famous US Women's Health Initiative study, which was published in 2002, showed that hormone replacement therapy using estrogen and progesterone or estrogen alone had serious potential side effects—including an increased risk of breast cancer and other problems like cardiovascular issues—there was an almost 50 percent drop in estrogen use and a 30 percent drop in progesterone use within 6 months. And a huge increase in the incidence of hot flashes, was seen! I believe lifestyle changes work best for mild to moderate hot flashes, and medication, such as hormone replacement therapy or venlafaxine, works better for severe to very severe hot flashes.

LIFESTYLE CHANGES

Note: I'm putting this section first because I believe these habits can make the biggest impact.

Improve your heart health. Several heart unhealthy changes, such as excessive weight gain, can exacerbate hot flashes. Plus, more women than men are now dying from cardiovascular disease, and these deaths occur mostly after menopause. As you improve your heart health, many menopausal symptoms and issues, like osteoporosis, can be significantly reduced. In addition, recent research suggests heart-friendly dietary changes may be associated with reduced frequency and severity of hot flashes (for

LOG YOUR FLASHES

You can purchase or make a diary to track hot flashes. Record the timing, severity (on a scale of 1 to 4), and what you were doing at the time (sleeping, eating, exercising, reading, stressing out, etc.).

1 = mild hot flash (usually lasts less than 1 minute and is mildly uncomfortable with no sweating)

2 = moderate hot flash (usually lasts less than 5 minutes and involves warmth over more of the body, sweating, and a need to take off clothing to feel better)

3 = severe hot flash (usually lasts more than 5 minutes and is more of a burning warmth; it disrupts normal activities, such as work or sleep, involves lots of sweating, and requires a thermostat adjustment to cool down)

4 = very severe hot flash (this completely disrupts activities and requires treatment)

Keeping a diary for just 3 days (research has shown it's just as accurate as a 7-day log) can give you insight into what triggers your hot flashes and how much they impact your life. Give the diary to your doctor and work with her to decide how to best treat them. I'm not a fan of keeping diaries for everything (sleep, sex, etc.) because it can become a full-time job, but I think this is one of the few places in medicine where it can make or break your quality of life.

example, eating 2 to 3 tablespoons of flaxseed or sesame seeds on foods or in beverages and 20 to 40 grams of soy products—not soy supplements!—or protein daily).

Avoid hot beverages, spicy foods, and excess alcohol and caffeine. Drinking colder liquids can be helpful. Use your diary (see "Log Your Hot Flashes" above) to identify foods and drinks that trigger or exacerbate flashes.

Do not smoke or inhale second-hand smoke. It's simply unhealthy and makes hot flashes worse due to circulatory and temperature changes. Not to mention, smoking can cause early onset of menopause.

Exercise and lose or maintain weight (it matters!). Excess weight acts as an insulator, keeping heat in instead of letting it dissipate (it's like having a hot flash with a sweater on versus a T-shirt). Women with higher body mass indexes (BMIs) report more frequent and severe hot flashes compared to those with a lower BMI. In addition to helping with weight loss, exercise (even low impact) can reduce stress, improve mood, and may even reduce hot flashes.

Practice stress-reduction techniques. Meditation, yoga, exercise (again), and other stress-busting activities can reduce the severity of hot flashes and help minimize the negative impact menopause has on other areas of life, such as on sleep. Breathing exercises can help, too: Practice controlled, deep, slow abdominal breathing (six to eight breaths per minute) for at least 15 minutes twice daily (morning, midday, or evening) or at the beginning of a hot flash. Also known as paced respiration, this can decrease blood pressure (temporarily), the number of hot flashes, and their severity. It takes some practice, but you'll get it.

Drink sage tea (lukewarm or cold, not hot). Based on a few studies, it might provide a benefit due to the unusually high amount of plant estrogens in sage.

Wear slightly loose clothing. This helps keep the body's core temperature lower and won't feel as constricting or intense when a hot flash occurs.

Get acupuncture (once or twice every week or two). There is fairly good research showing it may help with hot flashes.

WHAT *MAY* WORK

1. St. John's wort (potentially with black cohosh) 500 to 1,200 milligrams a day in divided doses

In studies, taking 500 to 1,200 milligrams of St. John's wort per day (in divided doses) over 4 to 12 weeks has shown some efficacy for reducing hot flashes. Look for an extract that's standardized to contain 0.25 to 0.3 percent hypericin, the active ingredient in St. John's wort. (In the Depression section of this book, page 166, I recommended 0.3 percent hypericin based on those clinical studies, but most of the studies of St. John's wort in combination with black cohosh to reduce hot flashes or overall menopause symptoms used 0.25 to 0.3 percent hypericin.)

St. John's wort is an extract of the plant *Hypericum perforatum*. Researchers haven't yet been able to determine the exact mechanism of action, but it seems to block serotonin uptake and alter levels of multiple brain neurotransmitters, including dopamine, norepinephrine, and gamma-aminobutyric acid (GABA). Many prescription antidepressants can also reduce hot flashes based on this same mechanism, so this helps build a case for St. John's wort's ability to reduce them.

Critics of St. John's wort often do not mention that side effects—including insomnia, vivid dreams, anxiety, dizziness, and skin sensitivity—have been very low in clinical trials. But they *have* mentioned St. John's wort's potential to interact with or reduce the effectiveness of almost half of all prescription drugs, including oral contraceptives. This is true, but prescription antidepressants also have significant side effects. Regardless, do not combine St. John's wort with prescription antidepressants, including SSRIs (selective serotonin reuptake inhibitors), tricyclic antidepressants, or monoamine oxidase (MAO) inhibitors; immunosuppressants; antiretrovirals (anti-HIV drugs); blood thinners, like warfarin; and certain chemotherapy and other cancer drugs. Talk with your doctor about the possibility of using St. John's wort; it has been inappropriately tagged as the poster child of why supplements cannot be combined with prescription drugs, and this is not entirely fair in my opinion.

Now, if St. John's wort doesn't work for your hot flashes, combining it with black cohosh (*Cimicifuga racemosa* or *Actaea racemosa*) might help, according to numerous clinical trials. It's one of the most tested dietary supplements for hot flashes; the research has always been mixed and controversial. Black cohosh has been tested with dosages ranging from 8 to 160 milligrams per day for anywhere from 4 weeks to a year. The most common amount is 40 milligrams for an average of almost 6 months, which has turned out to be as safe and effective as a placebo or slightly more effective than a placebo overall. There's some research to suggest black cohosh works by reducing pain and impacting neurotransmitters (like serotonin), but this needs more investigation. There's just not enough evidence to recommend taking it by itself, only with St. John's wort.

There has been some concern that black cohosh might increase the risk of liver problems, and while the number of reports has been small, this is still something to be aware of.

HONORABLE MENTION

Magnesium is a viable option. In a study with breast cancer patients having hot flashes, subjects took 400 milligrams daily of magnesium oxide for 4 weeks (escalating to 800 milligrams if needed). Hot flashes, fatigue, sweating, and distress were all reduced. A larger clinical trial against a placebo was conducted, and it appeared that magnesium supplements worked similar to the placebo. But the benefit outweighs the risk right now for most individuals because it costs a couple of pennies a day and it's safe. Diarrhea is the most common side effect.

WHAT'S WORTHLESS

Omega-3 fatty acids. These have shown minimal effects for hot flashes. I really wanted to believe that fish oil (EPA and DHA) could help, thinking that if it can lower blood pressure and heart rate, it might be able to reduce the intensity of a hot flash. But in a randomized trial of more than 350 women published in the journal *Menopause*, 1,800 milligrams of omega-3 fatty acids (including 1,275 milligrams EPA and 300 milligrams DHA) worked no better than a placebo. (There was no improvement in sleep or mood either.)

Black cohosh. As I said earlier, this supplement by itself is a big "no!"

THE GREAT HORMONE REPLACEMENT THERAPY DEBATE

Let's talk about natural versus synthetic hormone replacement therapy (HRT). This is one of the most unproductive and distracting debates for menopausal women. Both natural (often called bioidenticals) and synthetic (what traditional hormone therapy uses, some of which comes from the urine of pregnant horses) hormones have one thing in common: They're all manipulated in a lab to make the final product. However, the traditional hormones have to go through FDA approval and the bioidenticals, which are often pricier, don't.

When women stopped taking (or failed to start) HRT therapy (synthetic or natural) after the 2002 Women's Health Initiative study, one of the greatest reductions in breast cancer rates was seen. The idea that "natural" HRT has proven itself to be safer and better is a lie because only synthetic HRT has been adequately tested. If some doctors were honest, they would tell menopausal women that they can go on natural or synthetic HRT but both probably come with similar side effects—an increased cancer and cardiovascular disease risk—until someone proves otherwise. (On occasion I have found side effects to be more severe with bioidenticals because purity and potency are not guaranteed.) It really just comes down to cost, preference, and how much confidence you have in the quality control of the product you're buying. Why is it so difficult to tell women this?

Regardless, whatever form you take and whatever you're using it for, your risk for breast cancer is probably increased. You should always take the lowest dose you need for the shortest period of time.

Red clover. Okay, I'm on the fence with these supplements. Red clover at daily doses of 40 to 82 milligrams of red clover isoflavones have shown a minimal benefit in reducing hot flashes, which some experts would regard as clinically meaningless. However, later studies with higher doses (80 to 160 milligrams of isoflavones and more) are showing more promise, so I don't want to say they're completely worthless just yet.

Chasteberry. This supplement has clinical evidence for premenstrual syndrome or issues related to menstruation, but in the area of menopause it's begging for clinical studies. Chasteberry has been preliminarily tested with St. John's wort (1,000 milligrams of chasteberry plus 900 milligrams of St. John's wort) for hot flashes, and it did not help.

Soy pills. The pills (not soy protein powder or the soy in food) just have too many human studies showing they didn't work or barely worked better than a placebo for hot flashes. In addition, recent research continues to suggest that soy protein and isoflavones from traditional soy sources (protein powder, tofu, milk, tempeh, edamame, etc.) might slightly reduce hot flashes, cholesterol, and breast cancer risk. Many traditional food sources of soy are low in calories and very high in protein and have omega-3s and fiber, so they are heart healthy (see the "Lifestyle Changes" section on page 245). I would rather have people try to reduce hot flashes with 20 to 40 grams of soy protein daily than with an expensive soy supplement that doesn't have any data against hot flashes.

Amino acids. L-isoleucine, L-valine, and L-methionine have done nothing for reducing hot flashes in studies. Plus, you would have to take so many pills (up to 10).

Vitamin E. Regardless of the dosage (even up to 800 IU per day), E has failed to reduce hot flashes more than a placebo!

DIM (3,3'-Diindolylmethane). Another supplement I've been asked about recently is DIM, an antioxidant from cruciferous veggies. Despite all the hype, no one has completed a study that can get me excited enough to recommend it over something less expensive and safer. Some folks claim this supplement reduces the risk of breast cancer based on a few metabolism studies. Come on! It is now known that in menopause, losing weight and exercising definitely reduces the risk of breast cancer and helps put the kibosh on hot flashes, too. So put your hard-earned money toward that instead!

Miscellaneous. Maca and Panax ginseng have some positive research suggesting they may reduce some menopausal issues (sexual dysfunction, for example), but not hot flashes. Evening primrose oil and dong quai haven't been impressive for hot flashes either.

Hypertension and Prehypertension

Dr. Moyad Secret Hypertension, or high blood pressure, is becoming the number one cause of cardiovascular disease death, and it's an epidemic that is truly out of control (60 percent of the population has elevated blood pressure). Prehypertension (above normal blood pressure but not quite hypertension) is also a risk for stroke, like hypertension. There are a variety of drugs that can mean the difference between life and death, so attempting to use mostly unproven supplements is very dangerous in this category. There are a few supplements that stand out—where the benefit may exceed the risk— but overall the most impressive research in this area has been on how comprehensive lifestyle changes (not just sodium and alcohol reduction) could profoundly lower blood pressure and reduce the need for low-dose blood pressure medications. Clinical trials such as DASH (Dietary Approaches to Stop Hypertension), which our tax dollars helped fund, could finally help people realize that they have the power to reduce their risk of this disease. Just a 2 mm Hg (millimeters of mercury) drop in blood pressure can reduce the risk of death from stroke, heart disease, and all causes!

One more thing: If you're worried about hypertension, then you should buy a home blood pressure monitoring device (my favorite company is Omron), which you can use whenever you want. (I recommend taking your blood pressure once or twice every 3 months from both arms and giving the results to your doctor.) One of the most important health indicators ever discovered is blood pressure, and we take it only *once* a year! Come on, folks! (Having your own blood pressure device also helps you avoid "white coat syndrome," where your blood pressure shoots up at the doctor's office because you're stressed.)

WHAT IS IT?

When the arteries are damaged, they are less elastic, less compliant, taking more force to get blood to flow through them. That's high blood pressure. A consistent reading of 140/90 mm Hg is considered high, but if it's between 120 to 139/80 to 89 mm Hg, you have prehypertension, which increases your risk of developing full-blown hypertension. I think of this as a wake-up call. (The number on top is the systolic pressure and the number on the bottom is the diastolic pressure, both of which measure pressure in your arteries.)

Hypertension can be caused by stress, heart disease, tobacco, alcohol, family history, genetics, and more. Sometimes,

MOYAD FACT: Your blood pressure should be roughly equal in both arms. If there is a large difference, it could be an early signal of circulatory problems.

there is no easy-to-pinpoint cause. Regardless, it needs to be treated ASAP, starting with lifestyle changes.

WHAT WORKS

Note: If you are already taking a blood pressure–lowering medication, never add these supplements without talking to your doctor first because it could cause dangerously low pressure.

1. L-arginine 4 to 8 grams a day *or* L-citrulline 2 to 4 grams a day

L-arginine and L-citrulline increase blood levels of nitric oxide, which can dilate blood vessels and reduce blood pressure (see the Erectile Dysfunction section, page 186). It really is that simple. More than 10 randomized trials have shown that L-arginine can reduce systolic blood pressure an average of 5 to 6 mm Hg and diastolic by 2 to 3 mm Hg (some subjects were on blood pressure meds, while others weren't). The problem is knowing what dosage works, and this is not easy to predict. In studies, doses have ranged from 4,000 milligrams to more than 20 grams (much of L-arginine is inactivated soon after ingesting it). Based on three of the most credible trials, though, the average dose per day was 4 to 8 grams, and the most common side effect was diarrhea.

I believe L-citrulline would be a wiser and safer choice initially, but unfortunately it does not have enough clinical trials yet. My experience is that it can usually do what L-arginine can, but at half the dosage. If L-citrulline doesn't work in a month, then you can take more L-arginine.

2. Omega-3 fatty acids
2,000 milligrams or more a day

A review of 70 randomized trials (yes, I said 70), published in the *American Journal of Hypertension*, found that the active ingredients in marine omega-3s (EPA and DHA) could reduce blood pressure by an average of 1.5 mm Hg systolic and 1 mm Hg diastolic. Dosages as low as 1,000 to 2,000 milligrams per day could help, but many studies used 2,000 milligrams or more. Untreated hypertensive subjects (taking no meds) had average reductions of 4.5 mm Hg systolic and 3 mm Hg diastolic. Even subjects with normal blood pressure had an average reduction of 1.2 and 0.6 mm Hg. These effects may be as powerful overall as reducing sodium or alcohol intake or increasing exercise. Changing multiple lifestyle habits produces greater decreases than fish oil. Still, fish oil has been proven to reduce triglycerides (a measure of fat in the blood), and perhaps it has some role in blood pressure improvement by reducing blood vessel resistance and boosting function.

HONORABLE MENTIONS

L-theanine (100 to 200 milligrams a day) **and GABA** (50 to 100 milligrams a day) are stress-reducing supplements that could help stabilize blood pressure or lower it by several points (see the Stress and Anxiety section, page 414). In fact, one of the most commonly used drugs for stress or anxiety caused by public speaking is a blood pressure–lowering drug, a beta-blocker, which also controls or lowers your heart rate!

CoQ10 appears to provide some small benefit at dosages of 100 to 300 milligrams per day, but I'm skeptical based on the quality of the studies and my experience with patients. Stay tuned, though, because while I think it's overrated, I cannot deny that the preliminary research is looking good! It apparently reduces chronic inflammation and relaxes arteries. My prediction is that CoQ10 will not live up to the hype, but we will see.

WHAT'S WORTHLESS

Garlic and vitamin C. These have some minimal blood pressure–lowering effects but not large enough and consistent enough to recommend them or give a dosage.

Calcium and vitamin D. They just don't work. The VitDISH randomized trial looked at elderly people with isolated systolic hypertension (systolic is higher than 140 mm Hg but diastolic is normal). Participants received 100,000 IU of vitamin D_3 or a placebo every 3 months for 1 year, but there was no significant change in blood pressure.

There is some preliminary data that African Americans may get a modest decrease in blood pressure when supplementing with vitamin D at 2,000 to 4,000 IU per day (a potential 3- to 4-point drop in systolic blood pressure). Still, this data is not consistent enough to rely on vitamin D to lower blood pressure.

In the largest and best calcium supplement clinical trials in the world, the mineral has shown no impact—good or bad—on blood pressure at normal doses. But recent evidence suggests excess amounts (two to three times the 1,200-milligram Recommended Dietary Allowance) could increase calcification (hardening) of the arteries and the risk of cardiovascular disease. While this is controversial, there still isn't any good reason to take calcium supplements for blood pressure.

Miscellaneous. Bitter orange and licorice supplements can raise blood pressure. Some people claim ginseng can raise blood pressure, too, but this has generally been due to stimulants that have been added to the ginseng. Supplements with caffeine can cause increases in blood pressure in some cases.

MOYAD TIP: A blood pressure cuff that's too small; crossed legs; a full bladder; caffeine intake; unsupported back, feet, or arm; and not sitting quietly can artifically increase your number. A cuff that's too large can give you a lower than accurate reading.

LIFESTYLE CHANGES

Heart healthy = blood pressure healthy. Nuff said.

Exercise and drop pounds. At least once a week I hear how losing weight and exercising (both cardio and resistance training) has allowed someone to lower the dose of or stop taking blood pressure medication. So, yes, it works, people! Plus, when combined with a healthy diet, exercise can make losing weight easier.

Cut back on sodium and alcohol. Lowering your consumption of these while upping your intake of potassium and magnesium from dietary sources could have a substantial blood pressure–lowering effect.

Control your breath. Learning to slow your breathing can help reduce stress and blood pressure. In fact, any stress-busting activity—such as gardening, tai chi, or any hobby you find relaxing—can have a profound impact on high blood pressure. Google "Resperate"—a device that helps you control your breathing and can help lower blood pressure.

Follow the DASH diet. There are many books about it or just google it. The DASH diet includes lots of fruits, veggies, nuts, whole grains, healthy fats, lean meat and poultry, and low- or nonfat dairy. It's been shown to dramatically lower blood pressure.

WHAT ELSE DO I NEED TO KNOW?

- Never just pop an over-the-counter blood thinner, such as aspirin, if you have uncontrolled hypertension. This is because the higher your blood pressure, the greater the chance that very thin blood can seep into spaces in the body where it doesn't belong. This is known as internal bleeding, and last I checked, this is not a good thing!

- Cold and flu remedies are notorious for containing the drug phenylephrine. It's a decongestant that impacts a receptor in the body that can also increase blood pressure in some people. Based on the largest research reviews, these effects (both positive and negative) are questionable, so avoid products that contain this ingredient.

MOYAD TIP: Per new research, shingles may increase the risk of stroke by creating a large inflammatory response, so this is another reason to get vaccinated with this one-time shot (Zostavax) if you qualify for it.

Idiopathic Pulmonary Fibrosis

THE JURY'S STILL OUT

Dr. Moyad Secret Idiopathic pulmonary fibrosis (IPF) is a progressive inflammation of the lungs with no known cause. It's not curable, but it can be treated, usually with steroids. NAC (N-acetyl-cysteine) was a standard treatment for this disease and it's a dietary supplement, but a recent large study called PANTHER-IPF showed that 1,800 milligrams per day did not beat a placebo in terms of improving pulmonary function. However, it did improve mental well-being, and research from other studies suggests it may reduce the toxicity of conventional treatment. Ask your doctor if it still has a role in your treatment regimen. Studies haven't yet shown whether combining new potential drug treatments with NAC is beneficial.

Not smoking (and avoiding exposure to secondhand smoke) is critical to slowing the progress of this potentially fatal disease, as you might expect. Here's something surprising, though: Viagra-like drugs are being studied for IPF because they improve respiratory circulation. If vasodilator drugs are being looked at for this condition, then supplements like L-arginine and L-citrulline should get more research because they can also improve circulation (see the Erectile Dysfunction section, page 186).

There are two new breakthrough drugs for IPF that should immediately get more attention compared to any supplement, and they are Nintedanib and Pirfenidone. Ask your doctor about these now, as in, don't wait!

Incontinence

THE JURY'S STILL OUT

Dr. Moyad Secret Incontinence can be caused by different things, but it's often related to muscle weakness or damage or nerve problems. Stress incontinence can be brought on by conditions that challenge weak core or pelvic muscles (often weight gain). Urge incontinence, sometimes referred to as overactive or spastic bladder, can be caused by a strong urge to urinate. Weight loss and core exercises (like with a $20 stability ball) should be considered a first-line medical treatment for incontinence, depending on your symptoms and what triggers them. Strengthening your core (the muscles along the front and back of your torso) can help reinforce the pelvic area. And losing weight has been shown in major clinical trials to dramatically reduce incontinence. (See the Weight Loss section, page 448.)

If you suffer from an overactive bladder or other types of incontinence that do not respond well to conventional medicine, or if you have trouble with prescription drugs, ask about PTNS (percutaneous tibial nerve stimulation), which can be done in a doctor's office or at home and now has excellent clinical evidence.

Infertility/Subfertility (Female)

THE JURY'S STILL OUT

Dr. Moyad Secret There are so many dietary supplements that can help with male infertility but none for female infertility (which I also call subfertility)! The most recent *Cochrane Database of Systematic Reviews* analysis on antioxidants for female subfertility looked at 28 clinical trials with 3,500 women who were taking supplements along with conventional therapies, such as in vitro fertilization (IVF). Researchers found that although antioxidants weren't associated with a significantly increased pregnancy or live birth rate compared to a placebo, there was a hint that there may be some minimal (statistically insignificant) benefit, and there were no adverse effects with supplementation. Any low-cost option that can improve conventional therapy for fertility may be worth a try.

Half of fertility problems are associated with the female (ovulatory problems, egg quality, fallopian tube damage, endometriosis), and antioxidants—such as vitamins C and E, NAC (N-acetylcysteine), and L-arginine—may reduce the oxidative stress caused by some of these conditions. (Oxidative stress is the normal wear and tear that happens to all cells through the course of daily living and environmental factors, such as sun and loud noises, and toxins, such as lead or smoke.) For example, a closer look at the research suggests that NAC might improve female infertility in women with polycystic ovary syndrome (see the section for this condition on page 373), and it can be used with conventional infertility drugs, like clomiphene. This is preliminary stuff but well worth an ASAP discussion with your doctor.

Infertility/Subfertility (Male)

Dr. Moyad Secret Up to 80 percent of male infertility cases are related to oxidative stress. All those little daily assaults on the cells—both from normal wear and tear and toxins (tobacco, trauma, weight gain, etc.)—take their toll on the reproductive system along with the rest of the body. Antioxidants help prevent and repair this microdamage, like tiny garbage trucks picking up all the cellular trash. Based on this and the fact that supplements have improved fertility in clinical studies, I believe most male fertility experts should (and do) recommend supplements.

When my brother Andy, who's in his forties, and his wife were trying to have a baby, all of his specialists encouraged using supplements (and they had a beautiful baby boy). Research shows that taking folic acid during pregnancy can help prevent neural tube defects, while other supplements help improve male fertility. I think it's interesting that even with as much criticism as some supplements get, conventional medicine clearly relies on dietary supplements for men and women when it comes to the perpetuation of our species. I know of no greater endorsement in all of medicine! Every day desperate couples pay ridiculous amounts of money for assisted reproductive techniques (ART). So it's definitely worth working with your doctor to see if any of the cost-effective dietary supplements in this section can help, with or without ART.

WHAT IS IT?

Here's a quick physiology review: Sperm cells (spermatozoa) travel within the seminal fluid, which is rich in nutrients; the combination of sperm and seminal fluid is known as semen. When something abnormally impacts sperm or seminal fluid production, male infertility (I also call it subfertility, although other doctors may have slightly different definitions) can occur. Conversely, any nutrients that can help facilitate this process can improve male fertility.

Infertility impacts about 15 percent of couples trying to conceive, and experts expect these numbers to increase dramatically because men and women are waiting longer than ever before to have a baby (plus, obesity has a huge negative impact on both male and female fertility). Approximately half of infertility cases can be attributed to the male (women used to take the brunt of the blame, but once again, just like driving directions and remembering anniversaries and birthdays, the men got it wrong). Half of males undergoing evaluation for infertility have abnormal sperm measurements, and one of the most common findings is called oligoasthenoteratozoospermia (or simply, OAT). Essentially, it's a scary word for a trio of problems: low number of sperm, poor sperm movement, and abnormal sperm shape, and it can be traced back to oxidative stress. (Reduced sperm motility by itself is referred to as asthenozoospermia or asthenospermia.) Regardless, for many of the men diagnosed with infertility, there's no obvious or contributory cause.

The largest research review ever completed on dietary supplements for male infertility involved men/couples undergoing ART. The researchers looked at pregnancy rates and live births and concluded that oral antioxidant supplements could improve the chances of conception during fertility treatment. They didn't recommend specific supplements, though. Why not? So many different supplements help reduce oxidative stress and improve fertility that they weren't able to single out any specific ones. I would argue, however, that if you look at benefit versus risk, there are some standouts (and some I would avoid).

WHAT WORKS

Note: You should take these supplements for 3 to 6 months before deciding if they're working. It takes that long to make an impact.

MOYAD FACT: The lower limit of a "normal" sperm count is 15 million sperm per milliliter. Seems like a lot, but like chocolate, you can never have enough.

1. Multinutrient fertility supplement one or two pills a day, or simply one or two multivitamins per day

This is one of the only conditions in the book where taking two multivitamins or multinutrient fertility supplements a day makes some sense. You want to be replete with nutrients to help the fertility process. And since you're generally only taking these for a short time—not years and years—the benefit outweighs the risk.

ProXeed (manufactured by Sigma-Tau) is popular with physicians because there's some preliminary research showing men who take it have increased pregnancy rates with their partners. It contains several nutritional compounds that have also been shown to be beneficial for fertility (most are discussed in this section). It's a little pricier to buy this versus just buying the individual ingredients, but there is good quality control and research supporting it. ProXeed (according to one study) contains L-carnitine (145 milligrams), acetyl-L-carnitine (64 milligrams), fructose (250 milligrams), citric acid (50 milligrams), selenium (50 micrograms), coenzyme Q10 (20 milligrams), zinc (10 milligrams), ascorbic acid (90 milligrams), vitamin B_{12} (1.5 micrograms), and folic acid (200 micrograms). It's safe to

259

take two of these ProXeed pills or a general male multivitamin (the multi will add even more key nutrients) daily. Right about now you might be wondering what the difference is between fertility supplements and a multivitamin. Not much, but some of these combination fertility supplements contain more of the specific nutrients that have been tested against infertility in past clinical trials (like carnitine, CoQ10, and selenium).

2. (tie) CoQ10 200 to 300 milligrams a day

This fat-soluble antioxidant improves energy production and reduces oxidative stress, and since the male reproductive tract is susceptible to oxidative stress, it makes sense that it could be beneficial. In addition, levels of CoQ10 in the seminal fluid correlate with sperm count and motility. In one study, men with idiopathic (no known reason) reduced sperm motility who took 200 milligrams of CoQ10 per day for 6 months saw increased motility. Another study of 212 infertile men taking 300 milligrams over 26 weeks found significant improvements in multiple parameters, including sperm density, motility, and acrosome reaction (the ability of sperm to meet the egg).

More research is needed on pregnancy and live birth rates with CoQ10, but this supplement (also known as ubiquinone) has an excellent overall safety profile. I recommend men take 200 to 300 milligrams per day to help preserve fertility (take it with a meal that has some fat in it).

Be aware that it has the potential to reduce the impact of warfarin because it has vitamin K–like clotting properties, but it may actually increase blood thinning when used with other drugs (like clopidogrel), so talk with your doctor if you plan to take it with other drugs. It can be costly, though, so shop around.

2. (tie) Vitamin C (ascorbic acid) 500 to 1,000 milligrams a day

Seminal fluid is high in vitamin C, and there is a relationship between higher vitamin C levels in the fluid and a lower risk of male infertility and improved male sperm quality. In addition, smoking and environmental toxins can dramatically lower vitamin C levels and damage sperm cells. Smokers, ex-smokers, and people exposed to toxins (such as lead) seem to respond well to vitamin C in terms of improving their overall antioxidant status, especially vitamin C levels. Studies have shown that consuming 500 to 1,000 milligrams daily of vitamin C in combination with other common antioxidants improves fertility in men. It is unknown if taking vitamin C by itself is as beneficial as taking the combination supplements (see #1), but the upside outweighs the downside.

Taking more than 1,000 milligrams of C per day decreases absorption, increases side effects, and may be detrimental to fertility, so don't overdo it. In fact, it could be argued that 500 milligrams per day improves fertility almost as well as 1,000 milligrams per day. A study by this super-smart guy named Moyad showed people at risk of kidney stones should choose buffered vitamin C or calcium ascorbate.

3. (tie) NAC (N-acetylcysteine)
600 milligrams a day

The liver produces a compound called glutathione, an antioxidant that's found in very high concentrations in the body. Taking too much acetaminophen greatly reduces stores of glutathione, which leads to the formation of high concentrations of free radicals in liver cells, oxidative stress, liver injury, and in some cases failure (especially in combination with alcohol). In the emergency room, doctors will give you NAC for an overdose of acetaminophen; it increases the production of glutathione to protect the liver from going into failure. Since glutathione is the primary antioxidant in the body, increasing levels of it protects against oxidative stress—and remember, up to 80 percent of male infertility cases are related to oxidative stress. You could just take glutathione supplements—and many people do—but they are poorly absorbed in the gastrointestinal tract. Instead, you're better off taking NAC. One study showed taking 600 milligrams of NAC daily improved semen measurements, but more research is needed, especially for pregnancy and live birth rates. (NAC in combination with whey protein can boost glutathione levels as well.)

3. (tie) L-carnitine 2,000 to 3,000 milligrams a day

In every cell of your body, L-carnitine transports fatty acids from one area of the cell (cytosol) to another (mitochondria) as part of the energy production process. Multiple clinical trials have demonstrated the ability of L-carnitine (or other forms of carnitine) to improve sperm characteristics and, potentially, pregnancy rates. Several randomized trials have found that L-carnitine improves sperm count, motility, and normal shape of sperm better than a placebo in men with idiopathic (no known cause) infertility.

Most trials have used an average of 2,000 to 3,000 milligrams per day (with or without food) or in the form of acetyl-L-carnitine without significant side effects. This is already a large dose and going beyond it can cause gastrointestinal problems, abnormal body odor, and neurologic concerns (such as peripheral neuropathy or nerve damage). The reason I ranked it number three instead of at the top is that these dosages just aren't practical for daily use. Plus, a few independent US studies from researchers I know and admire did not show the same dramatic results the previous studies did. There are several minimally different forms of L-carnitine, so take whichever you like (price does not connote effectiveness). There haven't been enough studies yet to really identify adverse events or serious drug interactions with L-carnitine, so talk with your doctor.

HONORABLE MENTION

Tongkat ali (*Eurycoma longifolia*), a plant that grows in the Malaysian rainforest, might improve various aspects of male health—including sex drive, testosterone levels (minimally, if at all), and sperm quality and quantity—as well as pregnancy rates, based on preliminary research using 200 milligrams a day. The product that has the most research—and the only one with real clinical data—is the standardized water-soluble extract of *Eurycoma longifolia* root called Physta (from Biotropics Malaysia). The aqueous extract has multiple ingredients—including tannins, high-molecular-weight polysaccharides, glycoprotein mucopolysaccharides, and quassinoid alkaloids. It's one of the only herbal products I would recommend for fertility because it has some research and a good safety profile.

WHAT WORKS BUT ISN'T WORTH THE MONEY

Notice I've changed the section heading here. I don't have any concerns about the following nutrients in lower doses in a multivitamin or combination fertility product; it's the large doses I worry about. The supplements here are supported by evidence that is as good as or better than the evidence backing the ones in the "What Works" section, but the safety issues prevent me from endorsing them (first do no harm). It's worth having a discussion with your doctor, though, because as safety improves, these supplements could get back in the game.

Folic acid in large doses. This just isn't an ideal antioxidant for male fertility. The Recommended Dietary Allowance is 400 *micro*grams a day, and it's easy to get plenty of it from a bowl of cereal in the morning and a multivitamin. Excessive folic acid (1 milligram or more) in men has been linked to a higher risk of prostate cancer. This finding is controversial (not definitive), but there's just no need to take this risk when so many other supplements appear to work as well and are safer.

Selenium, vitamin E, and zinc. Large doses of selenium (200 micrograms or more) and vitamin E (400 IU or more) supplements should not be used to improve fertility in men. Selenium has a history of potentially increasing the risk of skin cancer recurrence at higher doses, and there may be a connection to an increased risk of type 2 diabetes as well. With higher doses of vitamin E, there is a potentially elevated risk of all-cause mortality, heart failure, and even hemorrhagic stroke. (Breaking news: The largest trial of vitamin E and selenium found a significantly increased risk of prostate cancer in both groups upon further follow-up.) Zinc in large daily doses (80 to 100 milligrams or higher) has also been associated with higher rates of prostate cancer as well as hospitalizations for a variety of urologic conditions (the Recommended Dietary Allowance is only about 11 milligrams).

LIFESTYLE CHANGES

Heart healthy = sperm healthy. Most heart-unhealthy behaviors negatively impact almost all areas of male health, including fertility, therefore heart health is tantamount to male fertility.

Lose weight. Besides being heart *un*healthy, obesity in men can increase estrogen levels, lower testosterone levels, and negatively impact fertility hormones. It can also reduce levels of a crucial compound involved in sperm support and production (inhibin B) and can increase testicular temperature, which can result in reduced sperm counts and motility and altered sperm shape.

Kick the habit. Smoking and tobacco use in general dramatically lowers sperm and seminal fluid nutrient levels and reduces the testicular production of sperm. Oh, and smoking can kill you in many other ways and cause chronic obstructive pulmonary disease, which dramatically reduces your ability to breathe.

Limit alcohol. In excess (more than a drink or two a day), alcohol can increase the risk of sperm damage in some people and alter hormone levels that may make it more difficult to get your partner pregnant.

Boost your omega-3 intake. While the research is still out on supplement sources of omega-3 fatty acids, dietary sources may improve fertility. Salmon, tuna, sardines, and whitefish are a few marine sources; plant sources include flaxseed, chia seeds, plant oils (like canola), and walnuts.

Mind your Fs and Vs. Fruit and vegetables (even a few servings a day) can raise antioxidant and nutrient levels in the blood and sperm by a large amount.

Cool your package. A lower scrotal temperature may be associated with an increase in sperm quantity and quality, so you might want to switch to boxers from briefs, avoid spending too much time in hot tubs or saunas, and keep your laptop on your desk instead of in your lap. I think the impact is minimal, but it may provide a small advantage.

WHAT ELSE DO I NEED TO KNOW?

Varicocele is arguably becoming one of the most common and treatable causes of male infertility. An abnormal enlargement of the veins leading away from the testicles, a varicocele is caused by a backward blood-flow (kind of like varicose veins of the testicle). It's generally harmless, but it can alter the sperm production environment. A specialist can fix a varicocele on an outpatient basis (ask for microsurgical repair if available).

MOYAD FACT: One commonly used drug that can reduce sperm count and make it difficult to conceive is testosterone replacement therapy. If you have low testosterone, ask your doctor about treatments that won't impact fertility. And avoid taking any male testosterone dietary supplements, with the exception of tongkat ali (see page 304), because if they work to raise testosterone, they can reduce fertility. (But most of them don't work.)

Inflammatory Bowel Disease
(Crohn's Disease and Ulcerative Colitis)

THE JURY'S STILL OUT

Dr. Moyad Secret When the body's immune system starts attacking cells in the small or large intestine, leading to chronic inflammation, pain, diarrhea, bleeding, and other symptoms, it's called inflammatory bowel disease, or IBD. One of the reasons omega-3 fatty acid sales took off in recent years was due to research about their potential benefits against IBD, which encompasses Crohn's disease and ulcerative colitis, especially along with conventional treatment. Since IBD is a chronic inflammatory disorder and fish oil may reduce inflammation, it was a perfect fit, right? The problem is, many clinical studies have yielded mixed results and have used pretty poor methods. And as better studies have come along, the results haven't been as impressive. Like vitamin D, omega-3s have been overhyped for almost everything (but at least bone health is critical in IBD, so vitamin D could be helpful).

One of the biggest problems with using dietary supplements for IBD is that newer immune-altering conventional drugs have had such dramatic impacts on treatment for some people that it's hard for supplements to compete. I think they should be studied more for some of the symptoms of IBD and drug side effects. (See the Low Energy and Chronic Fatigue section, page 293, and the Insomnia and Jet Lag section, page 266, for more information; fatigue and sleep issues are common in IBD.)

Curcumin. I'm watching the research on curcumin, the active ingredient in turmeric, to see if the anti-inflammatory effects will help IBD; the trials are just getting off the ground. The problem with curcumin is it tends to have a low solubility and the bioavailability is pretty poor, so higher dosages and a better delivery system are needed in future studies. Tiny preliminary studies have shown promise when tested either against older conventional medicines or with them (called an add on), but these drugs aren't used as often as the newer biologic therapies.

Probiotics and prebiotics. These have been touted as an add-on treatment for IBD, but the data is not there yet. For example, in a large French study, the popular probiotic yeast *Saccharomyces boulardii* (1,000 milligrams per day for a year) did not beat a placebo in terms of maintaining remission, but since side effects were similar to a placebo and nonsmokers appeared to have a lower risk of relapse, this probiotic should be studied further in nonsmokers. And the probiotic VSL#3, which contains eight different bacteria, has several studies with some preliminary positive results for IBD, but they have not been dramatic enough to change conventional treatment.

Iron. One of the most common complications of IBD is iron-deficiency anemia. It can occur in up to half of people with IBD, so supplement or even IV therapy could benefit many people. In the large PROCEED trial, which was published in the *American Journal of Gastroenterology*, researchers found that 200 milligrams of elemental iron worked well in anemic IBD patients who were in clinical remission or had mild IBD. More than 60 percent of the participants had a clinically relevant response in their hemoglobin of 2 or more g/dL after only 8 weeks.

Whey protein powder. Carrying extra weight can exacerbate IBD. In a university study from Brazil, whey protein improved lean muscle mass and reduced fat percentage, specifically in Crohn's patients. When patients lose excess pounds, they often report less fatigue and improved quality of life. (See the Weight Loss section, page 448.) The dosage used in the Brazilian study was 0.4 grams of whey protein concentrate per kilogram of body weight (there are 2.2 pounds per kilogram).

Heart healthy = intestine healthy! Fiber could play a role in preventing ulcerative colitis relapse, although fiber intake should be reduced during flare-ups. There has been some research suggesting a heart-healthy diet can be beneficial, but you should avoid any foods that can exacerbate symptoms, however healthy they may be. Low-fat diets have had some success as well.

MOYAD FACT: While ulcerative colitis (UC) happens in the large intestine, Crohn's disease can affect the entire digestive tract. The inflammation in Crohn's occurs in all layers of the bowel wall and in patches, whereas in UC it happens throughout the affected area and doesn't extend beyond the innermost lining. Irritable bowel syndrome, or IBS, is not considered an inflammatory bowel disease and doesn't cause permanent damage to the digestive tract.

Insomnia and Jet Lag

Dr. Moyad Secret We are a chronically sleep-deprived nation. Stress, hormones, poor sleep "hygiene," and technological overstimulation are some of the factors that contribute to this problem. It's getting harder to turn off at the end of the day, so people are turning to prescription and over-the-counter drugs. The issue is that while these medications do cause drowsiness, they don't necessarily promote deep sleep or improve the quality of sleep. They can also decrease cognitive skills and balance and cause dry eyes and mouth, weakness, headache, blurred vision, and urinary problems. Now for even worse news: Prescription sleep aids are the third leading cause of unintentional drug overdose resulting in death (pain killers and antianxiety meds are first and second on the list, in case you're wondering). Plus, they are insanely expensive—at least $5 to $10 per pill! Steps need to be taken *now* to reduce the dependency on these medications, to reduce the dosage (look up FDA and Lunesta), or to at least better educate the public and health care professionals about some of the safer effective dietary supplements.

WHAT IS IT?

Insomnia just means you have a hard time falling or staying asleep. It leaves you feeling tired and can lead to all sorts of sleep deprivation–related problems, including depression, anxiety, irritability, immune suppression (increased risk of infections), stress, weight gain, memory problems, and an increased risk of accidents. It's natural to occasionally have trouble sleeping, but if it's becoming a nightly issue, you should talk with your doctor (see "Dissect Your Sleep Habits," opposite). Insomnia can be a complex problem; there are many potential causes, including aging (hormonal changes), prostate and bladder conditions, pain medications,

stress, anxiety, depression, weight gain, diet, exercise, and the list goes on.

Humans have five different stages of sleep. The first two are where light sleep occurs, and the third and fourth are where deep sleep happens (this is also when the body and brain go to work repairing tissues). These four stages make up non-REM sleep. Dreaming occurs in the final stage, called REM (rapid eye movement) sleep, which you experience several times a night. Most deep sleep occurs in the early part of the night, and most REM sleep (dreaming) occurs in the early hours of the morning. Knowing these stages and when they happen can help you better evaluate sleep

DISSECT YOUR SLEEP HABITS

In order to pinpoint what aspect of your sleep pattern has changed, your doctor may ask the following questions.

- Do you have trouble falling asleep? How long does it take?

- Do you have trouble staying asleep?

- When do you wake up (after an hour or after several hours)?

- How do you feel when you wake up (are you stressed, thinking about work, worried about family, wide awake, still drowsy, hungry)?

- How long does it take you to fall back asleep, or is it impossible?

- Do you wake up to urinate?

- Why do you think you're having trouble sleeping?

- Have you tried any sleep remedies? Did you experience side effects?

- Do you sleep with pets or a partner? Do they snore? Do you snore?

- Do you watch TV or use your phone or tablet in bed?

- Do you go to bed and wake at the same time every night, or does it vary?

- Do you drink alcohol or take any medications?

- Do you exercise? What time of day do you usually work out?

supplements and prescriptions. Some help you fall asleep and increase your chances of getting more light sleep, while others help you stay in deep sleep longer.

Jet lag, a type of insomnia, occurs during travel when your body clock hasn't yet adjusted to the new time zone. It's considered a circadian rhythm sleep disorder because it stems from a sudden change in your internal body clock. Flying east is usually worse because you lose time: Going from Michigan to Europe or the Middle East, you lose 5 to 8 hours, which means bowel habits, meals, sleep, and other daily rituals get thrown off. Flying west you gain time, so it is usually easier to adjust because there's still time during the day for your body to take care of its normal rituals. The farther you go in either direction, the worse the jet lag.

WHAT WORKS

Note: Do not use any sleep aid if you're pregnant or breastfeeding, and do not give them to children without close monitoring by a doctor.

1. Melatonin 0.5 to 3 milligrams maximum 15 to 30 minutes before bedtime or when waking in the middle of the night (not both); for jet lag, 0.5 to 5 milligrams before bedtime until you adapt to the new time zone

Produced by the small pineal gland deep in the middle of the brain, melatonin helps regulate your circadian rhythms. Many factors, including stress and aging, can throw off production of this important hormone. The supplement can induce sleep, meaning it helps you fall asleep, but it won't necessarily help you stay asleep. Many conventional and alternative medicine "experts" recommend taking 3 to 5 milligrams daily, but that's way too high. I recommend taking just 0.5 to 1 milligram on average (3 milligrams maximum!) 15 to 30 minutes before bed. The brain produces less than 30 micrograms of melatonin per day to help with sleep and other functions (it may also work as an anti-inflammatory and immune-enhancing hormone), so this is another reason not to overdose on it. As with prescription sleep aids, taking too much melatonin can make you tired the next day and may interfere with your memory, so find the lowest dose of melatonin that works for you and take it for only as long as is needed (the shorter the better).

Melatonin has a great safety record, but it's still possible to develop a dependence on it; over time it can lose its effect (this is called tolerance or tachyphylaxis), prompting some people to turn to stronger sleep aids, which they develop a tolerance to as well! Melatonin can potentially (but rarely) be combined with certain prescription sleep aids; always talk to your doctor first, though.

When you're shopping for melatonin supplements, don't be lured by pricey combination products. The vast majority of human studies used plain, inexpensive melatonin. Today, so many companies combine it with two or more ingredients and claim that it works better than melatonin by itself, or they charge more for a different form of melatonin, claiming it's released more effectively in the body. Don't fall for it! If you believe these claims, then I have some swampland chock-full of oil and gold reserves to sell you. That said, there is a type of prolonged-release melatonin (2 milligrams) available, which you're supposed to take 1 or 2 hours before bed, and there is some research to suggest that if you don't respond to regular melatonin, this extended version may be worth a try. It appears to work well for older adults (age 55 or older) who produce less melatonin.

Keep in mind that melatonin can mildly impact blood pressure, and the controlled-release version may reduce blood pressure slightly more than regular melatonin. If you're taking antihypertensive medication (such as calcium channel blockers or beta-blockers), talk to your doctor about adding melatonin. Also ask your doctor about melatonin if you're on warfarin or have epilepsy.

Melatonin doses for jet lag are a little higher—0.5 to 5 milligrams. In studies, participants taking the higher dose tended to fall asleep faster, but doses above 5 milligrams were not any more effective. (Controlled-release melatonin didn't work any better than regular melatonin either.) The more time zones that were crossed, especially flying eastward, the better the benefits were. Timing is critical here; if you take it too early, you'll fall asleep too early and delay your adjustment to local time. Take it at bedtime every night until you adjust to the new time zone. You could also do this on the day you leave for your trip by taking it at your projected bedtime in the new time zone. For example, if I were flying from Detroit to Rome (oh man, this sounds awesome already), I would take my dose of melatonin ideally somewhere between 3 p.m. to 6 p.m. Detroit time (which is 9 p.m. to midnight Rome time) and get some rest on the plane. Then when I got to Rome, I would get a ton of exercise by walking all over the place and take my melatonin again when I went to bed between 9 p.m. and midnight.

2. Valerian (*Valeriana officinalis*)
200 to 600 milligrams 30 to 60 minutes before bedtime

Valerian affects the availability and transport of GABA, or gamma-aminobutyric acid, which has a calming effect on the brain. Some studies have shown that valerian can help people fall asleep and stay in a deeper, more refreshing sleep. Always look for valerian as a root extract with at least 0.8 percent valerenic acids, which are the active ingredient. There really isn't a commonly studied dosage, but the safest, most effective range is from 200 to 600 milligrams. Take it 30 to 60 minutes before bedtime, but realize that it can take 2 to 4 weeks to kick in, unlike melatonin, which generally works immediately (that's why valerian's not a good solution for jet lag). Personally, I would not mix it with other herbs because it has only been studied by itself, and the more ingredients you add, the more you potentially dilute the active ingredient.

Never combine this supplement with other sleeping pills or central nervous system depressants, such as strong pain medications, because it can cause serious breathing or other respiratory problems. And always ask your health care professional if there are any potential drug interactions with this supplement that you need to be concerned about. Side effects in clinical studies have been rare but include morning grogginess, headache, and vivid dreams (almost like nightmares).

Many experts say that the research just hasn't shown profound effects with this herbal, but my research analysis criteria— along with my experience—lead me to disagree. For example, in a large study at the Mayo Clinic, researchers gave cancer patients 450 milligrams of valerian a day or a placebo for 8 weeks. The herbal did

269

not appear to work better than placebo based on a sleep quality index score, but the valerian group did report less fatigue, drowsiness, and trouble sleeping. And it was as safe as a placebo. Studies with menopausal women have also showed a clinical benefit for improving sleep over a 4-week period. In other words, benefit is greater than risk here for many individuals, so it may be worth a try. Finally, nobody has studied valerian long term in humans, so, like with any sleeping pill, take the lowest dose that works and only for the shortest time needed. In my experience, patients really like valerian; if they stick with it for a few weeks, they really see an improvement. It's the people who want to believe it will magically work right away who are usually disappointed.

3. (tie) 5-HTP (5-hydroxytryptophan)
50 to 100 milligrams 10 to 15 minutes before bedtime

The amino acid 5-HTP is an intermediate step in the conversion of L-tryptophan to serotonin in the body. It gets transformed into serotonin, a neurotransmitter in the brain that helps initiate sleep and reduces the time it takes to fall asleep; it may also help improve the amount of time spent in REM sleep. The supplement 5-HTP is similar in structure to the supplement L-tryptophan. In 1989, a particular brand of L-tryptophan caused an outbreak of a potentially fatal neurological condition; close to 40 people died and more than a thousand others were left with permanent disabilities. At the time, I was one of the student investigators at the University of South Florida who interviewed people affected by the tainted supplement. It was pretty clear, based on the research available then, that L-tryptophan worked as a sleep aid, but it ended up with a black eye, even though the problem was caused by the manufacturer, not the supplement itself.

Regardless, 5-HTP is a far better alternative for sleep—whether for insomnia or jet lag—because it easily crosses the blood-brain barrier and is rapidly converted to serotonin. Based on the research, take 50 to 100 milligrams before bed. Researchers have used higher doses (200 to 300 milligrams) in clinical trials, but in my experience with patients, these amounts are very potent. Only consider them if you've had no success with lower doses, which rarely occurs. Higher doses can cause nightmares or vivid dreams, and 5-HTP should not be combined with any other medications that also impact serotonin levels, such as antidepressants.

3. (tie) L-theanine 100 to
200 milligrams a day 30 to 60 minutes before bedtime

This is a fascinating amino acid because it's found in green tea and may offset the stimulatory effects of caffeine (it's amazing the way nature balances itself, isn't it?). Researchers believe L-theanine (also known as N-ethyl-L-glutamine) has the potential to reduce stress because it increases multiple compounds in the brain, such as GABA, serotonin, and dopamine, all of which promote relaxation. As a result, it can improve sleep, especially if stress is keeping you awake (see the Stress and Anxiety section, page 414). In some areas of the world, parents add it to milk as a way to calm babies and young children (this does *not* mean I'm encouraging parents to do this). The standard dose is 100 to 200 milligrams daily 30 to 60 minutes before bedtime. I like it because it's safe and fairly inexpensive, plus I always like to see how antistress supplements can impact sleep. For example, GABA is a supplement used to reduce stress and anxiety that also helps some people fall asleep. I believe future clinical trials will find a benefit with GABA at a low dose (50 to 100 milligrams).

WHAT'S WORTHLESS

Kava or kava-kava. This antianxiety supplement, an extract from the roots of a Polynesian plant, is commonly used in the South Pacific to calm, relax, and promote well-being. It is even used as an aphrodisiac. It contains several active ingredients—including kawain, dihydrokawain, and methysticin—but the most interesting ones in terms of their potential benefits are the kava pyrones (better known as kavalactones); as many as 15 of them exist. In the United States, many people take kava as a substitute for Xanax or Valium. Not surprisingly then, some alternative medicine experts recommend using it as a sleep aid before bed (150 to 210 milligrams). In studies, kava has shown preliminary evi-

MOYAD WARNING! Sleep aid supplement companies are notorious for loading up on ingredients to make you feel like you're getting more for your money, but you're just getting more worthless ingredients. All you need, based on the research, is the correct dose of the active compounds. Nothing more, nothing less. As I explain in the Appendix, on page 470 "dilution leads to pollution," so be wary of unnecessary ingredients.

dence that it can be effective for insomnia, and side effects overall have been low (1 to 5 percent in most). That said, you may be wondering why it's on this list then. Well, the problem is that it's getting the reputation as a liver killer (yes, candid is my middle name). Regulators in the UK pulled it off shelves after several reports of users needing liver transplants and complaints of other liver problems. More than a decade ago, the FDA issued a warning about an increased risk of liver toxicity with kava, but it's still legal in the United States (so they can't be that concerned, right?).

It's possible that the kava toxicity is due to some contaminant or a gene metabolism deficiency (CYP2D6 for all the nerds reading this book; P.S. I am an official nerd, too) seen in a small percentage of the population. But every time I'm ready to recommend kava again something makes me nervous. For example, the National Toxicology Program is a well-known laboratory study group that tests supplements, especially if they're popular. They usually conduct 2-week, 3-month, and 2-year toxicity and carcinogenic studies in rats and mice. When they examined kava, there was some hint of liver problems when combining this supplement with other drugs or supplements. In other words, the risk exceeds the benefit for now.

Miscellaneous. These supposed sleep supplements are not worth your money: passionflower, hops, wild lettuce, Jamaican dogwood, California poppy, chamomile, lemon balm, skullcap, and *Patrinia* root. I can count the number of good studies that have been done with these supplements on one hand. Passionflower extract helps promote sleep in mice, so if you're a mouse, you might sleep well after taking it. The studies in humans have been weak, though. As for hops, there used to be a condition known as hop-picker fatigue, which may have been caused by inhalation of the volatile oils of the hop plant or transfer of the hop resin from hand to mouth, but this condition isn't seen anymore thanks to the advent of harvesting machines. Yet, using it in a supplement for sleep has no evidence. In some studies, hops combined with valerian demonstrated a benefit for sleep, but on closer examination, it's probably due to the valerian itself. As far as wild lettuce and Jamaican dogwood are concerned, I'll just say they have serious side effects and no good research. The California poppy should not be confused with the Oriental poppy, which is the source of opium and drugs such as morphine, heroine, or codeine. Regardless, there haven't been any clinical trials on the California poppy. Chamomile tea is supposed to be relaxing and sedating, but the studies on this are weak, too. Lemon balm has had a few small studies showing decreased alertness, but nothing related specifically to sleep, so it gets a Moyad rejection letter. I have always had concerns about toxicity with skullcap, including increased liver problems and seizures. *Patrinia* root has shown some benefit but also a lot of side effects, like nausea.

WHAT ARE THE OPTIONS FOR KIDS?

Researchers have studied melatonin in kids (ages 6 to 14) with ADHD (attention deficit hyperactivity disorder) and sleep problems. In general, 3 to 6 milligrams before bed seemed to improve sleep, but other kids might not require as much. In children with autism spectrum disorders, for example, 1 to 3 milligrams of melatonin per day was effective. There have also been a few clinical studies of 5-HTP in children, but the most interesting one helped kids (ages 3 to 11) with a history of sleep terrors. They were given 2 milligrams of 5-HTP per kilogram of body weight before bed.

LIFESTYLE CHANGES

Work out more. Regular daytime exercise can make you tired by the end of the day, especially if it's moderate to intense. Yet clinical studies have shown that all sorts of exercise, even less vigorous workouts like tai chi and restorative yoga, can help. Just avoid working out within an hour or two of bedtime as that can make it harder to fall asleep.

Stop smoking. Besides all the other health problems it can cause, tobacco products are stimulants.

Limit alcohol. It might make you drowsy, but alcohol reduces deep and refreshing sleep and even the REM (dream) stage. It causes fragmented sleep, which means you wake up many times throughout the night (even though you may not notice it) and you're still tired in the morning. It can also make you get up at night to use the bathroom, which is another way it interrupts deep slumber.

Ease up on caffeine later in the day. Caffeine stays in the body (in large amounts) for about 5 to 6 hours, so if you're reaching for a java jolt between 4 p.m. to 6 p.m. or later, you may still be feeling the effects at midnight. Caffeine also blocks adenosine receptors in the brain, which makes it harder to fall asleep.

Keep your cool. A drop in body temperature at night is one of the physiological triggers for sleep (as the sleep center in the brain cools down, it's easier to fall asleep). So the temperature in your bedroom at night should be slightly cooler than normal. Some people find that taking a warm bath helps (as they get out, the heat dissipates and they feel cold).

Unplug in the bedroom. Bright lights, alarm clocks, computer screens, and televisions can make it hard to fall asleep.

Calm down. Anything that promotes relaxation, such as acupressure or meditation, helps with sleep. I believe that massage helps with relaxation and sleep, and if science never proves it, who cares! I massage my wife's back every single night and she sleeps like a baby on large doses of melatonin, and I always toss and turn.

Stick to a sleep schedule. Taking naps in the afternoon can disrupt slumber at night. And sleeping in an extra hour or two on weekends can make it harder to get back to your normal schedule once Monday rolls around.

Check your meds. Many drugs—such as diuretics, decongestants, and even antipsychotics—can disturb sleep, so check with your doctor to see if you can alter your schedule to minimize the impact on your z's.

I

Interstitial Cystitis

Dr. Moyad Secret For most individuals with interstitial cystitis (IC), dietary supplements are safer, cheaper, and about as effective as the most commonly prescribed oral FDA-approved drug for IC, Elmiron (pentosan polysulfate sodium). This drug comes with numerous potential side effects (hair loss, diarrhea, blood in the stool, dizziness, headache, rash, abnormal liver enzymes, and bruising), and higher dosages have worked no better than lower dosages in studies, which is why I believe it isn't much more effective than a placebo. (Its original intended use was as a blood thinner, but it didn't work!)

WHAT IS IT?

Interstitial cystitis, or painful bladder syndrome, is a chronic, debilitating, inflammatory bladder disorder that occurs mostly in women (80 to 90 percent of cases). The cause is unknown, and there is no effective conventional therapy for it. Symptoms include chronic pelvic pain, pressure or discomfort, urgency and frequency of urination, and getting up repeatedly at night to urinate *without* having an underlying urinary tract infection. Some people even experience pain with sexual intercourse. It's not uncommon for those who have IC to also have allergies, asthma, irritable bowel syndrome, endometriosis, or fibromyalgia, and about 90 percent of sufferers report a sensitivity to certain foods, such as citrus fruits, artificial sweeteners, and spicy foods.

Dietary supplements and drug therapies work by targeting an area of the bladder known as the GAG (glycosaminoglycan) layer, which is damaged in people with IC. This tissue is made up of chondroitin sulfate and sodium hyaluronate, both of which are seen in increased amounts in the urine of individuals with the condition. Also, people with IC have higher numbers of mast cells (which play a role in allergic reactions) in certain areas of the bladder. As a result, treatment is aimed at restoring the GAG layer or controlling the allergic reaction in the pelvis.

WHAT WORKS

1. Calcium glycerophosphate two or three tablets or ¼ teaspoon twice a day or before high-acid meals

Acidic foods and beverages can trigger IC symptoms, and calcium glycerophosphate, found in the product Prelief and generic forms, is widely used to neutralize meal acidity. The best study ever completed with this supplement found taking two calcium glycerophosphate pills before each meal significantly reduced pain, discomfort, and urgency and improved quality of life.

There is a lack of placebo-controlled clinical trials with this supplement, but I've ranked it number one due to its outstanding safety record and high patient satisfaction ratings. Surveys of users mirror what was found in the study mentioned above: improved quality of life and reduced pain/discomfort and urgency. The only controversy (apart from a lack of placebo studies) is the issue of whether urine acidity really exacerbates pain. Researchers used to believe that it made pain worse, but studies have shown that's not necessarily the case. Calcium glycerophosphate reduces acidity, but maybe that's not how it works. Regardless, patients swear by it.

Only take calcium glycerophosphate as needed with acidic foods; overusing it could chronically reduce stomach acid, which can affect the absorption of critical nutrients and increase the risk of infections.

I know what you're thinking: *Can't I just take Tums or Rolaids?* This hasn't been tested; however, in one small, older study of women with painful bladder disease, those who took 300 milligrams of the over-the-counter drug cimetidine (an acid blocker) twice daily saw a significant improvement in symptoms, including decreased suprapubic pain and less nighttime trips to urinate. But there was no change in the GAG layer or other membranes of the bladder. It's possible that the antacid effects of cimetidine and calcium glycerophosphate have been profoundly underappreciated in IC treatment.

The recommended dosage is two or three tablets or ¼ teaspoon twice a day or before high-acid meals (it's available in pill or powder form). You may need more or less. Two tablets of calcium glycerophosphate contain 130 milligrams of elemental calcium, and this should count toward your total calcium intake for the day.

2. Osteoarthritis supplements, such as glucosamine and chondroitin sulfate dosages vary

Glucosamine sulfate, chondroitin sulfate, and hyaluronate sodium help build the GAG layer of the bladder and reduce pain. There has been some preliminary positive research with the dietary supplement CystoProtek, which contains chondroitin sulfate, hyaluronate sodium, quercetin, rutin, glucosamine sulfate, and olive kernel extract. In the study, 37 participants who took the supplement for 6 months reported a significant reduction of IC symptoms. A larger study involved 252 IC patients who had failed with other treatments. They took four tablets per day, and the male subjects saw pain scores reduced by 52 percent after 12 months of treatment, while female subjects experienced a 49 percent drop in pain scores. More rigorous placebo-controlled trials

275

are needed, but this data is encouraging. I'd also like to see research done with larger doses of a traditional glucosamine or chondroitin osteoarthritis supplement (1,500 and 1,200 milligrams a day, respectively) to see how it would perform against lower doses and other products in this section; I often recommend these dosages to IC patients. (Some doctors are now doing intravesical delivery of chondroitin or hyaluronic acid, placing the compound inside the bladder through the urethra. Cool stuff!)

3. Quercetin complex 500 milligrams twice a day

Quercetin is an anti-inflammatory compound and localized mast cell inhibitor, which means it calms or prevents inflammatory reactions in and around the bladder, reducing pain and improving urinary symptoms. In one small study, patients who took a quercetin complex product (with bromelain and papain for better absorption) called Cysta-Q experienced a significant reduction in scores on a problem index, symptom index, and mean global assessment (which is a geeky way of saying they felt better). They took one capsule (500 miligrams) twice a day for 4 weeks. There was no placebo tested (and this is needed), but it's widely prescribed by urologists around the world for other inflammatory issues, such as chronic prostatitis, so I think there's definitely promise for treating IC.

HONORABLE MENTION

Aloe capsules (up to 3,600 milligrams a day, containing 1,200 milligrams of polysaccharides) may help some people with IC, according to some preliminary research. The study was presented at a major meeting and still hasn't been published; I would be more comfortable taking this off the Honorable Mention list and listing it as a more concrete option if it were to be published. The polysaccharides may enforce the GAG layer, but I'd like to see more research on the safety and efficacy of it.

WHAT'S WORTHLESS

L-arginine and L-citrulline. I discussed these supplements and their limitations in the Erectile Dysfunction section, page 186. And the research for IC has not been effective, even with large doses. Perhaps this is because some patients with IC already have high levels of nitric oxide. Since L-arginine and L-citrulline supplements can dramatically increase nitric oxide, they could be exacerbating the problem.

Vitamin C. Its acidity can make IC worse, so if you need to take it, please choose a buffered vitamin C or calcium ascorbate.

LIFESTYLE CHANGES

Heart healthy = bladder healthy. This is just a theory of mine when it comes to IC. I believe it's one of the reasons there are

INTERSTITIAL CYSTITIS TRIGGER FOODS

What you put in your mouth *can* affect your bladder: Since the compounds (good and bad) in many foods and beverages get filtered from the kidneys through the urine, they come into direct contact with the bladder wall for significant periods of time.

Some common trigger foods for interstitial cystitis include citrus fruits and juices (grapefruit, lemon, orange, pineapple); cranberry juice; tomatoes and tomato products; coffee (both caffeinated and decaffeinated); tea (caffeinated); carbonated beverages (diet, regular, caffeinated, or noncaffeinated); alcoholic beverages (beer, wine, champagne); spicy foods; artificial sweeteners; MSG (monosodium glutamate); vinegar; and Mexican, Thai, and Indian food.

fewer cases of this condition in Japan. Staying heart healthy also reduces overall body inflammation, and since IC is an inflammatory condition, it just makes sense.

Log your meals. Keeping a food diary to determine what foods and beverages improve or worsen symptoms is one of the smartest things you can do when it comes to IC.

Go less frequently. If urgency and frequency of urination are a problem, "stretching" your bladder by increasing the time between bathroom visits may help. One study with IC patients who did not have severe pain had subjects increase the intervals between urinating by 15 to 30 minutes; after 3 months, many of the participants reported a large reduction in urgency and frequency of urination.

WHAT ELSE DO I NEED TO KNOW?

Physicians prescribe many off-label drugs for IC, from muscle relaxants to medications that impact a variety of neurotransmitters (such as the prescription drug amitriptyline). If your doctor only wants to stick with FDA-approved drugs for IC, please fire him and seek out an expert in the area of IC (usually an OB-GYN or urologist).

Irritable Bowel Syndrome

Dr. Moyad Secret There are two important things to note about this potentially debilitating condition. First, people with irritable bowel syndrome (IBS) are more likely to also have celiac disease and lactose intolerance than people without IBS. Recent research also suggests the rate of functional dyspepsia (abdominal fullness, pain, bloating, and heartburn) is higher in those with IBS, too. So if you've been told you have IBS, get checked for these other problems because treatment for these issues can sometimes improve IBS symptoms as well. People with IBS are *not* any more likely to have colon cancer or inflammatory bowel diseases, such as Crohn's or ulcerative colitis.

Second, there used to be a prescription IBS drug that helped alleviate constipation (by improving gut motility), but it increased the risk of cardiovascular disease and was removed from the US market. The name is not important (okay, you got it out of me: It was Zelnorm), but people ask me all the time if I have any contacts outside the country who can get it! The point is, IBS can be so life-altering that people would actually risk getting heart disease just to get some relief. However, I'm happy to report that there are heart-safe IBS supplements out there that are so widely used that they're part of the standard of care by doctors in many cases. So you don't have to risk heart disease. I'm hoping that physicians will begin to embrace the supplements in this section as a result.

WHAT IS IT?

If you talk to 20 different people with IBS, each person would probably have a different definition of it, but the description that doctors have generally agreed on is abdominal discomfort or pain (cramping or bloating) associated with changing bowel habits. It must have occurred at least several days per month for 3 months and cannot be attributed to some other organic disease or condition. Abdominal pain is definitely the most common (and bothersome) IBS symptom; if there's no pain, then in most cases it's not IBS. Other common symptoms include gas, malaise (feelings of serious illness), muscle pain, and urgency. Overall, IBS can have a significant negative impact on quality of life.

No one really knows what causes IBS, but it's most likely due to several factors, including gut hypersensitivity, abnormal gut movements, inflammation, genetics, serotonin neurotransmission, and intestinal bacteria. Stress, anxiety, and a hectic lifestyle can make symptoms worse, which is why IBS is sometimes called nervous colon or spastic colon.

Women suffer from IBS more than men (2:1 ratio), and they're more likely to suffer from the form of IBS where constipation is the predominant symptom. It's more common in developed countries, and India has one of the lowest rates of IBS (no one knows why).

Treatment is complicated because IBS can take different forms; that's also why it's a highly underdiagnosed condition. An estimated 10 to 20 percent of the *global* population could have some form of it.

There are four primary subtypes of IBS:

- IBS with primarily constipation (IBS-C)

- IBS with primarily diarrhea (IBS-D)

- Mixed IBS (IBS-M or IBS-A), with alternating constipation and diarrhea

- IBS un-subtyped (IBS-U), not enough stool consistency to meet criteria for IBS-C, IBS-D, or IBS-M

(See the Travelers' Diarrhea section, page 426, and the Constipation section, page 155, for more information.)

WHAT WORKS

1. Peppermint oil 450 to 1,100 milligrams a day before meals for all types of IBS

Peppermint oil (from the plant *Mentha piperita*) contains menthol, which is an antispasmodic. It reduces contractions of

MOYAD FACT: Fifty percent of IBS patients use complementary and alternative medicines to manage symptoms.

the gastrointestinal tract, resulting in less cramping and bloating. No supplement in the history of dietary supplements has more positive research for all types of IBS than peppermint oil capsules, but *only* if they're enteric coated and pH dependent. *This is the most important thing to take away about peppermint oil!* Pills that are enteric coated and pH dependent (delayed release) won't dissolve until they have passed through the stomach and have encountered an intestinal pH of 6.8 or higher. Without these two things, peppermint oil is not very effective for IBS, and it can make acid reflux, if you have it, worse (heartburn is a common side effect with nonenteric-coated brands).

Look for the product Colpermin, which was tested in several Swiss studies, and take it 30 to 60 minutes before meals. These clinical studies found that people with IBS who took peppermint oil experienced less abdominal pain (the most consistent finding), bloating, feelings of incomplete emptying, urgency, frequency, flatulence, and rumbling/gurgling noises. IBS-D patients might even see a greater benefit from peppermint oil because they tend to experience more abdominal pain and cramping. One caution for those people who have allergies to peanuts or soy: Check the ingredients in peppermint oil capsules because some may contain an oil (arachis) found in peanuts or soy.

2. *Bifidobacterium infantis* 35624
one capsule a day for all types of IBS

This particular bacteria strain is sold under the product name Align. Studies have shown that it's most beneficial for reducing abdominal pain and discomfort, bloating and distension, straining, feelings of incomplete evacuation, and bowel movement difficulty. Again, in my experience, IBS-D types get the most benefit since they have more pain, but mixed IBS sufferers can get some relief as well. Align did not impact stool frequency in studies, but it helps in many other ways, so it's worth it. (The rate of side effects was low or similar to a placebo.) It can be stored at room temperature, and it can be taken without a meal. One capsule contains 1 billion colony-forming units (or CFUs). If you want to increase to two capsules a day, talk to your doctor.

There are plenty of probiotic supplements on the market claiming benefits or being tested for IBS, but the studies have not been long term. Another individual probiotic strain beginning to get some good research right now with IBS is *Saccharomyces boulardii*, so keep your eye on this one, too.

3. (tie) Fiber supplements 10 to
15 grams a day in divided doses for IBS-C primarily

Fiber supplements are known as bulking agents because they absorb water into the intestines and encourage more contractions (peristalsis), which IBS-C type sufferers need. Psyllium powder (10 to 15 grams per day in two divided doses) has been shown to improve regularity and consistency of stools and lessen abdominal pain within 3 months. Each tablespoon usually contains 3 grams of fiber (2 of which are soluble); check to make sure the product is gluten free (less than 20 ppm gluten) just to ensure a smooth trial period. Other fiber supplements, such as methylcellulose (Citrucel) and polycarbophil (FiberCon), as well as dietary fiber (like the kind found in cereals and bars) may also be beneficial. Psyllium has the most support in terms of research and improvement of overall symptoms, though, so it is my first choice. Fiber is ranked third overall in this section because it has not been as consistently effective as peppermint oil, and in some cases it increases bloating, abdominal distension, and gas. Yet it can also provide numerous heart-healthy benefits, such as normalizing blood cholesterol and sugars and increasing the amount of healthy bacteria in the intestines. (This could worsen abdominal discomfort and bloating in IBS-D patients.)

3. (tie) Loperamide up to
16 milligrams a day for IBS-D primarily

For the sake of this book, I consider loperamide (Imodium) to be a dietary supplement; this is because it was potentially derived from natural sources and your body thinks it's a plant as well (it attaches to certain receptors in the intestines that normally bind other plant-based products). It works by blocking specific receptors in the GI tract, which slows the movement of the intestines so that more water is absorbed, thus reducing diarrhea.

It's typically used for IBS-D, and while studies have reported benefits for all subtypes (it can reduce pain and most other symptoms), I personally never recommend it for IBS-C types because it can make constipation worse. Patients generally take an initial 4-milligram dose, followed by 2 milligrams every 4 hours, with a maximum dosage of 16 milligrams daily. Loperamide can be taken for about 12 hours after normal stools begin again, but no longer than that; chronic use can alter the functioning of the GI tract. If you have trouble taking pills, 7.5 milliliters of liquid loperamide (usually for kids) supplies about 1 milligram of the medication.

A word of caution: Imodium is an opioid receptor agonist, so you don't want to take an opioid, such as codeine, at the same time because it can intensify the sedative side effects and cause a potentially serious drug interaction.

HONORABLE MENTIONS

Melatonin relaxes the intestinal tract, reducing pain and bloating and increasing or regulating motility, so it's probably better for IBS-C versus IBS-D types. It may also reduce anxiety and stress and have anti-inflammatory effects—all of which help IBS. Several trials have found that taking melatonin (usually 3 milligrams) before bed may reduce abdominal pain in people who suffer with IBS and sleep problems.

Artichoke leaf extract (*Cynara scolymus*) can significantly reduce multiple IBS symptoms, including abdominal pain, cramps, bloating, flatulence, and constipation, especially for people with mixed-type IBS. But in some people it can also *cause* flatulence. The typical dose is two 320-milligram capsules three times a day. This supplement appears to favorably impact colon bacteria, and it may also have antispasmodic effects, but I'd like to see more research on it.

Calcium glycerophosphate (Prelief brand and generic) is an acid reducer that you take immediately before or during meals (two capsules maximum or $\frac{1}{4}$ teaspoon of powder). It has helped many people with painful bowel and bladder issues whose symptoms are exacerbated by acidic foods.

WHAT'S WORTHLESS

Aloe supplements. It's supposed to reduce constipation and improve motility, but results have been inconsistent. Plus, many aloe products are now diluted. My experience with this product has been hit or miss and I say pass.

Common fumitory or earth smoke. This herbal supplement for IBS scares me because of its potential for toxicity. Plus, it hasn't worked better than a placebo in studies anyway.

Arrowroot. This plant-based supplement has helped some individuals with IBS-D, but it was a tiny study and the results were weak, so until the findings can be reproduced, I don't recommend it.

St. John's wort. People commonly take this for depression, and it might reduce pain and stress (which is why IBS patients are frequently given prescription antidepressants). In one of the best studies to date, however, St. John's Wort did not work better than a placebo for people with diarrhea- or constipation-type IBS.

Turmeric. Researchers have seen some reduction in IBS-related abdominal pain with anywhere from 72 to 144 milligrams of turmeric extract taken over 8 weeks, but they found no difference in effectiveness between the two doses. Plus, there have been no placebo-controlled trials published over the past decade, so I'm skeptical that it works any better than a placebo. In fact, even though it's an anti-inflammatory, I've had some people complain of abdominal pain when taking this supplement for arthritis. I'm much more excited about turmeric as a spice for cooking.

WHAT ARE THE OPTIONS FOR KIDS?

IBS increases in prevalence from elementary to junior high to high school, where some surveys suggest it is as common as it is in middle-age adults. Peppermint oil supplements may reduce abdominal pain in kids (8 to 17 years old) with IBS, based on previous studies where it was used for 2 weeks. One well-done study used 187 milligrams (or 0.2 milliliters) of peppermint oil in an enteric-coated, pH-dependent, hard gelatin capsule (Colpermin was one brand tested). Kids weighing more than 100 pounds received two capsules three times a day, and kids who weighed between 65 to 100 pounds received one capsule three times a day. Pain reduction and improvements were observed in about 70 to 75 percent of the kids taking peppermint oil and 20 to 45 percent of the kids taking a placebo. *Remember:* Peppermint oil can cause heartburn, and when used in higher dosages than recommended, it can cause abnormally slow breathing (respiratory depression), so the recommended dosage should never be exceeded and children should always take it under the guidance of a pediatrician.

Some small studies with probiotic supplements, including *Bifidobacterium infantis* and *Lactobacillus rhamnosus* GG, showed improvement in kids' overall IBS symptoms, like abdominal pain and bloating. However, talk to your doctor about the latest research because it's a moving target right now.

LIFESTYLE CHANGES

Get moving! In one of my favorite studies, people with all types of IBS who exercised three to five times a week at a moderate to vigorous level (20 to 60 minutes a session) showed an improvement in IBS symptoms. The biggest finding was that it prevented IBS from getting worse.

Work with a nutritionist who specializes in IBS. This specialist will likely suggest an elimination diet, which involves removing certain foods to see if symptoms improve (see the section about avoiding FODMAP foods below). These diets take 3 to 4 months to complete because they also involve a reintroduction phase, where potentially offending foods are slowly added back to see if symptoms return. In some cases, testing for food allergies might be appropriate, but they generally aren't a big contributor to IBS, except when it comes to gluten. I believe if you have IBS, you should be tested for celiac disease *and* nonceliac gluten sensitivity. Finally, studies have suggested that people with IBS tend to have diets that are low in calcium, phosphorus, magnesium, vitamin A, and vitamin B_2, so make sure you look for foods or a basic multivitamin that supplies these nutrients.

Manage stress. This can have a dramatic impact on IBS symptoms. Learning relaxation techniques and how to deal with daily stressors is hugely important, both for IBS and your quality of life in general!

Avoid FODMAP foods. These are **f**ermentable **o**ligosaccharides, **d**isaccharides, **m**onosaccharides, **a**nd **p**olyols, all of which are poorly absorbed carbohydrates. Fermentable carbohydrates are not absorbed well in the intestines, and they're active in the gut, causing bacterial fermentation, which can lead to excess gas, bloat-

ing, and loose stools. In other words, they can make all types of IBS worse. A gastroenterologist or nutritionist should be able to give you a list of FODMAP foods. Fermentable carbohydrates include:

- Fructo-oligosaccharides, which are found in wheat and onions

- Galacto-oligosaccharides, found in beans, peas, lentils, and chickpeas

- Disaccharides, such as the lactose in milk and other dairy products

- Monosaccharides, which include foods that have fructose in them, such as honey, fruit juices, some fruits (apples, pears, mangoes, and canned fruit), high-fructose corn syrup, and many processed foods

- Polyols, such as sorbitol in various fruits and veggies, polyol-sweetened "sugar-free" manufactured foods and medicines, and resistant starches (such as green bananas and cold or reheated potatoes)

WHAT ELSE DO I NEED TO KNOW?

You may have to experiment with all sorts of treatments—what I call guinea pig medicine—until you find the one product that makes a difference for you. For example, I have seen men and women have zero success with several different approaches and then respond to a product like Beano, an over-the-counter supplement that is an antifoaming agent in the intestines. You just don't know what might work, so you have to be willing to try anything. Here are some of the many conventional over-the-counter and prescription drug options that help reduce pain, constipation, or diarrhea for IBS patients.

- **Over-the-counter laxatives:** Polyethylene glycol can be used for IBS-C.

- **Antibiotics:** Rifaximin is a great newer option for IBS-D. It's not absorbed into the body; it stays in the GI tract and may work by resetting the gut bacteria (some people with IBS have altered gut flora, so it's kind of like a reboot button).

- **Antispasmodics:** Hyoscyamine and dicyclomine can be used for all IBS types.

- **Antidepressants:** These can be used for all types of IBS. Antidepressants impact receptors in the gut and perhaps in the spinal cord to reduce abdominal pain, but they also stimulate gut motility, so they may be better for IBS-C types.

- **Certain IBS drugs:** Lubiprostone and linaclotide are both FDA-approved for IBS-C. They affect a specific area of the intestines to promote fluid secretion, which allows stools to move more easily.

- **Serotonin (5-HT3) antagonists:** The generic drug alosetron has been used for women with severe IBS-D to slow intestinal movement or motility so more water can be absorbed from the stool, relieving diarrhea.

- **Stool softeners (like docusate):** These are also helpful for constipation from IBS, especially if you have to strain to go.

Itchy Skin

I

Dr. Moyad Secret Itchy skin (pruritis) is a common symptom of many diseases, including diabetes and dermatitis (skin inflammation). With all the talk of essential fatty acids (omega-3s and omega-6s) as anti-inflammatory agents, the research should be focused on using some of these topically to moisturize skin and reduce itching. Conventional topical acne treatments can control this condition. Taking pills (supplements or prescriptions) for it isn't as effective because the medicinal contents might not make their way to the affected part of the skin.

Chia seeds and omega-3s and 6s. Chia seeds have the highest known concentration of plant omega-3 fatty acids in the world! Although you normally eat chia seeds, researchers are currently testing a 4 percent chia seed topical oil that is showing early benefits. Dietary oral supplementation with omega-3s, such as fish oil, or omega-6s, such as evening primrose, has provided some modest benefit in studies and is worth a try as well.

Slather on oats. Colloidal oatmeal has historically been used to treat itching and skin irritation because it soothes inflammation. It's available over the counter, and there's minimal risk to trying it.

Kidney Stones

Dr. Moyad Secret Want to know how you can cut your risk of getting kidney stones down to almost nothing? Remember these three things.

1. Reduce your risk of heart disease to as close to zero as possible through lifestyle changes, such as eating a healthy diet, exercising, and staying trim.

2. Stay hydrated. Drink when you're thirsty to keep your urine a clear color.

3. Be careful when taking a variety of supplements, especially calcium, vitamin D, and vitamin C (ascorbic acid). (I'll discuss this further below.)

   This is one of the only areas of medicine where there are more dietary supplements that can cause the condition than can prevent or treat it! For that reason, "WHAT'S WORTHLESS" comes before "What Works" in this section.

WHAT IS IT?

Kidney stones impact 10 to 15 percent of Americans (global rates are rising, too). Some experts believe the increase has been driven by warmer weather (leading to dehydration) and the obesity and diabetes epidemics. Stones are hard mineral or acid salt deposits that form in the kidneys and travel to the bladder. There are four main types of stones based on their content, including calcium oxalate (75 to 80 percent of stones) or calcium phosphate, uric acid (see the Gout section, page 207), struvite (usually from an infection), and cystine (rare).

Small stones (only a few millimeters) pass spontaneously in 90 percent of people, but the large ones can cause significant pain because the ureters that connect the kidney and bladder are relatively narrow and full of nerves. Some men say the pain is so bad it's "equivalent to giving birth," while some women have been known to describe it as "nowhere close to giving birth." The pain usually occurs on one side of the back or body, can be severe and colicky (starting and stopping) or constant, and often radiates around to the groin. Blood in the urine, nausea, vomiting, and even low-grade fever are also common. The real problem with kidney stones is that they can block urine drainage, which is similar to a clogged pipe. If urine gets backed up for too long, it can increase the risk of kidney disease, infections, and kidney failure.

If you've had kidney stones in the past,

your chance of having a recurrence within 10 years is about 50 to 80 percent, according to most studies. The risk of having a recurrence within the first year is 10 to 20 percent, especially if you fail to follow your doctor's preventive advice to make healthy lifestyle changes (plus some people are more genetically predisposed to stones).

There are many causes of kidney stones, including:

- Anatomic abnormalities of the kidney, bladder, or urinary tract

- Cancer

- Gastrointestinal diseases

- Genetics/family history

- Gout

- High blood calcium

- High blood levels of parathyroid hormone

- High blood pressure

- Hyperthyroidism

- Immobilization or physical inactivity

- Insulin resistance

- Medications (steroids, anticonvulsants)

- Obesity (this increases your risk more than any other factor)

- Osteoporosis

- Rapid weight loss

- Sarcoidosis

- Urinary tract infections or urinary retention problems

WHAT'S WORTHLESS

High doses of calcium carbonate or vitamin D. The large Women's Health Initiative study—36,282 postmenopausal women ages 50 to 79—found that women who took 1,000 milligrams of calcium carbonate and 400 IU of vitamin D daily for an average of 7 years had 17 percent more kidney stone episodes than the placebo group. A total of 449 women in the calcium and vitamin D group and 381 in the placebo group reported a kidney stone during the clinical trial. What is interesting is that many of the women in the study were already getting 1,150 milligrams of dietary calcium and 365 IU of dietary vitamin D, meaning they were getting these nutrients from food. This just goes to show that many people do not need to take supplemental calcium and vitamin D, and there can be negative health consequences if they do. There is already plenty of calcium in a moderately healthy diet.

Aim to get 1,000 to 1,200 milligrams a day of calcium from food sources first and foremost, and then supplement only if you're not getting enough. If you need supplemental calcium and you're at high risk for kidney or other types of stones, consider taking calcium citrate if your last kidney stone was a calcium oxalate stone; this form of calcium does not appear to raise kidney stone risk. When it comes to vitamin D, avoid taking more than what is already in your multivitamin unless a blood test shows you're low in vitamin D (less than 30 ng/mL) and you're not able to increase it by eating wild salmon, losing weight, or exercising more.

Vitamin C (ascorbic acid or plain vitamin C). Clinical trials have consistently demonstrated that plain vitamin C supplements in higher doses (1,000 milligrams or more) increase blood and urine levels of oxalate and can increase the risk of kidney stones, both in people with a history of stones and those who've never had one. Studies have found that large doses increase oxalate excretion in the urine by as much as 60 percent. Let me put this in perspective: Consistent oxalate increases of just 10 percent or more could be enough to create kidney stones. Plain vitamin C also lowers blood levels of uric acid by increasing filtration of it through the urine, which might also increase the risk of kidney stones. If you're at a higher risk than normal for a calcium oxalate kidney stone (because you've had a previous stone), taking large amounts of vitamin C supplements is a bad idea. Another option is to take a "buffered" vitamin C tablet, such as calcium ascorbate, which does not appear to increase oxalate levels as much, if at all (its impact on uric acid has not been well studied).

Inosine (inosine monophosphate). Inosine helps with energy production in the body, which is why there has always been interest in determining whether supplementing it could boost athletic performance (so far the answer is no). Because it may help fight inflammation, it's being studied as a uric acid *increasing* supplement in relapsing-remitting multiple sclerosis and Parkinson's disease (see the Parkinson's Disease section, page 359). But it can also increase the risk of kidney stones.

Cranberry. Some cranberry dietary supplements contain high levels of oxalate, so if you need to take this supplement (maybe for preventing a urinary tract infection), check with different companies to find one that's low in oxalate (less than 1 milligram per pill or less than 1 percent oxalate). (You'll have to call or research it online, though, since it's not on labels.) The average normal intake of oxalate from the diet is about 150 milligrams per day, but in one study, two cranberry tablets contained more than 350 milligrams. Another problem with some cranberry supplements is that they can contain ascorbic acid (a.k.a. vitamin C)—a double whammy!

Turmeric and ginger. These popular supplements may contain high levels of oxalates, which can increase the risk of kidney stones. Oxalates in plants exist in two forms: the water-soluble salts and the insoluble salts attached to calcium, magnesium, and iron. The former get absorbed in the intestines and reach the urine; the latter aren't absorbed and get excreted in the feces. Plants high in soluble oxalates have a greater chance of increasing urinary oxalate. When researchers tested spices themselves (not the supplements), they found: Green cardamom had the highest concentration of soluble oxalates (99 percent), followed by turmeric powder (95 percent), ginger (87 percent), malabathrum leaf (59 percent), and black cardamom (59 percent). Cinnamon was the only spice that contained only insoluble oxalate.

A clinical trial with young, healthy men and women without diabetes, published in the *American Journal of Clinical Nutrition*, found that 2,800 milligrams per day of a turmeric supplement caused a significant increase in oxalate (about 8 percent) within 6 hours. The 24-hour urine oxalate level increased from about 20 to 25 milligrams with turmeric, which is below what defines real kidney stone risk (40-plus milligrams), but many people with a history or risk of kidney stones also have increased absorption or production of oxalate.

Silicon dioxide. Manufacturers add silicon dioxide to many supplements to keep ingredients from clumping together and to absorb moisture. If you have a history of kidney stones, check to see if it's listed as one of the primary ingredients because it could create a silica kidney stone (bizarre but true)!

WHAT WORKS

Note: The supplements mentioned here help to *prevent* calcium oxalate kidney stones, not treat them.

1. Calcium citrate dosage is based on need, up to 1,200 milligrams a day maximum, depending on how much you're getting in your diet

This is the ideal supplement for people who need to increase their calcium intake but want to reduce their risk of kidney stones. (The Recommended Dietary Allowance of calcium is mostly based on age, gender, and situation such as pregnancy, but for most people it is between 1,000 and 1,200 milligrams daily.) Calcium citrate has not been shown to increase the risk of stones, and in some cases it can decrease the risk because it provides citrate in the urine, a natural stone inhibitor, and if taken with meals, it binds with the oxalates in foods (which helps discourage stone formation). Calcium citrate supplements with a little magnesium (50 to 100 milligrams) can help reduce the risk of constipation (common with this form of calcium) as well as stones because magnesium binds with oxalate. (You can get a ballpark estimate of how much calcium you're getting in your diet by keeping a food diary and then checking the calcium content of all the foods online or having a nutritionist evaluate your food log.)

2. Vitamin B$_6$ 50 to 200 milligrams a day

This vitamin prevents too much oxalate from being formed in the body. Several studies suggest that individuals with higher vitamin B$_6$ intake from foods (40 milligrams or more daily) have a lower risk of kidney stones. The recommended daily dietary intake is approximately 1.2 to 1.7 milligrams per day in adults, however, to reduce high oxalate levels, you need to take 50 to 100 milligrams per day or slightly more. Some companies sell a more active form known as pyridoxal-5-phosphate (P-5-P), but studies have primarily used the inexpensive and simple form of B_6 (pyridoxine hydrochloride), so P-5-P is probably not worth the money.

Taking more than 300 milligrams per day can lead to severe sensory neuropathy, which is basically nerve damage, so more is not better. If you have a history of kidney stones due to high urinary oxalate levels, talk to your doctor about trying the lower doses of vitamin B_6 that were studied, along with dietary and lifestyle changes. If you don't have an oxalate problem and take high amounts of vitamin B_6, it could paradoxically *increase* oxalate levels. Finally, never combine antiseizure drugs, especially Dilantin, with vitamin B_6; check with your doctor or pharmacist for the latest drug interactions.

3. Magnesium 250 to 500 milligrams a day

The Recommended Dietary Allowance of magnesium from food sources is generally 310 to 420 milligrams, but that's not easy to get unless you're eating a very heart-healthy diet. Supplementing makes more sense for people at risk of kidney stones. Taking magnesium with or right after meals not only can reduce levels of oxalate absorbed from the gastrointestinal tract (so it doesn't end up in the urine) but also appears to independently discourage the formation of calcium and oxalate in the urine. Several preliminary studies have found that combining 250 milligrams of magnesium oxide twice a day with a con-

ventional prescription medicine for stones (such as potassium citrate) significantly increased the antistone environment in the urine, with even greater reductions in oxalate. A word of warning: Magnesium can increase the risk of loose stools and diarrhea, and high doses (above 600 milligrams) can cause a variety of health problems, including arrhythmias, muscle weakness, and confusion.

HONORABLE MENTIONS

Oxalobacter formigenes is a strain of healthy bacterium that can degrade and reduce the absorption of oxalate in the gastrointestinal tract (the GI tract is loaded with healthy bacteria), meaning less gets into the urine. By age 8, almost all children test positive for it, compared to only 60 to 80 percent of adults. I think the decrease is partially due to the overuse of antibiotics and unhealthy lifestyle choices. Now here's what's really interesting: Consuming foods or beverages with oxalate (which is usually restricted in people prone to kidney stones) can *increase* the chances that *O. formigenes* takes up residence in your gut! Makes sense; it goes where the food is. (Foods high in oxalate include spinach, Swiss chard, sweet potatoes, and many types of nuts.) That's one of the reasons I'm generally not a big fan of severely restricting high-oxalate foods if you're at risk for kidney stones (contrary to the conventional belief). So why is it only an Honorable Mention? It's not widely available commercially as a probiotic yet.

Omega-3 fatty acids (1,200 milligrams per day of the active ingredients EPA and DHA) can lower urinary calcium and oxalate by affecting something known as prostaglandin metabolism, which is involved in inflammation and may increase stone risk, according to a Cleveland Clinic study. Omega-3 fatty acids in fish oil may impact the transport of oxalate so that it doesn't get dumped into the urine in larger amounts. Another study that used 1,800 milligrams of EPA found that it helped decrease calcium in those who had high levels in their urine, but not in those who had normal levels. In fact, those famous studies of Greenland Eskimos that showed a lower risk of heart disease with a greater omega-3 intake from fish (5,000 to 10,000 milligrams daily) also found a lower risk of kidney stones in this population. Omega-6 supplements may have antistone effects, too, because they contain GLA (gamma-linolenic acid) and linoleic acid, which can become DGLA and then PGE1, both anti-inflammatory compounds.

WHAT ARE THE OPTIONS FOR KIDS?

The incidence of kidney stones in adolescents is increasing by 4 to 5 percent per year, according to a Mayo Clinic study, which is a dramatic change from just a few decades ago. Obesity, type 2 diabetes, and hypertension increase the risk of stones in kids, just like in adults, so adopting heart-healthy habits is the first step.

LIFESTYLE CHANGES

Heart healthy = kidney healthy. The Coronary Artery Risk Development in Young Adults (CARDIA) study followed 5,000 Caucasian and African American men and women for 20 years. Researchers found that those with kidney stones were more likely to also have some blockage of their arteries. Exercising and losing weight are key lifestyle changes that can improve heart health and decrease stone risk. Review the US government–funded DASH (Dietary Approaches to Stop Hypertension) study with your doctor because, although it has been shown to reduce blood pressure, it appears to also dramatically lower kidney stone risk. Basically, DASH is just a heart-healthy diet high in fiber, veggies, fruits, nuts, seeds, and beans; low in sodium; and low to moderate in meat and sugar.

Watch your sodium and normalize your calcium intake. A historic, randomized trial from Parma, Italy, published in the *New England Journal of Medicine*, was the largest and longest kidney stone clinical trial in the history of medicine. Over 5 years, men who received the intervention diet (which contained normal calcium and low protein and salt) reduced their risk of a recurrent stone by 50 percent compared to the control group who only ate a low-calcium diet. This trial really turned the medical world upside down because it started to become very clear that diet and lifestyle changes make a very big difference. Sodium likes to hide in processed foods; if a food comes in a bag, box, can, or fast-food container, you're probably getting large amounts of sodium. Excess levels increase the amount of calcium in your urine and decrease the amount of citrate, which helps discourage stone formation. I went over calcium in the "What's Worthless" on page 287 section, already.

Hydrate daily. Imagine a glass with a couple of tablespoons of powder in it. If you add a small amount of water, you get clumps, but if you add a lot of water, then the powder easily dissolves into the mixture. Stones are just like those clumps. You need to produce 68 ounces of urine (about 2 liters) per day to prevent a kidney stone; to do this, you should drink as much as 85 ounces of fluid a day (about 10 cups), depending on how much water you lose from other activities, such as exercise or digestion. *All* fluids and even some foods contribute to urine production. Let the color of your urine be your guide: Dark yellow means dehydration, and a very light color or clear means you're adequately hydrated.

Get your daily servings of fruit and veggies. They're loaded with water, potassium, and magnesium, which increases the pH of urine. And a favorable pH reduces the risk of stone formation. Also, citrus fruits have citric acid, which increases pH and citrate levels in the urine.

Get more citrate. Just a little freshly squeezed lemon or lime juice is a good source of citrate, which discourages kidney stone formation.

Cut carbs. Reduce your intake of refined carbohydrates or sugars; these can increase calcium in the urine.

WHAT ELSE DO I NEED TO KNOW?

The Academy of Nutrition and Dietetics recommends a dietary oxalate intake of 40 to 50 milligrams per day or less for people at risk of stones. Many nutritionists and doctors recommend restricting any food or beverage high in oxalate. I don't agree and here's why: Some foods that are high in oxalate are high in insoluble oxalate, which is not a concern because it doesn't get absorbed; it passes through the body and ends up in the feces. Plus, many of these restricted foods have heart-healthy benefits and other antistone compounds in them (this is why the DASH study mentioned earlier, which was higher in oxalate, showed lowered stone risk). Some commonly restricted high-oxalate foods are beets, buckwheat, cocoa powder and chocolate, nuts, okra, rhubarb, seeds, soybeans and foods made from them, spices (such as ginger and turmeric), spinach, Swiss chard, tea (black and green), and wheat bran. Now do you see why I disagree? There are better ways to reduce stone risk for some individuals.

Low Energy and Chronic Fatigue   L

Dr. Moyad Secret The next time you walk into work yell out, "Where is the 1,3,7-trimethylxanthine?" Your coworkers will think you're smart, and you can tell them Dr. Moyad said it's perfectly safe to have a moderate amount of 1,3,7-trimethylxanthine every day. This compound is known to help with memory and may even reduce the risk of type 2 diabetes, depression, a variety of neurologic diseases (including Parkinson's), and prostate cancer. It may work by improving nerve cell function and allowing for smoother communication and transmission of cell signals (like having a 4G or 5G network for your cell service). It's also one of the best things ever proven to reduce fatigue and improve energy levels, and it has an outstanding safety record in moderation. If you get too much of this good thing, though, you could become anxious, irritable, and have trouble focusing and sleeping. What is it? This weird-sounding compound is the chemical structure and official name for caffeine. Gotcha!

WHAT IS IT?

Aging, reduced metabolism due to muscle loss, inflammation and stress from countless diseases, and drug treatments can all drain energy levels and increase fatigue. Physical fatigue can lead to mental fatigue (lack of focus or attention, depression, stress, and anxiety) and vice versa, which is why a supplement that has the ability to help with both aspects is ideal. There are many different descriptions for fatigue, but they all revolve around a lack of energy. If you're spending more of your day in bed or in a chair, it's time to talk with your doctor about potentially having your fatigue treated.

Chronic fatigue syndrome (CFS) is severe and disabling fatigue, usually with a variety of other potential symptoms, including reduced concentration, sleep problems, musculoskeletal pain, and even headaches. The cause is unknown and experts have speculated it may be triggered by a variety of things—from a lingering infection to an autoimmune syndrome—but no single reason has been identified and no single supplement has consistently been recommended in clinical guidelines because of lack of research. But I believe this section could help people with CFS because when ranking supplements, I focused on what has worked for more extreme conditions, like cancer-related fatigue, which, like CFS, can impact physical and mental function. And I think this section

293

could potentially help with *all* chronic fatigue situations where the reason cannot be easily identified and corrected with a trip or two to the doctor. (For example, on rare occasions, fatigue can be the result of nutrient deficiencies, such as B_{12}, folic acid, or iron, which can lead to anemia; low thyroid or testosterone can also cause fatigue, and this is easily corrected as well.)

When you're dealing with fatigue that is more intractable to lifestyle changes, using stimulants to improve energy levels can be problematic. Too little of a stimulant takes a long time to work—if it does at all—while getting too much can be dangerous because it increases the risk of a cardiac event, such as an arrhythmia. Therefore, the supplements recommended in this section are mild to moderate and have a safe track record overall.

WHAT WORKS

1. (tie) American ginseng (*Panax quinquefolius*) or Panax ginseng

1,000 to 2,000 milligrams a day in at least two divided doses

In a very well-done Mayo Clinic study—similar to a Phase 3 drug trial—with 364 cancer patients, participants took either 2,000 milligrams of Wisconsin ginseng, a common type of American ginseng, or a placebo. By the end of the first month, both groups were experiencing reduced fatigue. After about 2 months, twice as many ginseng patients reported less fatigue. Side effects were similar to a placebo.

The ginseng used consisted of pure ground root from one production lot (manufactured by Beehive Botanicals) and contained 3 percent ginsenosides, which researchers believe are the active ingredients. Most ginseng products on the market have at least 3 percent; some go as high as 50 percent ginsenosides. The higher the concentration of ginsenosides is, the lower the dose you should start with (always look for at least 3 to 5 percent ginsenosides). The same research group at the Mayo Clinic saw some benefits for cancer-related fatigue at 1,000 milligrams per day with a 5 percent ginsenoside product in a previous clinical trial. Ginseng derived from water extraction or from pure ground root has shown the best results and safety; alcohol- or methanol-based extraction methods could be less effective and possibly even toxic with long-term use.

Ginseng may reduce the inflammatory process associated with cancer or chronic fatigue, which in turn impacts cortisol, reduces stress, and improves energy. Ginseng (Panax or American) has a long history of improving energy levels in healthy individuals, but the fact that it worked in the extreme case of cancer-related fatigue tells me it can also help with other types of fatigue. (As I was preparing this section, a preliminary clinical trial from MD Anderson Cancer Center found similar benefits in cancer patients with Panax ginseng at similar dosages.)

1. (tie) Guarana (*Paullinia cupana*)

50 milligrams twice a day (containing no more than 40 milligrams of caffeine per day)

This plant from the Amazon River basin has been used as a stimulant for ages because it contains caffeine, but it also has a high saponin and tannin content, which may also contribute to reducing fatigue and improving focus. Bayer sponsored a study that found 222 milligrams of guarana (containing 40 milligrams of caffeine) worked better than a placebo for reducing mental fatigue and improving focus and attention. Other clinical studies of 75 milligrams of guarana found it improved memory.

Yet, this data on its own isn't enough to convince me that guarana could be a real winner in the fight against fatigue. I want to see how it does for extreme fatigue, such as what you experience during cancer treatment, which is why I like this next trial: The most famous study with cancer-related fatigue and guarana was done in Brazil. Researchers used a standardized extract with a 6.46 percent caffeine content (not much) and a 1.7 percent tannin content. Essentially, patients in this study received only around 5 milligrams of caffeine a day from guarana (a standard cup of coffee has 50 to 100 milligrams). More than 70 patients took either a 50-milligram guarana supplement or a placebo for 3 weeks, then took nothing for a week, and then crossed over to the other group (the original placebo subjects took the supplement and vice versa). After 21 days, half of the guarana patients reported significantly reduced fatigue compared to about 10 percent of the placebo group.

Most other trials have also used guarana with a fairly low caffeine content. When I (and others) have tried it, the effects seem to be attributable to more than just the caffeine; the other compounds in this plant help increase energy—not so much that it makes you jittery, though—and allow you to maintain concentration and focus. Instead of a roller-coaster effect—with higher energy and then a crash—it's more of a consistent merry-go-round feel. While the participants in these studies did not report anxiety and insomnia (as you might expect with products containing caffeine), I wouldn't take it in the late afternoon because it could be too stimulating for some people. Pregnant women should not use guarana either; while it may just be a mild stimulant, guarana cannot be considered safe in pregnancy unless it receives more safety research.

Yerba mate is another plant containing caffeine, and it's beginning to show some benefits for improved energy when used in beverages. It may end up working as well as guarana supplements, but more research regarding safety is needed.

HONORABLE MENTION

D-ribose has shown good results in a few preliminary studies (not nearly as good as the ginseng studies, though). They suggest 5 grams of this supplement three times a day can help reduce chronic fatigue from unknown causes. But a large, well-done study that proves it can beat a placebo is still needed. Regardless, it seems to have a good safety record, and it's certainly worth trying for a week or two to see if it works.

WHAT'S WORTHLESS

B vitamins. B vitamins for energy or fatigue are a waste of money unless you have a specific type of really rare anemia caused by a deficiency. And B_{12} injections for energy? Save your money! The human body needs such small amounts of these vitamins, and then it's just so cells can carry out their normal functions. There are no credible studies showing B vitamins can improve metabolism or energy or reduce fatigue.

Caffeine pills/concentrated caffeine sources. I think a single energy drink can be helpful, but more than two a day is a lot of concentrated caffeine. Think of it this way: When you drink shots of hard liquor, you get drunk fast, but if you're downing more diluted sources like light beer, you need larger volumes to feel the buzz. Caffeine is somewhat similar. When you concentrate the amount in a very small volume of liquid, it's easy to overdose, resulting in anxiety and even skipped heartbeats (bad cardiovascular effects). That's why I don't recommend caffeine pills except in some rare situations where nothing else works. And you can become addicted to higher doses of caffeine and develop a tolerance, where you need even larger doses to get the same effect. Finally, withdrawal from these very high doses of caffeine provided by pills and energy drinks is tough, and it can cause moderate to severe headaches. (*Warning:* The high acidity of energy drinks can potentially cause serious tooth damage. Rinsing with water or chewing sugarless gum after drinking them could help—or just don't drink them.)

L-carnitine. This dietary supplement had a lot of researchers excited because it just makes sense that it would help reduce fatigue. L-carnitine has a transport function in the body. It shuttles fatty acids into the cells, which helps produce energy (again, I'm talking energy on a cellular level, not on a run-a-marathon level). However, clinical trials haven't supported the fatigue-reduction theory. There have been a few small studies suggesting that getting 1 to 2 grams (1,000 to 2,000 milligrams) per day of L-carnitine may reduce fatigue in some individuals, but a recent large Phase 3–like study of 2,000 milligrams per day of L-carnitine over 4 weeks did not show a benefit in cancer patients compared to a placebo. Some might argue that the study wasn't long enough, but in my book, 4 weeks *was* adequate to see a hint of efficacy in cancer-related fatigue. And if it doesn't work for cancer-related fatigue, I'm skeptical that it can help for other types of serious fatigue. In my experience working with countless cancer patients, I haven't seen it do anything.

However, if you have lower levels of L-carnitine, which may be the case in some people with chronic fatigue syndrome, supplementation might make a difference. In one 2-month study, CFS patients who took L-carnitine reported significant improvements in fatigue. I'm still on the fence, but it might be worth trying a minimum dose of 2,000 milligrams per day (this is not a small dose). Most of the positive research from L-carnitine has come from a group of researchers in Italy, and I'd like to see other trials from outside the country confirming the results before I jump on the L-carnitine bandwagon.

LIFESTYLE CHANGES

Heart healthy = healthy energy levels. By lowering blood pressure, weight, and stress, you can reduce chronic inflammation, which can sap energy!

Work out more. While it didn't earn a place in my "What Works" section, my prediction is resistance exercise with protein powder supplementation will appear in that section in the next edition of the book. Exercise (both aerobic and resistance training) has been shown in numerous clinical trials to improve energy levels and reduce fatigue. In fact, weight lifting just twice a week (upper and lower body) for 15 to 20 minutes continues to show excellent results. It's simple: Increase your muscle mass and your metabolism increases, which also increases energy levels. If you're experiencing extreme fatigue, it's best to exercise every other day

(versus daily) because it takes longer to recover from exercise when you're that worn down. Many patients have told me how much better they feel when they cut back on daily exercise. Do aerobic ("cardio") exercise every other day for approximately 30 minutes (moderate to vigorous intensity), and on the other days perform a light activity, such as a short walk. Now, for those of you without fatigue issues or who are just tired at the end of the day, regular daily (or almost daily) exercise can make you feel better. Regardless, consistent exercise can keep you at your peak both physically and mentally!

In chronic fatigue patients, graded exercise therapy (doing 30 minutes of easy exercise 5 days per week) has shown some of the most compelling evidence yet of how exercise can improve fatigue and help patients get back to normal social and work activity.

Dial in your diet. Talk to a nutritionist about calculating an adequate daily calorie and nutrient intake. Eating too much or too little—or not enough nutrients—can create fatigue. On average, you should consume approximately 15 calories for every pound that you weigh, meaning if you are 150 pounds, you should eat about 2,250 calories a day to *maintain* your weight. This is a very general guideline; everyone's metabolism is different. A nutritionist or a good personal trainer can perform testing to determine your actual daily metabolic rate (how many calories you're burning a day).

Eat adequate protein. You require

adequate amounts of high-quality protein to rebuild and repair body tissues, including muscles, which contributes to good energy. The best sources are from dairy, eggs, fish, meat, and poultry, but if you're vegetarian, there are also soy, brown rice, and hemp protein powders as well as dietary sources, such as beans, lentils, and quinoa. The average daily protein requirement is about 0.8 gram of protein per kilogram of body weight (1 kilogram = 2.2 pounds), so a 150-pound (68 kilograms) person needs about 54 grams of protein a day. This might sound like a lot, but one small protein drink and one small serving (mini-can) of tuna fish, for example, gives you about 40 to 50 grams of protein. Two eggs give you 12 to 15 grams; a steak, 40 grams; a chicken breast, 30 grams; 3 ounces of fish, 20 grams; 1 cup of milk, 8 grams; 1 cup of yogurt, 8 grams; and so on. Protein is everywhere! In the next few years, I think the recommendation will be to consume a maximum of half your body weight in grams of protein per day to maintain muscle mass and energy. So, a 200-pound person would need to eat up to 100 grams of protein per day. This becomes a little harder, which is why I love to recommend taking 25 to 50 grams per day of whey protein isolate (powder that only contains protein, no fat or sugar—or only very small amounts of fat and sugar) to improve energy levels. One of my favorites is the Jay Robb brand (it comes in strawberry, vanilla, and chocolate flavors), but there are so many options, so look around.

Low Testosterone

L

Dr. Moyad Secret The number one culprit behind low testosterone (also called low T, male menopause, andropause, or male hypogonadism) in men is weight gain! This is never mentioned in the commercials, though. Overweight men experiencing symptoms of low testosterone should always try to drop pounds first. Some men can become dependent on testosterone drugs and may not be able to produce the hormone naturally again after they come off of them. In other words, the cells in the testicles that produce testosterone could shut down permanently and the testicles could shrink (yikes!). One other reason to be conservative: Testosterone may increase the risk of heart disease (this is controversial, but it's better to be safe than "respiratorially challenged," in other words, dead). Don't get me wrong, testosterone replacement therapy is a great option for some people, but the drug is overprescribed to overweight and obese men. Also important: Men getting a testosterone blood test should get it early in the morning (before 10 a.m.) when levels are at their highest. It is also important to fast for 9 to 12 hours beforehand; recent research shows that eating before the test (which almost every Web site still says is okay) can artificially and dramatically—by as much as 50 percent—lower testosterone values for 1 to 2 hours! Also, testosterone levels should not be measured by a saliva test because they're not always accurate.

Full disclosure: I hate this category of supplements and do not believe they compete with conventional prescription drugs at all, except when it comes to price and in really rare situations where it may only take a slight increase in testosterone to feel better. No supplement has ever come anywhere close to working as well as prescription testosterone, which can boost levels by 200 to 500 ng/dL within days. If a supplement could accomplish an increase of 100 ng/dL over 3 months, it would be universally hailed as a miracle. Unless an abnormally low testosterone level can be raised to a normal range, I'm skeptical that the product works. Keeping a normal testosterone count in the normal range doesn't impress me. This kind of small change can be due to sleep, exercise, and many other reasons that have nothing to do with a pill. The recommended options in this section can increase testosterone by 25 to 50 points, not a big boost at all. So why am I including supplements that lead to such small improvements in this section? Because this category was the largest-selling supplement category on TV last year. The prescription testosterone business is a billion-dollar industry, and the supplement testosterone segment is arguably a billion-dollar industry, too. Testosterone is so overprescribed, but people are desperate for options.

WHAT IS IT?

Testosterone is the male sex hormone. It's just as important for men as estrogen is for women. At puberty, boys experience a sharp rise in testosterone, which helps increase muscle mass, exercise capacity, and the number of red blood cells in the body by 15 to 20 percent (maybe this explains the term *red-blooded male*). It also deepens the voice, increases sex drive, and causes spontaneous erections (those were always interesting, especially when I had to read a book report in front of the class and decided to wear tight pants to school that day—bad move, Moyad!). This is all driven by the brain, of course, which sends a hormone signal (luteinizing hormone or LH) to the testicles to make testosterone. If the signal is disrupted in any way or if the Leydig cells in the testicles, which make testosterone, are damaged, less of the hormone may be produced. Aging, genetics, lifestyle changes (weight gain!), medications, and certain diseases (like diabetes) can reduce testosterone count. However, adding more testosterone to normal "T" levels can increase the risk of stroke.

The symptoms of low testosterone are diverse (see "Low T Q&A," opposite), so a blood test is the easiest way to tell if you have a problem. Depending on your situation, your doctor will usually look at three things in the blood first.

1. Free testosterone or percent-free testosterone (testosterone that's not bound to anything else)

2. Total testosterone (free T plus T bound to two proteins)

3. Bioactive/bioavailable testosterone (free T plus T attached loosely to one protein)

There are numerous other blood tests that may help your doctor decipher the cause of low testosterone, including SHBG (sex hormone-binding globulin) protein level, prolactin, and LH and FSH (follicle-stimulating hormone).

The same concerns and contraindications that apply to prescription testosterone replacements apply to dietary supplements. For example, individuals with prostate enlargement, a history of prostate or breast cancer, or urinary issues or who are at greater risk for prostate cancer should not use these products because testosterone can increase the risk of these cancers and exacerbate urinary and prostate problems. People with a history of liver or kidney problems or breathing issues while sleeping (sleep apnea) are not necessarily good candidates for testosterone replacement either. You'll need regular blood tests to monitor testosterone, cholesterol, hematocrit (red blood cell count), and liver function, even if you're taking a supplement versus a prescription. Finally, testosterone replacement can reduce the size of the scrotum and inhibit mature sperm development, so if you're trying to have a baby, this is not a good option, nor is it a reliable method of birth control! (Men with low T who want to increase it and maintain their fertility should talk to their doctors.)

LOW T Q&A

Low testosterone manifests in many ways, so way back in 2000 a bunch of experts got together to develop a questionnaire known as ADAM (Androgen Deficiency in the Aging Male). But the questionnaire has become synonymous with low-T supplement and drug advertising. In other words, a man will most often see it on a low-T drug or supplement Web site, take it, and then, depending on his answers, ask his doctor about low-T drugs or supplements. My problem with this questionnaire is that it leads men to believe that the answer to all of their problems lies in a dietary supplement or prescription testosterone replacement therapy, when the issue might just be due to aging, lifestyle, or a crazy busy day or week! Also, diet and exercise might easily fix the problem.

Here are the questions:

1. Do you have a decrease in sex drive?
2. Do you have a lack of energy?
3. Do you have a decrease in strength or endurance?
4. Have you lost height?
5. Have you noticed a decrease in your "enjoyment of life"?
6. Are you sad or grumpy?
7. Are your erections less strong?
8. Have you noticed a recent deterioration in your ability to play sports?
9. Are you falling asleep after dinner?
10. Has there been a recent deterioration in your work performance?

If you answer "yes" to question 1 or 7, or any other three questions, you may have low testosterone, according to the questionnaire. However, depending on the hour or day or month, your answers may vary. I personally would answer "yes" to questions 1 and 7 on Monday after a 10-mile run and after eating a large meal, but not on Tuesday after resting! I also could have answered "yes" to questions 3, 6, and 9, depending on the week, while I was writing this book. My point here is that this questionnaire should not make or break the decision to get treatment. I think it's more helpful as a way to bring attention to the problem. By the way, it is possible to have low testosterone and not experience any of the above symptoms.

HOW DO LOW T DRUGS AND SUPPLEMENTS *REALLY* WORK?

There are five primary ways that dietary supplement companies will try to convince consumers that their products increase testosterone. These mechanisms are physiologically possible, but I've yet to see most supplements work anywhere remotely like them. Here's my take on each method, including the benefit-to-risk ratio.

1. By blocking the conversion of testosterone to a more potent form of testosterone known as DHT (dihydrotestosterone). This creates a dam effect so that more testosterone builds up. (Saw palmetto is supposed to work this way, but it does not increase testosterone.)

2. By blocking the conversion of testosterone into estrogen, which also creates a dam effect so that more testosterone builds up. (Fenugreek is supposed to work this way, but I don't believe it has much of an impact.)

3. By providing a compound that is a building block of testosterone that the body then turns into the hormone. (For example, the body produces DHEA, or dehydroepiandrosterone, which gets converted into testosterone. You can buy it as a supplement, but the problem is it can also get converted into estrogen, and which way it goes can't be controlled!)

4. By directly stimulating the Leydig cells in the testicles to produce more testosterone. (The herb tongkat ali, page 304, may do this a little or produce DHEA.)

5. By improving overall mental (mood), sexual, and physical health (by promoting weight loss, improving exercise capacity, and so on), which results in an increase

WHAT WORKS

1. DHEA (dehydroepiandrosterone)
25 to 300 milligrams a day

Note: I cringed when making this my top supplement because it's not only inconsistent in raising testosterone, it also has safety issues. Unfortunately, it has the most favorable clinical research. I do believe that some men who are nervous about prescription testosterone's side effects and cost may want to try this for 3 to 6 months to see if it makes a difference.

DHEA is converted into testosterone in the body, so the thinking is that if you give the body more of the building blocks of the

in testosterone production because there's less stress and other factors that can limit it. (The combination of L-arginine and Pycnogenol or using an L-arginine substitute, such as L-citrulline, can accomplish this.)

Options 1 and 2 are a waste of money and can be dangerous. Researchers have tested the first option with prescription drugs, such as finasteride and dutasteride, but they reduce sex drive and can cause erectile dysfunction. You should also save your money when it comes to a class of drugs called aromatase inhibitors, which block the conversion of testosterone to estrogen (option 2) in women with breast cancer and in men. In males, it can cause general weakness and accelerate bone loss (like women, men need some estrogen for bone health). Recent research published in the *New England Journal of Medicine* demonstrated that men also need a little estrogen to reduce body fat and improve or maintain sexual health. In other words, men need to have some estrogen to keep their masculinity! How interesting is that?

Option 3 can help a little, but only if testosterone is really low, and it can still have side effects (liver problems and reduced good cholesterol levels). It can also lead to increases in estrogen that could cause breast enlargement or pain or an increased risk of breast cancer in some men.

Options 4 and 5 are the Holy Grail for both efficacy and safety reasons. Researchers have not been able to identify a dietary supplement that can actually *perform* option 4, unfortunately. I'm sure it's just a matter of time, though. Option 5 is promising, but it needs to be tested in men with low testosterone and not just in those with normal levels.

hormone, you get more of the hormone. That's generally true, but it's also a building block for estrogen. Small to large quantities (25 to 300 milligrams a day) of this fairly inexpensive dietary supplement can increase a man's testosterone if it's low, but it can also cause liver toxicity and potentially increase estrogen levels, and large increases in estrogen can be problematic. I have watched so many men take this stuff and see only a slight bump in testosterone with very little symptomatic benefit.

In one of the better randomized trials, which was done at the Washington University School of Medicine and published in the *American Journal of Clinical Nutrition*, older men and women took 50 milligrams of DHEA daily for 1 year. By the end, total testosterone in the men had increased from 420 to 491 ng/dL on average, but the placebo group also saw increased T, from 420 to 448. Free testosterone and growth factors also increased, as did estrogen levels. Women in this study saw HDL (good) cholesterol levels drop more than 4 points. A 2-year randomized trial from the Mayo Clinic (published in the *New England Journal of Medicine*) showed no increase in testosterone in men who took 50 milligrams of DHEA daily. And HDL levels dropped 6 points in men and 8 in women.

2. L-arginine aspartate

2,800 milligrams a day and **Pycnogenol** 80 milligrams a day **combined** or **L-citrulline by itself** 1,500 to 3,000 milligrams a day

L-arginine gets turned into nitric oxide in the body, which can increase bloodflow to the penis. It can also stimulate the production of creatine, which body builders use in supplement form to boost strength, and growth hormone. (L-arginine is discussed in detail in the Erectile Dysfunction section, page 186.) What's up with all the Arnold Schwarzenegger talk, you ask? Since L-arginine does many of the same things that testosterone does, such as impact growth hormone and increase muscle strength, some researchers believe it can also increase testosterone. Unfortunately, the conversion of L-arginine into nitric oxide just isn't very efficient; the liver and intestines get rid of most of it, so

higher doses are needed to see a small impact. *However*, when you combine L-arginine with Pycnogenol, the results are much better, and in fact, two well-done clinical trials have found that the combo raised testosterone in men.

One of the studies was a 6-month clinical trial comparing Prelox, the best-selling L-arginine-Pycnogenol combination product, to a placebo. While the main focus was its impact on erectile dysfunction, participants also significantly increased testosterone by almost 75 to 100 points. The dosage of L-arginine was 2,800 milligrams per day and Pycnogenol was 80 milligrams daily. Other trials have revealed some potential safety issues—including increased cardiovascular risk in people with a history of heart attack or peripheral artery disease—when taking L-arginine by itself, so I only recommend the combination product.

L-citrulline—a compound found naturally in watermelon rind—also gets turned into nitric oxide in the body, and that pathway is much more efficient, so you can take smaller dosages (1,500 to 3,000 milligrams per day). The research on L-citrulline and testosterone is ongoing, though, so I'm keeping an eye on it and you should, too; you can speak with your doctor about it.

3. Tongkat ali (*Eurycoma longifolia*)

200 to 300 milligrams a day in divided doses

Many years ago I spent almost 2 weeks in Malaysia speaking to various groups about supplements, and almost every store I walked into was selling this stuff. I also noticed it everywhere when I was in Singapore. This is a dietary supplement (taken from a plant or a common shrub found along the slopes of hilly areas in the Malaysian rainforest) to keep your eyes on because it has preliminary human data showing it might improve various aspects of male health, including sex drive, testosterone levels, and sperm quality—at only 200 to 300 milligrams divided into two daily doses.

The tongkat ali product that has the most research—and the only one with real clinical data—is the standardized, water-soluble extract of *Eurycoma longifolia* root called Physta (manufactured by Biotropics Malaysia). The company's aqueous extract has multiple ingredients—including tannins, high-molecular-weight polysaccharides, glycoprotein mucopolysaccharides, and quassinoid alkaloids—that may play some role in testosterone production. The company is currently funding many clinical studies, and results from the last one showed an increase in testosterone of 76 ng/dL in men with very low testosterone, which is not much, but for a supplement it's as good or better than DHEA. The only problem is that, while it was a well-done study, it did not include a placebo group.

A better study (published in the journal *Evidence-Based Complementary and Alternative Medicine*) followed men who took 300 milligrams daily of either Physta

or a placebo for 12 weeks. The participants reported improved erectile function and libido, but did not increase their testosterone significantly (50 points) compared to the placebo. I believe this supplement can potentially directly stimulate some testosterone production, and I will be keeping my eye on further studies with it. So far, I haven't been able to identify any significant side effects or drug interactions with tongkat ali, which is also referred to as Malaysian ginseng.

I am often asked whether the inexpensive tongkat ali sold in many health food stores is similar to what has been used in the clinical trials, and the truth is that no one knows, but I do not have confidence in them. The Physta product has batch-to-batch consistency and quality control studies, which basically means I trust this company more than other suppliers of tongkat ali.

WHAT'S WORTHLESS

Tribulus terrestris. This has to be one of the most overhyped dietary supplements for raising testosterone that I have ever come across in my career. Tribulus contains a compound called protodioscin that, along with other ingredients, is supposed to act like DHEA. This sounds good in theory, but the research—and my experience with it—hasn't panned out. It's a dud, in other words. One Australian study with rugby players found no increase in testosterone with it.

305

POTENTIAL "T" BUSTERS

All of the following can reduce testosterone either in the long or short term (which could potentially impact a blood test).

- Alcohol in excess (three or more drinks a day) can cause weight gain, increase estrogen levels in men, and negatively impact cells that produce testosterone.

- Abnormally low cholesterol levels—LDLs between 20 to 50 mg/dL—(which can happen with statin overuse) can decrease testosterone because cholesterol is needed to make the hormone. But that's not to say high cholesterol makes for more testosterone! Keep your LDLs in the Moyad range (100 or below).

- Diabetes or prediabetes can impact testosterone because insulin resistance and weight gain lower testosterone production.

- Eating—especially foods containing sugar—can create insulin spikes, which can dramatically lower testosterone in some men for up to several hours, which is why I generally recommend fasting before getting a blood test for testosterone.

Fenugreek. This is a popular ingredient in testosterone-enhancing supplements, and there's some research to suggest it can increase testosterone by itself or when combined with other supplements, but the research has not been consistent. "Experts" claim fenugreek works by blocking the enzyme aromatase, which converts testosterone into estrogen. I don't believe it, but if it really does this, I don't recommend it anyway because, as I mentioned earlier, men need some estrogen to support their bones (and even sex drive). Without it, they can experience accelerated bone loss, as seen with drugs called aromatase inhibitors. I find it interesting that fenugreek used to be sold as a female breast enlargement supplement and is used in some areas of the world to improve breast milk production! And now somehow it's a magical product for testosterone? One of the best studies to look at fenugreek actually found it significantly *lowered* free testosterone levels in healthy men compared to the placebo group.

Zinc. There are so many "experts"

- HIV infection and especially the drugs used for treatment involve metabolic changes, including weight gain, that can commonly lead to low testosterone.

- Lack of regular exercise (aerobic and resistance training) can lead to increased weight gain and reduced testosterone levels. Both cardio and resistance training are key for weight management. Strength training using the largest muscle groups—legs, butt, back, chest, and abs—increases testosterone for 1 to 2 hours post-workout. In other words, a squat releases more testosterone (temporarily) than a biceps curl will. However, excessive exercise can temporarily reduce testosterone levels. Regular aerobic exercise (along with strength training) helps keep weight normal, which allows for healthy testosterone production.

- Pain medications (especially prescription opioids) can substantially reduce testosterone levels.

- Lack of sleep—getting just 5 hours a night, for example—can reduce testosterone by 10 percent or more.

- Weight gain has the biggest negative impact on testosterone.

who continue to support the idea that zinc increases testosterone levels. The truth is that there may be a small benefit, but this really only applies to those individuals who are profoundly deficient in zinc, which is rare today. However, the so-called experts will take results with a very specific population, such as people with chronic kidney disease, and try to say oral zinc will raise testosterone for all men. Don't believe it!

D-aspartic acid. This amino acid is advertised as being able to promote higher testosterone levels, but based on my experience and a recent study, I'm skeptical.

Saw palmetto. Simply put, the largest randomized studies ever done with saw palmetto showed no increase in testosterone. (Please refer to the Benign Prostatic Hyperplasia section, page 98, for more information.)

Panax ginseng. Sorry, it may help with erectile function, but researchers haven't seen any consistent increase in testosterone in clinical trials.

Miscellaneous. Here are some other

supplements that just don't have adequate evidence.

- Boron (this particular supplement should get more research)
- Cordyceps
- Potency wood
- Truffles
- Vitamin D
- Wild oats
- Wild yam
- Yohimbe

LIFESTYLE CHANGES

Heart healthy = testosterone healthy. Again, excess weight is a huge cause of reduced testosterone. Exercising and eating a healthy diet will help you control your weight and will improve your cardiovascular disease risk. Here's some scary info: Obese male teenagers appear to have 25 to 50 percent less testosterone than their healthy-weight peers. This is stunning research because in the past it was thought that it took time for weight gain to impact testosterone production, but these newer studies with children clearly show that teens are just as vulnerable as older adults.

Lung Cancer

THE JURY'S STILL OUT

Dr. Moyad Secret Former and current smokers should avoid beta-carotene supplements because they could increase the risk of lung cancer, according to the large CARET, ATBC, and AREDS 2 trials. If you're being treated for lung cancer, stay away from these supplements. In addition, selenium supplements do not prevent the recurrence of lung cancer, and they may increase the risk of it returning. Here is a classic example of individualizing how we "prescribe" supplements, just like we do with drugs; some supplements may be very good for a condition, but not for every person with that condition. Lung cancer prevention and treatment with supplements is a case of less is more—and more is really bad for you!

Lupus

Dr. Moyad Secret Lupus is a chronic autoimmune disease that primarily affects women, but it also carries a higher risk of cardiovascular disease (CVD) due to the chronic inflammation that occurs. In fact, CVD is the number one cause of death in lupus patients, so they should try to reduce their CVD risk factors by lowering cholesterol, blood pressure, and blood glucose through lifestyle changes. New research has found that weight loss can significantly reduce fatigue in lupus patients—even those on steroids. It's been suggested that low vitamin D levels contribute to the risk of CVD, especially in lupus patients, but I think it's far more important to reduce your traditional CVD risk factors than to rely on this vitamin D theory. Normalizing vitamin D is a good idea for general bone health, but not for improving CVD risk. Lupus also causes inflammation of the kidneys (called lupus nephritis).

NAC (N-acetylcysteine). Taking 1,800 milligrams per day may reduce protein levels in people with lupus nephritis, but a larger trial is needed. (Protein in the urine, especially high amounts, is an indicator of disease severity and progression.)

Turmeric. It's showing up in clinical trials in lupus nephritis patients, and it can potentially lower protein and blood levels in the urine at dosages of 500 milligrams three times a day with meals (each dose contains at least 22 milligrams of the active ingredient curcumin). Turmeric does have anti-inflammatory potential, but I don't know if it will be enough to help with this condition.

Fish oil. Taking 3 grams, or 3,000 milligrams, per day appeared to slow disease activity and may reduce heart disease risk factors, according to a 24-week trial from Ireland, but unfortunately these results haven't been confirmed yet in further studies.

WHAT'S WORTHLESS

DHEA (dehydroepiandrosterone). This hormone-precursor to estrogen and testosterone had some initial excitement about its potential to improve fatigue and quality of life and reduce bone loss in lupus patients, but randomized trials of 200 milligrams or more have now failed to show a benefit. It has also lowered good cholesterol (HDL) in studies, which is another reason I'm generally not a fan of it.

Macular Degeneration

Dr. Moyad Secret A primary treatment for intermediate to advanced (a.k.a. late) stages of age-related macular degeneration (AMD) includes dietary supplements, and these supplements have the ability to prevent some individuals with AMD from losing their vision! However, 8 out of 10 people are either taking the wrong dose or shouldn't be taking the supplement at all, according to some research. Two surprising factors that determine which supplements are safe to try are smoking status and history of urologic problems, and both of these will be discussed in more detail. If you're worried about AMD, get a dilated eye exam—it could save your vision.

Individuals with intermediate to advanced stages of dry (geographic atrophy) and wet (neovascular) AMD are now candidates for the AREDS 2 supplement (Moyad #1 recommendation) and AREDS 1 (Moyad #2 recommendation). This represents one of the most dramatic clinical findings for a supplement in the history of medicine because of the potential of these pills to now prevent vision loss.

WHAT IS IT?

AMD is the primary cause of blindness in adults 55 and older worldwide; in the United States, it's responsible for 50 percent of all vision loss. It's caused by the deterioration of the central portion of the retina (also known as the macula), which is responsible for seeing what is directly in front of you (near or far) and also detailed vision and color perception. More than one-third of individuals over age 75 have AMD, which can take two forms: The "dry" type (80 to 90 percent of all cases) occurs when cells in the macula break down slowly and gradually blur central vision. The wet (a.k.a neovascular) form occurs when an abnormal overgrowth of blood vessels leaks blood and fluid at the back of the eye, leading to a loss of central vision. It is less common but more frequently results in profound vision loss.

Major risk factors for AMD include family history, smoking, advanced age, hypertension, and low macular pigment (it protects the eye from damaging rays), but other factors include a poor diet, obesity, unprotected exposure to the sun, and light-colored skin or eyes. (The color of your iris is not the same as your macular pigment.)

There really aren't any symptoms in the early stages of macular degeneration, but an ophthalmologist will be able to spot small, yellowish metabolic waste deposits known as drusen during an eye exam (all the more reason to get regular

311

exams). As the disease progresses, there are large areas of retinal pigment epithelial cell loss, which leads to central vision decline. So, the first noticeable symptoms don't occur until later in the disease process, and these include blurring of central vision; visual distortion; lines that appear wavy (for example, even telephone poles can appear crooked) or are missing; and difficulty reading, driving, and recognizing faces. The Amsler grid (page 313) is part of a basic eye exam that you'll get at your doctor's office (or you can do it at home). If the lines are wavy or missing, you might have AMD.

WHAT WORKS

Note: You'll notice that my recommendations for this condition are a combination of vitamins and minerals. This is because the best research on AMD centers around two landmark studies that tested specific formulations of several vitamins and minerals. These studies were called the Age-Related Eye Disease Study (or AREDS) 1 and 2. All three recommendations (including the Honorable Mention) should be taken with meals to reduce side effects, such as stomachache, and improve absorption. The supplements that have worked in AREDS 1 and 2 have only benefited those with intermediate to advanced AMD.

FOR CURRENT, FORMER, AND NEVER SMOKERS

1. Combination product (you can buy this exact mixture or something close to it from many companies)

500 milligrams vitamin C (as ascorbic acid)

400 IU vitamin E (as dl-alpha-tocopheryl acetate)

80 milligrams zinc (as zinc oxide)

2 milligrams copper (as cupric oxide, to prevent potential anemia from the high intake of zinc)

10 milligrams lutein (water-soluble triglyceride form)

2 milligrams zeaxanthin (water-soluble triglyceride form)

This formula came out of the AREDS 2 study, and, as with the first study, it's been shown to potentially slow the progression of macular degeneration, especially the intermediate to advanced forms. AREDS 2 was a very complicated but wonderful clinical trial that replaced beta-carotene with the carotenoids lutein and zeaxanthin, and it found that they were safer than and perhaps as effective as beta-carotene. The result: A formula that's better for current and former smokers. The other interesting observation was that the 80-milligram dose of zinc *may* have worked better than a lower dose (25 milligrams) tested in this study. Keep in mind that almost all of the participants in AREDS 2 also took a

(continued on page 314)

AMSLER GRID

If you usually wear reading glasses, put them on to take this test.
 Instructions:

1. Hold the grid approximately 12-14 inches from your face.

2. Using only your left eye (with your right eye closed), look at the dot in the center of the grid and make sure you can see the whole grid.

3. If any of the lines on the grid look blury, distorted, or are missing, write down exactly what you see.

4. Repeat with your right eye (keeping your left eye closed this time).

5. Share any abnormalities with your eye doctor.

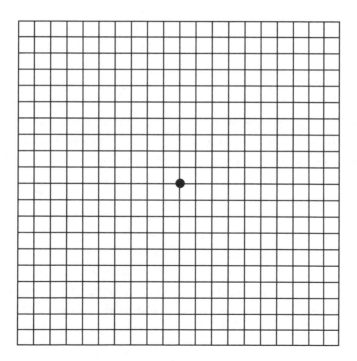

Centrum Silver, which I also recommend. Ask your doctor whether you should be taking the formulation on page 312 or a modified version with less zinc (25 milligrams).

FOR NEVER SMOKERS

2. Combination product

15 milligrams beta-carotene

500 milligrams vitamin C (as ascorbic acid)

400 IU vitamin E (as dl-alpha-tocopheryl acetate)

80 milligrams zinc (as zinc oxide)

2 milligrams copper (as cupric oxide, to prevent potential anemia from the high intake of zinc)

This formula (in a specific Bausch & Lomb formulation sold as PreserVision Eye Vitamin and Mineral Supplement) was used in the AREDS 1 study, and it has been shown to slow the progression of age-related macular degeneration, especially in those with intermediate to advanced AMD. It reduced the risk of progression to advanced AMD by 25 percent, and it reduced the risk of moderate vision loss by 19 percent. It's *only* for people who have never smoked. Former or current smokers should *not* take it because beta-carotene in supplement form (it's okay in food) can increase the risk of lung cancer in individuals with a smoking history. It has not been shown to restore vision loss, prevent AMD, or help people in the earliest stages.

When the retina absorbs light, as it does day in and day out, it also produces free radicals, which cause cellular damage over time. But certain nutrients, like those listed above, can reduce exposure of the retina to these and other harmful particles. If antioxidants from food or supplements have an impact anywhere in the human body, it seems that the eye is one of the best places to study this effect, especially the retina, because it is very susceptible to damage as we get older. The researchers didn't study the effect of each individual supplement on the eye, only the combination. However, the trial did show that even patients with adequate healthy diets could benefit from this supplement combination.

There were some significant side effects of this formula, though: The dose of zinc was linked with a higher risk of yellowing of the skin and a higher risk of being hospitalized from genitourinary problems, such as prostate enlargement, urinary tract infections, and kidney stones (this was compared to the formula without zinc). In all fairness, other eye health studies, including AREDS 2, have not found this risk to be serious, and if the trade-off is preserving your vision, it might be worth it. In addition, while it wasn't looked at in the AREDS studies, taking 400 IU of vitamin E daily has been found to increase the risk of prostate cancer. And former and current smokers or anyone who's been exposed to asbestos should not take beta-carotene supplements because they increase the risk of lung cancer. What it boils down to is this: Ask your doctor whether you should be taking the formulation on page 314 or a modified version with less zinc (25 milligrams). Keep in mind that almost every participant took a Centrum multivitamin in addition to the formula, which I also recommend.

HONORABLE MENTION

FOR CURRENT, FORMER, AND NEVER SMOKERS

Lutein (10 milligrams a day) **and zeaxanthin** (2 milligrams a day) may be beneficial in preventing AMD or keeping it from progressing past the early stages. It's also a viable option for people who may be concerned about taking large doses of zinc or vitamin E. The high concentration of lutein and zeaxanthin, known as carotenoids, in the macula gives it a yellowish color (the Latin word for yellow is *luteus*, and the Latin word for Moyad is *Moyad*). Where do you think that yellow color in egg yolks comes from? Yup, lutein! The two supplements work as photoprotectants, meaning they help filter or absorb potentially damaging light rays as they enter the eye. The body cannot make lutein or zeaxanthin, so they must come from diet or supplements. Manufacturers only recently developed the ability to make them, otherwise this duo probably would have been used in the original AREDS study. So, the idea here is simple: If you can increase the macular pigment of the eye with lutein and zeaxanthin, then you can reduce the risk of age-related eye disease, but this still needs some more research.

You can increase absorption by taking these with a meal that has some fat in it. Naturally then, any medications that block the absorption of fat (such as the weight loss drug Orlistat) may reduce absorption of lutein and zeaxanthin. Do not take these supplements when pregnant or breastfeeding because this has not been studied.

Be warned that lutein can cause yellowing of the skin (this is called bananadermosis—just kidding, it's called carotenodermia). It's harmless and temporary and should go away when blood levels of the carotenoids drop. Before supplementing with lutein and zeaxanthin, work with your eye doctor to determine if you even need it. He'll check your macular pigment optical density (the greater the concentration of lutein and zeaxanthin, the lower the potential risk of AMD) and then track it over 6 to 12 months with the supplements to see if there's any improvement.

WHAT'S WORTHLESS

Beta-carotene supplements for anyone with a history of smoking. They have been found to increase the risk of lung cancer in former and current smokers in three major clinical trials. The beta-carotene you get in foods like sweet potatoes, kale, spinach, and carrots is safe, though.

Omega-3 fatty acids. When these omega-3s were added (1,000 milligrams per day) to the AREDS 2 formula, they failed to slow the progression of AMD. Sorry, folks! They can help with dry eye (see the Dry Eye section, page 181), though.

But, eating two servings of omega-3-rich fish per week (like salmon, sardines, anchovies, mackerel, halibut, trout, whitefish, and tuna) and using plant-based cooking oils, walnuts, flaxseed, and chia seeds *might* work to help prevent AMD because the compounds may be better assimilated as part of a varied nutrient-rich diet than supplements are.

Blueberry extract (or *any* berry extract). I've never seen them work, and they have not had adequate testing for AMD, so stick with getting berries the old-fashioned way because there *may* be some benefit to berries in their whole, natural form due to other compounds yet to be discovered. In fact, whole blueberries are getting a lot of research attention, and these studies seem to suggest that they may lower the risk of eye diseases, including AMD, and other berries are also being studied.

Astaxanthin. This carotenoid (it contributes to the red color of cooked shellfish and salmon) is being studied and getting a lot of hype, but I believe it will end up being one of the most overrated supplements of my time! It has been combined with lutein and zeaxanthin in a few studies, but I don't see how the results are any better than those with lutein or zeaxanthin by themselves—or couldn't be improved simply by changing the dose of lutein and zeaxanthin.

Vitamin A. This is a fabulous eye health supplement, but the amount found in most low-dose multivitamins and in food is outstanding. In other words, you don't need a special supplement.

Vitamin D. I believe any relationship between higher vitamin D blood levels and lower risk of AMD has more to do with weight than anything else. As you gain weight, your vitamin D level goes down and your risk of eye disease goes up. When you lose weight, vitamin D in the blood rises and your AMD risk drops. In other words, vitamin D supplements are getting way too much credit!

LIFESTYLE CHANGES

Heart healthy = eye healthy. Normal cholesterol, blood pressure, and blood sugar levels are all associated with a lower risk of AMD, as is exercise. I hope you are sitting down for this one: Some recent studies are showing up to 70 *percent* reductions in AMD in people with better diets who exercise and don't smoke. Those who are obese have twice the risk of developing more advanced macular degeneration than normal-weight people do. It is also interesting that lower levels of inflammatory blood markers, such as CRP (C-reactive protein), are also associated with a lower risk of AMD.

Quit smoking. Smoking is the undisputed major risk factor for AMD, and it has been found to increase the progression of AMD to the more advanced stages.

Wear shades. Sunglasses appear to reduce the risk of AMD, according to several studies. Look for a pair that blocks UVA and UVB light.

Add eye-boosting nutrients. Multiple studies have suggested that getting more lutein and zeaxanthin from food (6 milligrams or higher total) has been

FOODS HIGH IN LUTEIN AND ZEAXANTHIN

FOOD SOURCE	APPROXIMATE LUTEIN AND ZEAXANTHIN AMOUNT (MG PER SINGLE SERVING)
Kale (1 cup cooked or raw)	20 to 24
Spinach ($\frac{1}{2}$ cup cooked)	15 to 20
Lettuce (1 cup raw)	2.5 to 3
Broccoli ($\frac{1}{2}$ cup cooked)	2.2 to 2.5
Sweet corn ($\frac{1}{2}$ cup cooked)	1.5 to 2
Green peas ($\frac{1}{2}$ cup cooked)	1 to 1.5
Brussels sprouts ($\frac{1}{2}$ cup cooked)	1 to 1.3
Egg yolk (one yolk)	0.5 (actually one of the best sources because absorption is so efficient)
White cabbage (1 cup raw)	0.3 to 0.5

Note: Other respectable sources of lutein and zeaxanthin include arugula, basil, collard greens, parsley, radicchio, and watercress.

associated with a lower risk of cataracts and AMD. The foods in the table above contain high quantities of both nutrients (they're usually found together).

WHAT ELSE DO I NEED TO KNOW?

- The prescription drugs for the less common "wet" form of AMD are fabulous but also more expensive than gold. One effective option is ranibizumab (Lucentis), but it can cost $2,000 per injection! Another drug, bevacizumab (Avastin), is FDA approved for treating cancer and has a similar structure to Lucentis, but it costs just $50 per injection. They had equivalent results in a head-to-head study for wet AMD, yet there was an unexplained increase in the number of people on Avastin who experienced infections and stomach disorders that required hospitalization. Regardless, it's worth asking your doctor about them.

- Folic acid and vitamins B_{12} and B_6 are currently being studied for their ability to slow the progression of AMD, and honestly, this caught a lot of experts off guard, including me! A large Harvard study was evaluating whether high dosages of these vitamins can lower the risk of cardiovascular disease but failed to find a connection. However, in the process, the researchers discovered that the supplements appeared to reduce the risk of AMD or the progression of the disease in earlier stages. Remember, there are no supplements that have been proven to do this yet. But, as is often the case, more research needs to be done since this was not an AMD or eye-related study.

Memory Loss

Dr. Moyad Secret How is your hippocampus today? This funny-sounding yet very important structure deep in your brain is your memory center, and it's very vulnerable. When it thins (atrophies), it may lead to memory loss, mild cognitive impairment (MCI, a kind of pre-dementia), and possibly even Alzheimer's. So being good to your hippocampus is important. As we get older, the hippocampus shrinks, and it appears that obesity, diabetes, brain injury, sleep apnea, depression, and many other factors contribute to the shrinkage. Yet exercise and other heart-healthy behaviors as well as mental stimulation could make it grow! Some supplements may be able to protect your hippocampus from shrinking, but there isn't a single pill out there right now that works better than making aggressive heart-healthy changes. The combination, however, has the potential to prevent memory loss. (Please also see the Alzheimer's Disease, Dementia, and Mild Cognitive Impairment section, page 65.)

WHAT IS IT?

The memory issues that someone with MCI or dementia experience are usually chronic and very noticeable to others, while the memory loss discussed in this section is the type that is occasional and more subjective. It's forgetting where you put your keys, the name of your neighbor, or your doctor's appointment. Most people experience these lapses as they get older, and some might have them more frequently or to a larger degree than others. Aging is the primary culprit, but medications, a heart-unhealthy lifestyle, alcohol abuse, depression, head trauma, genetics/family history, illness, low thyroid levels, HIV infection, and many as yet unknown factors can contribute to it. Even if you always know where your keys are, you can probably still benefit from reading this section!

WHAT WORKS

1. (tie) *Bacopa monnieri* (Brahmi or bacopa) 300 milligrams a day

This is an alternative Ayurvedic medicine that in preliminary clinical trials reduced stress and anxiety better than a placebo. Although this plant has been used in India and Pakistan for various ailments (especially related to the lungs and vascular system), the real focus lately has been on its potential for memory enhancement.

Many of the components of bacopa were isolated years ago and include alkaloids, saponins, sterols, bacopa saponins, and bacosides. The bacosides appear to be involved in nerve cell repair, production, and signaling, and they also appear to have some antioxidant benefit in different areas of the brain, including the hippocampus, frontal cortex, and striatum. The specific compounds garnering attention and research for their effect on the brain are bacosides A and B.

In one 12-week trial, a 300-milligram daily dose (55 percent combined bacosides, meaning a combo of A and B) resulted in a significant improvement in memory, learning, and speed of information processing. The results were observed in the latter weeks of the study, suggesting it needs to be taken long term to potentially see a change; no benefits have been seen in studies lasting fewer than 12 weeks. In a study published in the *Journal of Alternative and Complementary Medicine*, Australian researchers reviewed six clinical studies and found that bacopa extract at 300 to 450 milligrams per day (containing 40 to 55 percent bacoside content) appeared to improve memory, but not other areas of cognition. (Always look for a product that has been standardized to a minimum of 25 percent bacoside A or ideally 50 percent bacosides.)

There are two products that have an impressive history of clinical studies and quality control. The first is BacoMind, which is an alcoholic extract of bacopa (20:1 herb-to-extract ratio) and one of the only bacopa products to be tested in older adults *and* children. At 225 milligrams

twice a day, researchers found significant improvements in short-term and long-term memory in older adults and in kids (225 milligrams once per day) there was a significant improvement in working and logical memory, as well as memory as it relates to personal life. The other is Keen-Mind (also known as CDRI 08), another bacopa extract product that appears to help improve the processing and storing of new information. (It's standardized to a minimum of 55 percent total bacosides and is extracted with 50 percent ethanol.)

The most common side effect of bacopa, especially at higher doses, is mild gastrointestinal upset, such as abdominal cramps, increased stool frequency, and nausea, so take it with a meal.

1. (tie) Panax ginseng (extract G115) or Korean red ginseng 200 to 400 milligrams a day

The primary active ingredients in ginseng are ginsenosides, and there are seven main ones found in many dietary supplements: Rb1, Rb2, Rc, Rd, Re, Rf, and Rg1. Some of them have shown an ability in the laboratory to reduce levels of a compound called amyloid beta peptide, which is found in the brains of patients with Alzheimer's. Ginsenosides can also reduce the production of some inflammatory compounds and improve bloodflow. One trial using 4,500 milligrams of Panax ginseng per day (ginsenoside content of about 8 to 8.5 percent) showed cognitive improvements within 12 weeks that were significantly better than a placebo. A smaller trial with Korean red ginseng found that 9,000 milligrams per day over 12 weeks worked better than 4,500 milligrams to improve cognition in Alzheimer's patients.

Although these doses would be appropriate for patients with MCI or Alzheimer's, I would never recommend such high amounts for healthy individuals who just want to improve memory; I just included them to make a point. At least five randomized trials (from a meta-analysis published in the *Cochrane Database of Systematic Reviews*) have found improvements in cognitive function with low daily doses of ginseng—200 to 400 milligrams. Many of the trials were done with a product called G115 from Pharmaton (a.k.a. Ginsana), a 4 percent ginsenoside extract. The quality control with this product is very good, which is another reason I like it. Gastrointestinal side effects are rare, but you should still take it with food to minimize them. Also, in my experience this supplement can increase energy levels and reduce fatigue (this was demonstrated in a large Mayo Clinic clinical trial with cancer patients), so taking it in the late afternoon or evening could disrupt sleep.

2. Huperzine A (*Huperzia serrata*)
50 to 100 micrograms a day

Derived from club moss (a well-known Chinese herb), huperzine A is used to treat Alzheimer's disease in China and other countries. More studies are needed, but there have been at least 20 randomized clinical trials with this herb, so it's worth looking at. Researchers believe it works in a variety of ways, including increasing acetylcholine levels in the brain, which is also how some of the prescription drugs for Alzheimer's and MCI work (that's why it's been called a natural cholinesterase inhibitor), and improving bloodflow to areas of the brain that impact memory (reduced bloodflow is a leading cause of dementia). Preliminary results in clinical studies (both in China and the United States) suggest that at dosages of up to 400 micrograms per day it can improve mental health, including memory, and other symptoms of Alzheimer's.

Huperzine A has also been used in a combination supplement in some preliminary trials looking at former NFL players with brain injury and cognitive impairment. It appeared to increase bloodflow to specific areas of the brain, but whether this leads to an improvement in memory needs more study. Regardless, memory loss is becoming an epidemic in former football players, and since there are very few treatment options, this is one (along with others in this section) that needs more attention. Now, the clinical evidence compared to bacopa and ginseng is much weaker, but since it has a track record with dementia, it's possible that small amounts of this product (50 to 100 micrograms per day) over time could improve memory in people who have had some noticeable memory loss, or up to 200 micrograms for those who have been diagnosed with MCI or dementia.

Side effects in clinical trials were low, but nausea, dizziness, gastrointestinal symptoms, headaches, and reduced heart rate have been reported. Drug interactions are not well known, so this may be a supplement to watch instead of try until more research is conducted. This herb should not be combined with FDA-approved cholinesterase inhibitors (donepezil, galantamine, rivastigmine) because the side effects in combination could be serious.

WHAT'S WORTHLESS

Ginkgo biloba (also known as EGb 761 in Europe). I know ginkgo is prescribed in some parts of the world to help preserve memory, but I'm skeptical for a couple of reasons. First, there are serious quality-control issues with it. And second, as the clinical trials have become more rigorous, the results with ginkgo have become less impressive. The largest US study of this supplement, called the Ginkgo Evaluation of Memory (GEM) trial, looked at whether ginkgo could reduce the risk of Alzheimer's in elderly patients with either normal cognition or MCI. The researchers found *no* impact despite using one of the finest ginkgo products available in terms of quality control and research. What they did notice is that the ginkgo group had *twice* the number of hemorrhagic strokes. Even though this was not statistically significant, it emphasizes a point about this supplement that definitely worries me: It has extreme blood-thinning potential. Researchers saw similar results (including the increased incidence of strokes and no impact on memory) in the second-largest

ginkgo and memory study, known as GuidAge, which was an Alzheimer's prevention study.

Phosphatidylserine and phosphatidylcholine. These tongue twisters are fatty compounds found naturally in cell membranes, especially in the brain. Lots of "experts" recommend these supplements for improving memory or cognitive function, but based on my experience and the lack of good research, I say save your money. (Choline, which is a primary component of phosphatidylcholine, is essential for brain development, but supplementation beyond diet has not been effective.)

High doses of B vitamins. These actually made depression worse in patients with Alzheimer's in the large Alzheimer's Disease Cooperative Study (published in the *Journal of the American Medical Association*). Researchers tested 5 milligrams of folic acid, 25 milligrams of vitamin B_6, and 1 milligram of vitamin B_{12} over 18 months and found that the combination reduced a blood marker called homocysteine that had been associated with cognitive decline (when it's at high levels). However, this is a case where improving the blood test results doesn't necessarily translate to improving the actual symptoms (the homocysteine levels dropped, but researchers didn't see any cognitive improvement). It was also concerning that almost 28 percent of patients in the B-vitamin group experienced depression, compared to 18 percent who took a placebo. If it has no hint that it helped, and even made things worse, with

Alzheimer's patients, I can't get excited about it for memory loss.

Vinpocetine. This extract from the periwinkle plant increases bloodflow to the brain, which could be helpful, but there is no adequate research that the supplement by itself improves memory. It's begging for more research, though.

LIFESTYLE CHANGES

Heart healthy = memory healthy. Almost anything that has been found to reduce the risk of cardiovascular disease (exercising and maintaining normal cholesterol, blood sugar, and blood pressure levels and a healthy weight) can also help lower the risk of memory loss. A leading cause of dementia is reduced bloodflow to the brain, so lowering your stroke risk is hugely important in preventing vascular dementia.

Find the right protein, fat, and carb balance. New studies are suggesting that a diet high in lean protein and healthy fats may protect against MCI, while a high-carbohydrate diet may promote it. I think what's really going on is that people who have problems controlling their blood sugar, such as those with prediabetes and diabetes, may have a greater risk of memory loss in general. There is a theory that the brain may experience its own diabetes-like condition, where its ability to absorb sugar (your noggin's number one fuel source) is compromised, increasing the risk of memory problems.

Be more active. New exercise studies demonstrate that as you lose weight, you also experience dramatic changes in bloodflow to the brain and improvements in cognition. Research has shown that aerobic exercise actually expands the hippocampus and staves off the shrinking seen with age (it typically shrivels by 1 to 2 percent per year). A 1-year study of non-exercisers versus more active people found that the couch potatoes had a 1.4 percent reduction in hippocampus size. The walking group, who hoofed it for 40 minutes 3 days a week, increased hippocampus size by 2 percent! The walkers with the biggest boost in hippocampus size also had the best rise in test scores. And here's a case where more *is* better: More intense or frequent exercise appears to have even more profound effects on hippocampus size (a 10 percent size difference). Of course, exercise also reduces depression, stress, and anxiety, which is also good for memory.

Flex your mental muscles. Cognitively demanding exercises—such as crossword puzzles, Sudoku, playing cards, and reading—appear to reduce the risk of memory loss for some people. Activities that challenge the mind also help strengthen and protect it. In fact, that "use it or lose it" saying was initially coined in this area of research.

Take time to de-stress. Chronic stress can increase the amount of stress steroids produced in the body, which can block brain activity and may increase the risk of memory loss. Whether this turns out to be true is not so much the issue because it is already known that chronic stress is damaging to the human body in general, so you should minimize it as much as possible.

Java up. Caffeine is your friend—in moderation. It stimulates a variety of areas in the brain, including memory centers, and protects the hippocampus from damage that can be caused by stress or aging. We usually only hear about the dangers of ingesting massive amounts of caffeine; it just never gets the credit it deserves.

WHAT ELSE DO I NEED TO KNOW?

Because there are so many causes of memory loss, it is important to see your doctor or a specialist if you've noticed consistent memory problems. Some are easily fixed, and some can result in permanent losses if untreated. Here's a partial list of potential causes.

Alcohol abuse

Cholesterol (too high or too low)

Chronic renal failure

Depression

Diabetes

Head injury

HIV infection

Hydrocephalus

Hypertension

Hypothyroidism

Medication side effects

Obesity

Syphilis (untreated)

Testosterone deficiency

Tobacco use

Vitamin B_1 and/or B_{12} deficiency (get tested)

Migraine

Dr. Moyad Secret Migraine drugs are expensive and potentially toxic, but people who get these debilitating headaches are desperate for anything that can help. No supplement can reverse a migraine once it has started, but some can help *prevent* migraines or reduce the number, intensity, or frequency of attacks. More and more doctors are becoming aware of how supplements can help migraines. And in some cases, they're part of the standard treatment protocol (per the American Academy of Neurology, or AAN), which is very exciting and one of the reasons I love the world of dietary supplements, because when handled appropriately, they can really improve someone's life!

WHAT IS IT?

A migraine is an intense, one-sided, throbbing headache that often recurs and is usually accompanied or preceded by sensory changes and other physiological symptoms. Scientists haven't pinpointed the exact cause of migraines yet, but they involve vascular and neurological changes in the brain. Some speculate that these headaches may be caused by an overactive "switch" in the brain that triggers the release of compounds that can cause significant pain. Researchers believe there may also be an inflammatory element to migraines. They're often triggered by stress, hormonal fluctuations, weather changes, and food (see page 329 for a list of common triggers). What's more, an amazing 70 percent of migraine sufferers have a family history of these headaches, so there could be a genetic link.

Common symptoms include throbbing head pain that is incapacitating; sensitivity to light, sounds, and smells; nausea and vomiting; runny or stuffy nose; eye tearing; and vision changes. Movement often makes the pain worse, so many people prefer to rest in a quiet, dark room until the headache subsides. About 20 percent of migraine sufferers experience "auras"—visual changes such as flashes, zigzags, splotches, shimmering colored lights, or even blind spots—before or during a migraine. (Some studies have shown that people who experience migraines with auras have a higher risk of stroke, and this is an active area of research.)

WHAT WORKS

Note: Do not use the supplements here in combination, and give whichever one you're trying at least 3 months to see a difference.

1. Butterbur (*Petasites hybridus*) up to 75 milligrams twice a day

This plant, which grows in wet marshy areas, contains chemicals called petasites (petasin and isopetasin) that may have anti-inflammatory properties. Taking 75-milligram dose of butterbur (the Petadolex brand has the most research) has been shown to reduce the frequency of migraine attacks by about half (start with this dose and slowly work up, if necessary, to a max of 150 milligrams per day). The maximum response was achieved after 3 months with a product that contained at least 15 percent petasins (always look for this on the label). Mild gastrointestinal upset, especially burping, was the most common side effect reported.

I gave this herbal supplement a high ranking for three reasons: First, the quality of evidence backing it is better than it is for the other suggestions here. Second, it can be standardized to an active ingredient. Finally, the AAN and the American Headache Society now consider this a Level A recommendation, meaning it has more evidence for prevention than any other supplement. This means you can go to the store and buy a product that contains the exact ingredient researchers studied in the clinical trials, which isn't always the case when it comes to herbal products. Butterbur also has a positive clinical history of helping with another inflammatory condition, allergies. In other words, it has a fairly long track record of efficacy and safety in multiple areas of medicine.

Cautionary notes: Butterbur contains dangerous compounds known as pyrrolizidine alkaloids (PA), which are toxic to the liver and lungs and increase the risk of blood clots, but these are supposed to be removed in commercial supplements. Regardless, make sure you purchase only butterbur supplements that are certified and labeled "PA-free." Additionally, pregnant women should not use butterbur because its effects on the fetus are unknown. Also, never consume this plant in any other form (in other words, don't go foraging for the plant and make a tea out of it).

2. Vitamin B_2 (riboflavin) 25 to 400 milligrams a day

Most conventional medical treatment guidelines recommend this vitamin as an option for migraine prevention. In one study, 56 percent of participants who took 25 to 400 milligrams of B_2 per day for a 3-month period cut their migraine frequency in half. Researchers believe the vitamin may speed up brain metabolism by improving how cells use oxygen, which enhances normal brain function. There is a low rate of side effects, but diarrhea, stomachache, and increased urination have been reported. (Don't be alarmed if your urine turns fluorescent yellow—it's harmless.) Always take vitamin B_2 by itself—never in a multivitamin or B-complex supplement—so you don't ingest a toxic dose of other vitamins in the process. Most treatment guidelines recommend aiming for 400 milligrams per day (either all at once or divided into two or three doses) for 3 months, but research has shown taking as little as 25 milligrams per day can be beneficial. Just increase the amount gradually if you don't get relief.

Now, is B$_2$ a groundbreaking preventive treatment? No. The evidence is good, not amazing, but since the cost and side effects are so low, it makes sense to recommend it.

3. Magnesium 300 to 600 milligrams a day

A deficiency of this mineral can trigger migraines. When magnesium is low, the body generates a compound called substance P, which stimulates sensory fibers in the brain and can lead to headaches. People taking acid reflux medication (especially proton pump inhibitors), those eating a diet high in meat or low in carbohydrates (or both), and women with heavy periods (magnesium is part of the blood) are at risk for magnesium deficiency. If you're curious about your levels, ask your doctor for an ionized magnesium blood test; it will give you a clearer picture than the standard total magnesium blood test. (Magnesium supplements may also be helpful for menstrual-related migraines even when levels are adequate because the mineral may not be utilized appropriately.)

Magnesium supplements are available in many forms, but study subjects who took 600 milligrams of magnesium citrate daily experienced a reduction in both migraine frequency and severity (the study included only people who had

migraines without auras). Some data supports taking a daily 400- to 600-milligram dose of elemental magnesium in the form of magnesium oxide, slow-release magnesium, or chelated magnesium, all of which are cheaper than magnesium citrate. However, I think 300 milligrams of magnesium citrate twice a day is the best option because it's been widely studied, and you can take it with or without food.

The most common side effect is soft stools or diarrhea, so if you suffer from constipation *and* migraines, you'll be set! Also, taking more than the recommended amount won't work better than normal doses. Megadoses (research varies on this, but I say more than 600 milligrams per day) can cause abnormal heartbeat or breathing problems. Individuals with kidney problems (magnesium is excreted by the kidneys) or a history of soft stools and diarrhea (those with IBS-D, for example) should avoid magnesium, unless your doctor clears it.

HONORABLE MENTIONS

CoQ10 boosts brain energy metabolism and could cut headache frequency by 50 percent. In one study, a total of 150 to 300 milligrams per day (in up to three divided doses) over 3 months reduced the frequency and severity of migraines as well as nausea, and subjects saw improvements within the first month. If money isn't an issue (this is an expensive supplement), opt for the higher dose as it appears to be more effective, and always take it with a meal. There were some rare reports of gastrointestinal side effects, such as stomachache and cramping, and skin allergy, but overall CoQ10 has a good safety record.

Alpha-lipoic acid at 600 milligrams per day provided some benefit in a preliminary clinical trial, but more data is needed. Yet, since it is so safe at this dosage, it gets somewhat of a free pass. Give it a try.

Vitamin B_{12}, B_6, and folic acid are crucial vitamins that help the body process homocysteine, an amino acid that has been linked to an increased risk of cardiovascular disease. Extremely high levels of homocysteine may be especially dangerous in people who experience auras, since they're already at higher risk of stroke. One human study found that 25 milligrams of B_6, 400 micrograms of B_{12}, and 2 milligrams of folic acid reduced homocysteine levels by almost 40 percent and decreased the frequency and severity of aura-related migraines. Keep in mind: Homocysteine has been tied to a lot of diseases, and research hasn't shown yet that lowering levels will significantly impact health, but there does appear to be a benefit when it comes to migraines.

So, what does this all mean? If you have migraines, especially those with auras, ask your doctor for a homocysteine blood test. Also, there is a test available (for the MTHFR gene) that may be useful in determining other potential migraine treatments.

WHAT'S WORTHLESS

Feverfew. This herb is frequently touted for migraine prevention, but not for long if this book has any impact. Feverfew has an active ingredient known as parthenolides, which researchers believe might work for migraines by keeping platelets from sticking together, promoting the release of serotonin, and fighting inflammation. The problem is that there are just as many studies (and some higher-quality ones, at that) showing no benefit as there are showing a positive effect on migraines. In other words, although many experts recommend it for migraine prevention, I do not. (Sorry, folks. Let the hate mail begin!) Besides inconsistent study results, the side effects—gastrointestinal upset, mouth ulcers, and joint aches—make me nervous when I look at the benefit-to-risk ratio. Finally, the variation in active ingredients among the different brands is huge, so you don't really know what you're getting.

Melatonin. Melatonin at 2 milligrams per day was tested for migraine prevention in a small but good-quality trial with no benefit found over the placebo. It's great for sleep and jet lag and maybe some other things, but I'm not ready to get excited about it for migraines.

Probiotics. Asking me if probiotics can prevent migraines is like asking me if gummy bears can lower cholesterol. No! Don't get me wrong. I'm excited about some of the probiotic research, but not when it comes to migraines.

A SURPRISING CAUSE OF MIGRAINES

During my 25 years in medicine, I've seen many cases where dietary supplements have *triggered* migraines, especially when a patient is taking several different kinds. I cannot tell you how many times patients have told me that they not only feel better but have fewer migraines after reducing the number of supplements they take per my recommendation. I believe this is due to two things. First, supplements can contain everything from caffeine to preservatives to other irritants, and all of these can trigger headaches. And second, taking a lot of pills—whether prescription medications or supplements—is stressful. It takes time and costs money, and the resulting stress is also a trigger for migraines. So, is it time to cut back on your pill-popping habit?

WHAT ARE THE OPTIONS FOR KIDS?

Migraines affect up to 5 percent of children, and there are some good supplement options out there to help them.

Butterbur (the Petadolex brand) was tested in a small study of children and adolescents with migraines, and it appeared to reduce headache frequency. Children between 8 and 9 took one 50-milligram capsule per day and those between 10 and 12 took two per day (100 milligrams total) for 8 weeks. Another study in children showed similar results over a 4-month period with dosages between 50 to 150 milligrams per day (6- to 9-year-olds received the lower dosages and 10- to 17-year-olds received the higher ones). Butterbur extracts in these studies contained a minimum of 15 percent petasins.

Magnesium supplements (400 milligrams per day) along with either acetaminophen or ibuprofen were given to children ages 5 to 16 who reported at least four migraine attacks per month. In this study, magnesium appeared to improve the effectiveness but not the toxicity of acetaminophen and ibuprofen over an 18-month period.

CoQ10 helped kids (average age 13) at a dosage of 1 to 3 milligrams per kilogram of body weight per day in a liquid gel capsule in one study. Reduced headache frequency and disability were reported.

LIFESTYLE CHANGES

Log it. Identifying your triggers—and avoiding them—is crucial in preventing migraines (See "Common Migraine Triggers," opposite). Keeping a headache diary (you can easily make one yourself or find one online) can help you track and pinpoint potential culprits. In one study, more than 75 percent of sufferers were able to identify a trigger just by analyzing their diaries.

(continued on page 330)

COMMON MIGRAINE TRIGGERS

- Aged or strong cheeses
- Alcohol
- Allergies (histamine can be a trigger)
- Artificial sweeteners, like aspartame
- Beans
- Bright lights or similar visual stimulation
- Caffeine (consuming more than 300 milligrams per day or withdrawing from a 100- to 200-milligram per day habit)
- Chocolate
- Citrus
- Dairy products (including milk, cheese, yogurt, and sour cream)
- Dehydration
- Dietary supplements
- Eggs
- Fatigue
- Flying
- Infections
- Medications taken or missed
- Menstruation (dramatic hormone changes)
- Missed or irregular meals
- MSG (monosodium glutamate)
- Neck pain
- Nitrites (found in cured, processed, or preserved meat)
- Nuts
- Onions
- Perfumes or other strong odors
- Sexual activity (increases and decreases)
- Skipping meals
- Sleep (poor quality or too much)
- Smoking
- Spicy foods
- Stress/anger
- Weather (especially temperature increases and even nearby lightning strikes)
- Weight changes, especially gaining
- Yeast extracts

Lace up. Being overweight or carrying excess belly fat increases migraine risk because it creates a state of internal auto-immunity and inflammation, which can lead to migraines. In one study, aerobic exercise (specifically indoor cycling for 40 minutes three times a week) reduced headache frequency as well as relaxation techniques or the prescription drug topi-ramate did.

Get lean. A low-fat diet (anywhere from 28 to 66 grams of fat per day) is associated with significant reductions in headache frequency, intensity, and duration as well as medication intake. However, was it the reduction in fat, weight loss, or improvement in cholesterol that deserves the credit? Who cares? Heart healthy = headache healthy.

Cool down. Applying a cold compress to your head can reduce pain (it's an anti-inflammatory), but heat can make it worse.

De-stress daily. Relaxation techniques—including meditation, massage, yoga, tai chi, and acupuncture—can reduce tension and might reduce suscepti-bility to migraine triggers.

Watch your meds. Be careful about overusing pain medication, even over-the-counter products, for headaches. Always follow the dosing and frequency recommendations on the label (often, you shouldn't take them for more than a few days a week). You can develop a resistance to them over time, which can bring on headaches more frequently, known as rebound headaches.

WHAT ELSE DO I NEED TO KNOW?

After taking one of the supplements recommended in this section for up to 6 months, have a discussion with your doctor about your symptoms. She may want to adjust your dosage or have you quit or switch the supplement you're taking. If it reduces the number of migraine attacks you suffer by half, you know you're on the right track.

MOYAD WARNING: If you have any of the following symptoms, it may be a medical emergency, not a migraine.
• Change in vision, slurred speech, problems moving your arms or legs, confusion, loss of balance, or memory loss could indicate a stroke.
• Fever, stiff neck, nausea, and vomiting could be meningitis.
• Severe headache after a head injury or strong blow to the head could be a concussion or internal bleeding.

Multiple Sclerosis

M

Dr. Moyad Secret A chronic autoimmune disease, multiple sclerosis, or MS, is characterized by demyelination, destruction of the protective myelin sheath or coating that surrounds the nerves. Loss of myelin makes it harder for nerve signals to travel back and forth to the brain. One of the most exciting areas of research in dietary supplements for MS suggests that inosine may slow the destruction of the myelin covering around the nerves. Variable dosages (500 to 3,000 milligrams per day), depending on uric acid levels, can increase uric acid and potentially slow the progression of MS, but it also increases the risk of a uric acid kidney stone. Uric acid functions as a free-radical absorber and may inhibit the damage caused by this autoimmune disease up to a point. Most people, especially those with or at risk for gout, should *not* take this supplement because it can dramatically raise uric acid levels and increase the risk of kidney stones. Yet, in MS these supplements may actually help because MS patients have been known to have lower uric acid levels. It's currently being studied in relapsing-remitting MS (2,000 to 3,000 milligrams per day) and even Parkinson's disease. Again, this is preliminary, but it's interesting enough to discuss with your doctor.

Vitamin D. Higher vitamin D levels in individuals with MS have been correlated with less MS activity. In the BENEFIT trial, MS patients who had vitamin D blood levels of 20 ng/mL or higher in the first 12 months following their first episode had a significantly lower risk of new active lesions and relapse, lower increase in lesion volume, and lower disability during the following 4 years than those who had a vitamin D blood level less than 20 ng/mL. I'm not convinced that the higher vitamin D levels improved the MS prognosis, but rather that less severe MS is associated with higher vitamin D levels. I recommend MS patients work with their doctors to normalize their vitamin D levels because of its known benefit for bone health.

Red yeast rice. This supplement, which is used to lower high cholesterol, may also slow the progression of later-stage MS; studies of cholesterol-lowering statin drugs, such as simvastatin, have shown recent promise in slowing progression or reducing brain shrinkage rates in secondary progressive (chronic) MS patients (red yeast rice contains a compound that's very similar to what's found in simvastatin, hence the possible connection). If you cannot tolerate this statin or other statin drugs, ask your doctor about taking red yeast rice.

Narcolepsy

THE JURY'S STILL OUT

Dr. Moyad Secret Excessive daytime sleepiness (EDS) is the primary problem for people with narcolepsy, even when they're taking prescription stimulant medications. There is preliminary research from Duke University suggesting that a low-carbohydrate diet (less than 20 grams of carbs per day) along with plenty of fluids and a daily multivitamin (for deficiencies that could occur while dieting) could modestly improve symptoms, including EDS. Carbohydrates can cause an insulin spike and sluggishness, which can trigger a narcoleptic episode. I think it's worth a try, especially since narcolepsy patients have a higher risk for obesity, type 2 diabetes, and abnormal cholesterol.

Narcolepsy usually begins in the teens or twenties, and symptoms include excessive sleepiness; cataplexy (sudden reduction or loss of muscle tone after an emotional trigger—usually laughter or at times anger or surprise); hallucinations upon falling asleep or when awakening; and sleep paralysis (inability to move or speak during sleep-wake transitions).

L-carnitine. A novel preliminary study from the University of Tokyo in Japan discovered some patients with narcolepsy have lower blood levels of carnitine, so researchers conducted a preliminary 8-week study of 510 milligrams of L-carnitine a day compared to a placebo. Subjects reported spending less time dozing off during the day with the supplement (the primary endpoint). The study suggests that some narcoleptics may have abnormal fatty acid metabolism, which means they're not able to supply various body tissues with the energy they need to conduct normal activity, leading to narcoleptic symptoms. L-carnitine may improve this metabolism. More research is needed.

Nausea and Vomiting

Dr. Moyad Secret Any supplement that helps with severe nausea caused by pregnancy or cancer chemotherapy will usually work for nausea from other reasons, such as motion sickness and medication, too. Most medical experts and clinical treatment guidelines are beginning to recommend at least one supplement for nausea, but unfortunately this is another area of the dietary supplement world that does not receive enough credit. There needs to be more education for both health care professionals and patients.

WHAT IS IT?

Nausea is the feeling of being sick to your stomach, as if you're going to vomit. It can be a subtle, low-grade feeling or a strong, almost overpowering sensation.

There's a specific area of the brain called the vomiting center that controls emesis (a fancy word for throwing up). When it receives a signal—often through the neurotransmitter serotonin—from other areas of the brain, the gastrointestinal tract, or even the inner ear, the vomiting center triggers your stomach to send everything back up. Many antinausea medications (also known as antiemetics) work by blocking receptors for serotonin so the message doesn't get through. Here's another example where "everything in moderation" applies. While serotonin does many good things in the body (it's the "happy" neurotransmitter), a large increase can *cause* nausea, vomiting, and other GI issues, such as diarrhea.

WHAT WORKS

1. (tie) Ginger (*Zingiber officinale*)
500 to 1,500 milligrams a day in divided doses

This common supplement may block serotonin receptors in both the central nervous system and the gastrointestinal tract, and it might also have a calming and antispasmodic impact on the GI tract. In one National Cancer Institute study (the University of Rochester Cancer Center and the National Cancer Institute's Community Clinical Oncology Program, which is just known as URCC CCOP), conducted with 576 cancer patients (primarily breast cancer) at 23 medical sites around the United States, subjects took 500, 1,000, or 1,500 milligrams a day of ginger supplements along with conventional prescription medicines for nausea and vomiting or a placebo (along with conventional meds). The 500- and 1,000-milligram ginger groups experienced a 40 percent reduction in nausea. This was a large trial, so it should be standard practice now to recommend 500 to 1,000 milligrams of ginger (equivalent to $\frac{1}{4}$ to $\frac{1}{2}$ teaspoon of ground ginger) daily for several days before and after chemotherapy. Higher doses (1,500 milligrams per day) did not work better in this study, but they have in other studies, especially in some individuals with higher weights. Chemotherapy-induced nausea and vomiting is very difficult to alleviate, so if ginger works in this situation, then it should work in other cases of nausea and vomiting.

Ginger supplements are also effective for nausea during pregnancy. (Talk to your OB-GYN, though. Although most doctors agree it works, some feel it has not had enough safety testing.) About 75 to 80 percent of women experience nausea early in their pregnancy (about 50 percent have vomiting and nausea). In a small percentage of women, it can be so severe that it causes significant weight loss, electrolyte imbalances, and dehydration. The nausea and vomiting in pregnancy is associated with levels of the hormone hCG (human chorionic gonadotropin), which stimulates estrogen production in the ovaries; estrogen increases the risk of nausea and vomiting. Ginger supplements at these dosages: 350 to 500 milligrams three times a day, 125 to 250 milligrams four times a day, and 500 to 1,000 milligrams total per day for 4 days to 3 weeks have all noticeably reduced nausea and vomiting in patients in the first trimester of pregnancy. Higher dosages are not better, and you run the risk of causing side effects, including uterine contractions and heartburn. Most important, past clinical trials of ginger in pregnancy showed no greater rate of birth defects, miscarriages, or deformities compared to pregnant women who didn't take the supplement.

I recommend using real ginger root–based dietary supplements, not flavored products, like ginger ale or ginger tea, which are not as concentrated. If you have trouble taking pills, you can find purified ginger candies, gum, and other options at most health food stores. The active ingredients in ginger are probably gingerols, zingerone, and shogaols, and I think they'll soon be standardized in many dietary supplements so you can look at the label and know exactly what you're getting. In the best clinical trial ever conducted for ginger (the cancer study mentioned on page 333), the capsules contained a purified liquid extract of ginger root (250 milligrams in each capsule) with 8.5 milligrams of concentrated gingerols, zingerone, and shogaol. So when buying a ginger supplement, first make sure it's from ginger root and then see if it's standardized to any amount of gingerols, zingerone, and shogaol. I would never buy a ginger supplement with more than 5 percent gingerols because this increases the risk of gastrointestinal side effects, such as acid reflux and stomachache.

Note: There is a moderate risk of

increased self-reported bleeding events, especially when combining ginger with other blood thinners, such as aspirin or warfarin. This is why people on prescription blood thinners or with a low platelet count were usually not candidates for ginger supplements in clinical trials.

1. (tie) Vitamin B$_6$ (pyridoxine) 10 to 25 milligrams every 8 hours or 25 to 50 milligrams once a day

It's well known that a low level of vitamin B$_6$ is associated with a higher risk of severe nausea in pregnancy, and it may contribute to other types of nausea as well. Clinical studies with B$_6$ for severe nausea in pregnancy have been almost as impressive as those with ginger. (The American College of Obstetricians and Gynecologists recommends B$_6$ as "first-line pharmacotherapy" for nausea in pregnancy.) There are many theories about how it works to reduce nausea. One is that it functions as a coenzyme to help reduce the ability of hormones (like estrogen) to cause nausea. It also may play a role in the production and balance of important neurotransmitters—such as serotonin, dopamine, norepinephrine, and GABA (gamma-aminobutyric acid)—preventing excesses or deficiencies of these compounds from causing nausea.

Ginger and vitamin B$_6$ are really almost standard medicine to relieve nausea and vomiting during pregnancy, so if one doesn't work, try the other. (Some pharmaceutical companies offer higher doses of B$_6$ in prescription or medical food form.) Vitamin B$_6$ hasn't been well tested for nausea outside of pregnancy, but I believe it should be helpful. The most commonly recommended dosage (in the form of pyridoxine hydrochloride) is 10 to 25 milligrams every 8 hours (for a total of 30 to 75 milligrams per day), but some effective studies also used as little as 25 to 50 milligrams total per day. You can take it with or without food for several days.

2. Whey protein powder isolate 25 to 50 grams a day

A combination of whey protein powder and ginger is showing an even greater benefit for nausea than either one alone in some recent studies. In one trial, 32 grams of whey protein powder and four 250-milligram doses of ginger supplements daily for several days after chemotherapy led to a large reduction in nausea. This is not a surprise (to me, at least) because concentrated protein has been shown to reduce nausea better than carbohydrates and fats. This was first tested in pregnancy, and now it seems to be holding true for other causes of nausea, too, such as motion sickness and chemotherapy-related nausea.

How does it do this? The GI tract can have what are known as dysrhythmias, which essentially means the normal flow or movement is altered by some kind of internal (drug or hormone) or external (high waves on the ocean) stimulus. Protein reestablishes that normal rhythm. (Ginger can do this as well, but it works differently.) Concentrated protein sources, such as powders, also slow the rate of gastric emptying, which reduces nausea as well. There are so many concentrated protein sources out there—including whey, casein, egg white, soy, rice, hemp, pea, chia, and flax—but it's the "isolate" derivatives, or pure protein products without much fat, carbohydrates, or lactose, that appear to be the most helpful. Even though these preliminary nausea studies looked at whey protein, I think any protein isolate is worth a try. (See the Weight Loss section, page 448, for more information.)

Now for the catch! High-protein diets that include too few carbohydrates can also increase the risk of constipation and, yes, *nausea*. That's not to say you shouldn't increase your protein intake; you just need to find a nutrient balance that works well for your body.

WHAT'S WORTHLESS

Antidepressant dietary supplements. Products like 5-HTP or other supplements that increase brain levels of serotonin can cause nausea much like prescription antidepressants do. Participants in clinical trials who took increasing doses (the dose was gradually upped) as well as high doses of 5-HTP (up to 900 milligrams per day) had a greater risk of nausea. St. John's wort has also caused nausea in clinical trials, although the number has been small.

Miscellaneous. The following have caused gastrointestinal side effects or nausea in clinical trials.

- Black cohosh
- Capsaicin
- Glucosamine and chondroitin
- Iron
- Omega-3 or fish oil supplements (usually 3,000 milligrams or more triggers nausea, but it can occur at lower doses, too)
- Selenium in high doses (more than 200 micrograms a day)
- Vitamin C in high doses (1,000 milligrams or more)
- Zinc

WHAT ARE THE OPTIONS FOR KIDS?

Ginger is being tested for children with chemotherapy-related nausea, and it's demonstrating benefits preliminarily, so talk to your child's doctor. It should not be surprising that what works for nausea and vomiting in adults can also work in kids, but at lower dosages.

LIFESTYLE CHANGES

Use acupressure. Over-the-counter wristbands place light pressure around the lower forearm in a spot that helps prevent and reduce nausea and vomiting (called P6 or Pericardium 6). The bands have a stud in the middle that pushes down slightly on a point between the two tendons on your inner forearm. For maximum benefit, wear the wristbands on both arms. There are many similar devices, so look for them in any drugstore.

Get needled. In addition to acupressure, there's very good evidence that acupuncture can help reduce nausea and vomiting from chemotherapy. Practitioners use the same forearm point mentioned above, among other points.

Make nice with your stomach. When you are feeling nauseated, drink beverages and eat foods that are gentle on your stomach (like what your mother used to give you when you had the flu: ginger ale, drinks that have lost their fizz or gone flat, bland foods, sour candy, and dry crackers). Cold drinks and foods should be easier to tolerate than warm foods. Also, eat five or six small meals daily versus two or three large ones when nausea strikes (it's easier for your stomach to digest smaller meals). It should be obvious, but I'll say it anyway: Avoid spicy, fatty, fried, or very sweet foods. I tell patients to eat as if they were a baby when they're nauseated. Cut food into tiny pieces or mash it so

MOYAD FACT: In lab tests, ginger (2,000 milligrams per day for 1 month) appeared to kill abnormal cells while sparing healthy ones. It's just begging to be tested in humans, especially people with a higher risk of colon cancer since the intestines come into direct contact with ginger before it's absorbed.

it's easier to swallow and easier for your digestive tract to process.

Stay nourished. If you have chronic nausea or vomiting due to pregnancy or chemotherapy, make sure you're getting enough nutrients. Try nutritional shakes or drinks, which may be easier to keep down than a solid meal.

Protect your teeth. Did you know that the watery-mouth feeling you get before throwing up is your body's way of protecting your tooth enamel? If you're vomiting frequently, brush your teeth at least twice a day to remove acid and food residue and gargle with mouthwash; even slightly abnormal mouth odors can increase nausea.

Nonalcoholic Fatty Liver Disease and Nonalcoholic Steatohepatitis

Dr. Moyad Secret Nonalcoholic fatty liver disease (NAFLD) is the third most common cause of liver transplantation in the United States (behind alcoholism and hepatitis C), but I believe in the next 10 to 20 years it will take over the number one spot unless the obesity epidemic is reversed. The good news is that lifestyle changes, especially weight loss, are very effective, and often they're the first line of treatment. For many people these changes are inexpensive (especially compared to drugs and medical care) and easy to make. When it comes to combating this disease, doctors need to be more open to trying several different types of therapies, including a variety of dietary supplements, to reduce liver enzymes and damage. The truth is, supplements work as well as most prescription drugs, if not better in some cases, and they can be taken with pharmaceuticals as well.

WHAT IS IT?

Nonalcoholic fatty liver disease is exactly what it sounds like: Fat gets deposited within and around the liver due to a poor diet, excess calories, and some bad luck (some people are more susceptible due to a family history). So when you gain weight, it's not just showing up on your belly, backside, or arms; it's also impacting your organs. The liver is a particularly dangerous spot for this to happen because the extra fat affects its ability to function normally, and this organ is responsible for so many things in the body—from immunity to cholesterol regulation to digestion. If NAFLD is left untreated, it can progress to nonalcoholic steatohepatitis, or NASH (*steato* means fat, and although *hepatitis* is a disease, it really just means inflammation of the liver). This occurs when the fat accumulation becomes so pervasive that liver cells start dying and the liver becomes scarred (fibrotic), leaving it unable to carry out its normal functions, which can lead to cirrhosis, liver failure, cancer, and the need for a transplant.

Here's the really shocking news: About one in three adults in the United States has NAFLD, and about one in 20 has NASH! Even worse, experts believe one in 10 children now has it, too. That one-in-three stat should sound familiar because it's the approximate rate of obesity in the United States as well. See the connection? The risk of NAFLD rises as body weight increases. About 67 percent of people with a body mass index (BMI) of 30 or higher and more than 90 percent of individuals with a BMI greater than 39 (considered morbidly obese) have NAFLD. The condition is so tied to obesity that many physicians, including myself, now consider NAFLD as one of the factors contributing to metabolic syndrome, a constellation of health problems that includes increased waist size (abdominal obesity), high triglycerides, low good cholesterol (HDL), high blood pressure, and high blood glucose or insulin resistance. Metabolic syndrome increases your risk of cardiovascular disease, diabetes, and cancer.

Most people with NAFLD don't have any symptoms, but elevated ALT and AST liver enzymes on a blood test are a tip-off that something's affecting liver function. Some patients will complain of fatigue and right upper quadrant pain or a feeling of fullness in that spot, though, and as many as 50 percent of patients will have an enlarged liver due to the extra fat. If your doctor suspects NAFLD or NASH, she will likely conduct a NAFLD fibrosis score (which looks at your age, BMI, liver enzymes, and other blood test results; you can even do it yourself online) or order an ultrasound, CT scan, or MRI. In severe cases, a biopsy may be needed.

WHAT WORKS

Note: All of the following have been studied in NAFLD or NASH patients. Again, lifestyle changes are first-line therapy for NAFLD, but supplements can also help. For more aggressive NASH, dietary supplements can safely be used along with lifestyle changes and drug therapy. At least 3 to 6 months of supplementation is needed to determine if liver enzymes, liver fat, inflammation, and fibrosis are being reduced.

1. Vitamin E (as d-alpha-tocopherol or RRR-alpha-tocopherol) 800 IU a day

Also known as the natural form of vitamin E, d-alpha was tested in a large clinical trial known as PIVENS (Pioglitazone versus Vitamin E versus Placebo for the Treatment of Nondiabetic Patients with Nonalcoholic Steatohepatitis). The 2-year study compared the drug pioglitazone (30 milligrams per day), vitamin E (800 IU once a day), and a placebo in nondiabetic NASH patients who did not have cirrhosis. Get this: Researchers were looking for a two-point improvement in subjects' conditions (based on a clinical rating system), which occurred in 34 percent of the drug group, 19 percent of the placebo group, and *43 percent* of the vitamin E group. Both the drug and vitamin E also reduced liver enzymes, liver fat, and inflammation (there was no improvement in fibrosis).

This is a classic example of why dietary supplements should be a specialty in medicine and not a part-time job or hobby! Vitamin E supplements are never recommended for anything today, and that is generally appropriate because of the increased risk of prostate cancer they cause in some men (at 400 IU daily). (In the PIVENS trial, the side effect rate was similar to a placebo and there was no increased risk of more serious problems with vitamin E.) But here's a case where it can be helpful for people who have a potentially fatal disease with few remedies. In fact, current guidelines from the American Association for the Study of Liver Disease, American College of Gastroenterology, and American Gastroenterological Association recommend the use of vitamin E as *first-line therapy* in nondiabetic NASH without cirrhosis. Supplements like vitamin E should be treated like a drug. Only certain people qualify to take certain drugs (they're not right for everyone), and the same holds true for vitamin E. You and your doctor should look at the research and your individual situation. It's all about risk versus benefit.

2. Omega-3 fatty acids (EPA and DHA) 800 to 2,000 milligrams a day

There is some excitement about using fish oil—either in a more concentrated and expensive prescription or in supplement form—for NASH. (I think the supplement is better because it is cheaper, safe, and the quality control of most fish oil products right now is excellent.) Interestingly, a review of nine clinical studies using omega-3 supplements (involving 355 people with NAFLD) found an improvement in liver enzymes, especially AST, and a reduction in liver fat. Some of the studies used much higher doses than I'm comfortable with recommending, so stick to between 800 and 2,000 milligrams daily.

Fish oil does have side effects, including stomachache, increased ease of bleeding or bruising, fishy aftertaste, itching and rashes, and adverse blood sugar and LDL changes. You may have to play with dosages to find a level where side effects are tolerable or eliminated.

3. (tie) NAC (N-acetylcysteine) 1,200 milligrams a day

NAC increases production of an antioxidant called glutathione, which protects the liver. There has been some favorable clinical research showing a reduction in liver fat and fibrosis in NASH patients taking NAC, but another reason I'm recommending it is my (and my colleagues') experience using it to treat liver damage from toxins, such as overuse of acetaminophen. In fact, emergency room doctors frequently use it to reduce damage to the liver from acetaminophen overdose.

3. (tie) Whey protein isolate 20 to 25 grams a day

Whey protein isolate (which you can buy as a powder or find in protein bars and other products) works similarly to NAC. Its high levels of cysteine may increase glutathione, which protects the liver. Some early studies show that just 20 grams per day for 3 months may help reduce elevated liver enzymes. But protein powder, specifically whey, may also work because it can help promote weight loss when used as part of a healthy diet and exercise program. High-protein diets are beneficial for weight loss because protein takes longer to digest (meaning you don't get hungry as quickly as you do with simple carbs), and it helps you maintain or build muscle (if you're resistance training) even while losing weight. The more muscle you have, the higher your metabolism is. Protein powders are one of the most concentrated forms of protein with the lowest amount of calories. Plant-based protein powders—such as soy protein isolate, pea, brown rice, and hemp—may help also, but they have not been as well studied for NAFLD (and the taste factor is still an issue—many of them taste like dirt!).

HONORABLE MENTION

Betaine (TMG or trimethylglycine), originally derived from sugar beets, may reduce liver enzymes at larger daily doses (up to 10 to 20 grams) in people with NASH. The results so far have been mixed; they were positive initially, but subsequent research wasn't as good (there are just not enough studies yet). Regardless, it's worth discussing with your physician.

WHAT'S WORTHLESS

The following supplements can potentially increase liver enzymes, so they should be avoided if you have NAFLD or NASH.

- Chaparral leaf
- Ephedra
- Gentian
- Germander
- Kava
- Red clover

- Senna
- Shark cartilage
- Skullcap
- Vitamin A (in excess, such as 25,000 IU or more a day)

Vitamin D. It's completely overhyped for NAFLD due to misinterpretation of the research. Weight loss can benefit NAFLD patients, and when you lose weight, vitamin D levels go up. That doesn't mean vitamin D is *causing* the weight loss. So don't spend money on D if you haven't been told you have low levels. Just lose weight!

Folic acid and vitamin C. These have both been used as treatments for NAFLD, but the research doesn't show any benefit, so save your money.

WHAT ARE THE OPTIONS FOR KIDS?

Thanks to skyrocketing rates of childhood obesity, NAFLD is the most common liver disease in children and adolescents in the United States. Of course, losing weight through diet and exercise is the best treatment option, but the most promising supplement that I've come across so far for kids is vitamin E. Although the biggest research trial (called Treatment of NAFLD in Children, or TONIC) didn't find a statistically significant difference between a placebo, the diabetes drug metformin, and vitamin E, a daily 800 IU dose of vitamin E (d-alpha-tocopherol) did reduce liver enzymes (ALT) better than the others.

After 96 weeks, 28 percent of the kids taking a placebo improved, 41 percent of those on metformin showed improvements, and 58 percent of the children on vitamin E got better.

Vitamin E deserves more credit (and research) here, especially since there are so few official treatments for kids with NAFLD, apart from lifestyle changes. Plus, five children in the placebo group developed diabetes while nobody in the vitamin E group did, and side effects of vitamin E were similar to the placebo. Daily doses between 400 to 1,200 IU have been found to improve liver enzymes, so talk with your child's doctor about the appropriate dose.

LIFESTYLE CHANGES

Heart healthy = liver healthy. Dietary changes that improve heart health (and help you lose weight) also benefit your liver. Increasing the consumption of polyunsaturated fats (such as omega-3 fatty acids), reducing sugar intake (including sodas and fruit juices), increasing your fiber intake (20 to 30 grams daily), reducing red meat and processed meats and fast foods, and increasing fish consumption can improve your liver enzymes.

Shrink your waistline. Weight loss and exercise are the *most* effective lifestyle changes you can make to improve NAFLD. These are the first things your doctor will tell you to do because they help reduce insulin resistance and visceral abdominal fat (the kind that settles around your organs, including your liver). Imaging studies have shown positive changes (reduced fat) in as little as 6 to 12 weeks of losing 1 or 2 pounds a week. (More rapid weight loss can sometimes make the condition temporarily worse, so be careful.) I have seen liver enzymes return to normal in individuals who have dropped 5 to 20 pounds or more. Even just exercising, without losing weight, will help reduce liver fat and improve the organ's ability to repair itself. And don't forget weight lifting: Adding lean muscle improves your metabolism and reduces fat.

Reduce your carbs. So far, there isn't one particular eating plan that works better than others for NAFLD, but many doctors (myself included) like to recommend low-carbohydrate diets, especially for patients who have diabetes. Preliminary studies with the Mediterranean diet (high in vegetables, beans, fish, fruit, fiber, and "good" fats and low in meat and sugar) appear to show a benefit as well. Bottom line: Any reasonable, healthy program that helps you cut calories as well as lose weight and keep it off can be helpful.

Reduce or eliminate alcohol. Alcohol is toxic to the liver, and when it's processed, it can damage liver tissue—especially if you drink in excess. Cutting back or quitting altogether can make a big difference, bringing those liver enzymes back to normal!

Go high octane. Are you ready for this one? Caffeinated coffee—two to three cups a day—may reduce the risk of NAFLD or NASH. Research over the past

20 years has suggested that consuming coffee can reduce the negative effects of toxic substances, like alcohol. The jury is still out over whether it's the caffeine or other compounds in coffee (it's high in antioxidants) that deliver the protective effect, so caffeine in general or decaf may not be beneficial.

Eat more choline. Some research suggests that diets higher in this B vitamin, which is found in all human cells, can improve liver function by reducing inflammation. The PIVENS study showed that it may even reduce scarring (fibrosis) in some individuals. The best way to get it is through diet, especially protein, such as chicken, eggs, turkey, fish, nuts, and seed oils.

WHAT ELSE DO I NEED TO KNOW?

Talk with your doctor about these drugs and supplements, which show some promise in treating certain aspects of NAFLD.

- Metformin, a low-cost generic drug commonly used in people with diabetes, is not a standard treatment, but it has helped reduce liver enzymes slightly, and it may also help with weight loss and diabetes risk. It doesn't reduce inflammation or the amount of fat in the liver, though.

- Orlistat, an over-the-counter and prescription weight loss drug, could theoretically be beneficial if it helps a patient lose weight, but it's controversial because there have been some reports of liver disease associated with its use. Two newer weight loss drugs approved by the FDA (lorcaserin and phentermine-topiramate) might also help.

- Cholesterol-lowering drugs (statins) have appeared to be mostly safe when used for NAFLD, and they may help prevent further fatty deposits (such as triglycerides) in the liver.

- Preliminary studies suggest that 140 milligrams per day of silymarin (milk thistle) might reduce liver enzymes (AST and ALT) in individuals with NASH, but this needs more research. If silymarin helps, it's most likely going to show the most benefit early in the disease process.

- Alpha-lipoic acid (ALA) is being studied for weight loss and improving glucose levels in people with diabetes, and since these two factors are often found in fatty liver disease, it's likely that there would be some benefit for NAFLD. It has an excellent safety record, especially between 600 and 1,800 milligrams per day, so ask your doctor about it. Just divide the total into two or three separate doses and take it 30 minutes before meals (that's how it was studied for weight loss).

Osteoarthritis and Joint Pain

Dr. Moyad Secret Dietary supplements for osteoarthritis (OA or degenerative joint disease) are the most underappreciated supplement category. First, let's look at the conventional medical options for pain. Acetaminophen can increase the risk of liver toxicity; in fact, it's the number one cause of acute liver failure in the United States. Ibuprofen and similar drugs can increase the risk of cardiovascular disease, internal bleeding, kidney damage, gastrointestinal problems (ulcers), and now probably sexual dysfunction. Opioids, the strongest prescription pain medicines, are now the number one cause of unintentional prescription drug overdose leading to death in the United States. Not such great options, right?

Dietary supplements for OA might not work as well or as fast as over-the-counter or prescription painkillers, but they have an outstanding safety record *and* they may also help reduce the progression of OA. However, the American College of Rheumatology (ACR, the leading educator of health care professionals in the area of OA) recently revised its treatment guidelines for osteoarthritis and recommended against the use of chondroitin sulfate, glucosamine, and topical capsaicin for knee OA. This is a good organization, but it continues to be enamored with expensive and potentially toxic options—and closed-minded when it comes to dietary supplements. I thought the Hippocratic oath was to "first do no harm." Other international organizations are still recommending both conventional medicine as well as dietary supplements for the treatment of OA. (In slight defense of the ACR, they did overwhelmingly endorse exercise and weight loss for OA of the knee.)

WHAT IS IT?

Osteoarthritis is one of the most common and disabling chronic diseases that impact us as we age. It's the erosion or reduction of joint cartilage and eventually the underlying bone; the resulting inflammation contributes to further cartilage breakdown. Joints (and muscles) can become sore and stiff, sometimes to the point where it's difficult to carry out daily activities or even sleep. The elbows, hips, knees, ankles, shoulders, neck, and even the tiny joints in the hands and feet are all prone to osteoarthritis. Imaging tests or x-rays may reveal areas of bony outgrowth called osteophytes, which are created by the bone in an effort to stabilize the joint.

Age is the biggest risk factor, but others include inflammatory joint disease (gout, rheumatoid arthritis, and infection), obesity (the strongest modifiable risk factor), occupation (a job that requires repetitive knee bending, for example), and previous injury to the area (such as a torn knee ligament).

WHAT WORKS

Note: Some of the remedies for joint pain overlap with remedies for muscle soreness and pain, but it's critical to first determine with your doctor what the exact source of the discomfort is (joint, muscle, bone, nerve, or a combination).

1. (tie) SAM-e (S-adenosylmethionine)
600 to 1,200 milligrams a day

SAM-e is widely used in Europe as a prescription for a variety of conditions, especially osteoarthritis and depression (see the Depression section, page 166), and it's enjoying a resurgence in the United States, too. Researchers aren't sure how this naturally occurring compound controls pain, but it does play a primary role in several pathways in the body, including transmethylation, transsulfuration, and aminopropylation, which basically means it helps to reduce pain in multiple ways.

A recent review of numerous clinical trials comparing SAM-e to a placebo or NSAIDs (nonsteroidal anti-inflammatory drugs, such as ibuprofen, aspirin, and naproxen) concluded that SAM-e is at least as effective as NSAIDs for osteoarthritis but with fewer side effects; in fact, people taking SAM-e were almost 60 percent less likely to experience a side effect compared to NSAID users. It takes longer for SAM-e to kick in, but after a month or two, its effect is similar to NSAIDs. SAM-e may reduce morning stiffness, swelling, pain at rest and in motion, and even the popping or cracking sounds associated with OA, and it may improve range of motion and walking ability.

Effective dosages range from 600 to 1,200 milligrams per day for at least 30 to 90 days, usually on an empty stomach. Most trials tested SAM-e for between 10 days and 3 months, with the most common trial period being 30 days, so how it will perform long term is unknown. Plus, more safety data is needed. One enduring concern with SAM-e is that it may increase blood levels of homocysteine, which might be an indirect marker of cardiovascular risk, but recent studies show this is not as much of an issue. Regardless, please talk to your doctor about using SAM-e. If a jump in your homocysteine level is observed, you may be instructed to take more B vitamins.

Be careful when you're taking over-the-counter NSAIDs along with SAM-e; this hasn't really been studied. In addition, most of the research with SAM-e and pain has been for knee and hip OA; that's not to say you couldn't try it for other types of chronic pain, but let your doctor know. Finally, the biggest side effect of SAM-e, in my experience, is on your wallet; it can be ridiculously expensive, so shop around.

1. (tie) Glucosamine sulfate
1,500 milligrams a day and
chondroitin sulfate 800 to
1,200 milligrams a day

Glucosamine is a basic building block for the production of glycosaminoglycans and proteoglycans, which are important components of joint cartilage. Although the body produces it naturally, glucosamine supplements are generally derived from crab shells or the shells of other sea creatures. (Vegetarians are in luck because there are now some corn-based sources of glucosamine; perhaps in the future the supplement will be called glucornsamine.) If you have a shellfish allergy, do *not* take it unless you know it comes from a non-shellfish source. Glucosamine is often combined with chondroitin sulfate, another component of joint cartilage. It helps retain water in the cartilage and may help support the joint and slow disease progression. Chondroitin supplements usually are made from shark, pig, or cow cartilage, but now there are some algae sources as well.

Recently, the much-anticipated results of the large LEGS (Long-Term Evaluation of Glucosamine Sulfate) study from Australia—one of the largest and best supplement trials ever—came out. After 2 years, researchers found a combination of 1,500 milligrams of glucosamine sulfate and 800 milligrams of chondroitin sulfate daily significantly and favorably impacted joint space narrowing (less narrowing equals healthier joints), especially in people with mild OA. The results suggested the supplements were slowing the progression of OA compared to the placebo (half the rate—wow!). Now, all groups reported a reduction in pain, but no group was significantly better after 2 years. Three-year trials are showing more impressive reductions in pain, though, so perhaps this trial was too short or there weren't enough participants with moderate to severe OA (only 5 percent). Still, the LEGS trial is remarkable in the sense that it suggests the earlier you use it, the better; it also shows that the combination of glucosamine and chondroitin sulfate is better than either alone. Another significant finding of the LEGS trial was that side effects of the supplements were similar to the placebo.

Like SAM-e, this is another supplement that you have to take for several weeks to see results. There have been reports of blood thinning (do not combine with warfarin), stomach upset, and excess gas in other studies. If you're following a low-sodium diet, check the label on your glucosamine supplement; many contain 20 to 50 milligrams (or more) of sodium per one or two capsules.

On its own in studies, 500 to 1,500 milligrams per day of glucosamine sulfate resulted in a greater reduction in pain and a greater improvement in function than a placebo. Longer-term trials with chondroitin by itself have found it may help reduce cartilage volume loss and reduce pain (800 to 1,200 milligrams a day). So either one works on its own, but I think the combination is most powerful. I would love to see a study of glucosamine sulfate, chondroitin sulfate, and SAM-e taken together! Of course, you could try this yourself and ask your doctor to monitor your progress. (I don't currently recommend another form, glucosamine HCL, based on results of the Glucosamine/Chondroitin Arthritis Intervention, or GAIT, and other trials.)

2. Capsaicin cream (0.015 to 0.075 percent) applied up to four times a day

Over-the-counter joint creams or gels, such as capsaicin (an ingredient from cayenne and other hot peppers), seem to work well for hand and knee arthritis, but not so much for the hip because they just can't penetrate that deeply. In several clinical trials, participants used 0.025 percent capsaicin four times daily for 4 to 12 weeks. In other trials, people applied 0.015 percent capsaicin once a day for 6 weeks and 0.075 percent four times a day for 4 weeks. In all of these clinical trials, capsaicin was significantly more effective for improving pain than a placebo. The longer the study, the greater the reduction in pain severity (there was no hint that it slowed progression). Be warned, redness and a burning sensation are common because of the way this herbal topical works. You can also buy capsaicin in pill form, but there's no research yet on how it impacts OA, so stick with the cream for now.

HONORABLE MENTIONS

Note: There are so many potentially effective and safe OA dietary supplements that it was almost impossible to just pick the top three!

Avocado/soybean unsaponifiable (ASU) supplements, a phytosterol extract from avocados and soybeans, reduce inflammation and stimulate repair. Several clinical studies are suggesting that these may be especially helpful for knee pain (less so for the hip). Although they are an approved prescription medication for OA in some countries, more research is still needed. Studies have looked at daily doses from 300 to 600 milligrams and both work well. Obviously, if you are allergic to avocados or soy, you should not take these.

Boswellia (Indian frankincense), an herbal extract taken from the *Boswellia serrata* tree, also appears to reduce inflammation and compounds that increase joint damage. Most of the research for it has been in small studies, but the results have been consistent. In one trial, a 333-milligram dose, given three times a day, reduced pain and swelling and improved function over 8 weeks of treatment. And another study, which administered the same dosage and was conducted over 6 months, showed similar benefits. An extract of *B. serrata* enriched with 30 percent 3-O-acetyl-11-keto-beta-boswellic acid (called 5-Loxin) reduced pain and improved function over 90 days at 100 or 250 milligrams daily. Side effects in most studies were the same as a placebo. Overall, it improved some components of OA but not others. I don't think it would hurt to try it for a month and see if you notice a difference; you can always go back to NSAIDs.

Omega-3 companies claim that their products—which may come from sardines, anchovies, mackerel, krill, or even the New Zealand green-lipped mussel— are somehow different than their competitors' products, but in my opinion, it's all BS (bogus science)! While the dosage may vary slightly from form to form, the active ingredients EPA and DHA are going to be the same, so first give the least expensive product a try and see if it helps. Omega-3s are natural anti-inflammatories, and the research shows that the standard dose of 1,000 to 2,000 milligrams per day of EPA and DHA may reduce aches and pains in the back, knee, hip, and other joints. Higher doses might even work better, but you should discuss that with your doctor.

Warning: Prescription omega-3 oil is a big waste of money, and too many doctors push it because they don't realize that fish oil dietary supplements have great quality control (in other words, mercury and most other contaminants aren't an issue).

Fish oil has also shown a modest benefit for rheumatoid arthritis, a chronic inflammatory autoimmune disorder of the joints and bones. If you experience gastrointestinal problems (like nausea, diarrhea, or discomfort), skin abnormalities (itching, eruptions, allergies), or easy bleeding, then your fish oil dose is either too high or just not for you.

Hyaluronic acid is a component of joint fluid, and preliminary clinical trials are beginning to show that taking it in supplement form (80 to 200 milligrams daily) may strengthen the area around the cartilage, known as the joint matrix or joint support system, and may stimulate certain cells to produce more hyaluronic acid. More research is still needed, but the benefit outweighs the risk right now. A word of warning for vegetarians or anyone who's allergic to poultry: It's usually derived from chicken cartilage.

MSM (methylsulfonylmethane) supplements contain sulfur, which occurs naturally in joints. A few small studies of 1,500 to 6,000 milligrams a day for 12 weeks have demonstrated a small reduction in pain and improvement in function. I think it might work best combined with glucosamine or chondroitin or both; I wouldn't use it alone unless my top picks in this section were a bust.

Pycnogenol, an extract from the bark of the French maritime pine tree, helped reduce OA-related joint pain and stiffness by 35 to 55 percent in two clinical trials. Participants were also able to cut back on their pain medications. The trials lasted about 3 months, and the most effective dose was 50 milligrams two or three times a day (100 to 150 milligrams total) taken after meals. It's pricey though, and there haven't been enough clinical trials to warrant using this before you give some of the cheaper and better studied supplements here a try.

WHAT'S WORTHLESS

Vitamin D. Normalizing low blood levels of vitamin D (35 to 40 ng/mL) has been shown to provide minimal relief from muscle discomfort in some people, but the same doesn't hold true for bone. A recent 2-year study of moderate-dose vitamin D supplementation to reduce OA pain did not work better than a placebo.

Rose hip. There have been several weak studies with this herbal, which has shown some benefit for pain relief. The problem is that you would have to take five capsules twice a day to get the dose that was studied, and this is simply too costly and unrealistic.

Curcumin. This yellow coloring agent, which is derived from turmeric, is the anti-inflammatory du jour. But we need more clinical trials ASAP. Of course, I am excited about the preliminary data showing curcumin can reduce the pain of OA, but with such a crowded field of potentially beneficial supplements, you have to prove yourself. Very high doses of curcumin in some studies have caused abdominal fullness and pain, and the bio-availability (ease of absorption) of this supplement is just not that good.

Bromelain. An extract from pineapple, it's been tested at 800 milligrams per day over 12 weeks in small clinical studies, but did not beat a placebo. Bromelain combined with trypsin and rutin has shown some benefit, but again, the study design and results were not exciting enough to bump this supplement into the effective category.

Eggshell protein or natural eggshell membrane (NEM). Preliminary research with this new supplement, which is made of proteins (similar to those found in human joints) that can build and support cartilage, suggests it may reduce joint pain and improve flexibility at 500 milligrams per day. However, there are egg protein powders that are wonderful sources of protein, and they might be worth a try while the eggshell membrane supplement gets more research.

Ginger. It's better known for its ability to combat nausea, but it may also have anti-inflammatory effects. Studies have shown modest to zero benefit, though. It has a good safety record, but why experts tout it as having good human evidence is beyond me.

Cat's claw. There are two species of this vine from the Amazon River basin that are used in South America as general anti-inflammatories, but there just haven't been any good clinical studies. Nobody has been able to explain how it might work (the mechanism of action) to slow the progression of OA either. These supplements aren't magic, folks.

Devil's claw. The active ingredient in this African plant appears to be iridoid glycosides, especially something called harpagoside, but I don't believe the mechanism of action has truly been discovered yet. Some compounds in this plant act as COX-2 inhibitors, which are heart unhealthy (remember Vioxx?). Preliminary laboratory data has been encouraging, and some of the clinical studies are also positive, but in terms of methodology they've been weak, which makes me question the results. Side effects have been rare, but gastrointestinal upset, diarrhea, skin reactions, and loss of taste have occurred. It would be a sin to try this until better safety and efficacy are proven.

Collagen hydrolysate. This is obtained by extracting collagenous tissues from animals. It's an amino acid mixture high in glycine, proline, hydroxylysine, and hydroxyproline, which are also found in human cartilage. A trial of 10 grams daily of collagen hydrolysate for 24 weeks found some reductions in pain that beat a placebo, but the average dropout rate at most of the clinical trial sites was very large. Give me more data!

DMSO (dimethyl sulfoxide). This is a sulfur-containing compound made from wood pulp that comes in a gel, liquid, or roll-on form. There was a favorable older study using a 25 percent DMSO topical product, but it has not been replicated. Some people develop a rash or itching with it.

White willow bark. Some osteoarthritis and pain supplements contain salicin, or white willow bark, which is just a copycat of aspirin. The makers of these products may claim that their expensive product is working by some miracle or unique mechanism to reduce pain (or thin the blood), when in reality you're just getting another version of cheap aspirin. But aspirin has 100 times the research of white willow bark, and I always recommend spending your hard-earned money on that instead. I wish these companies would test their products against aspirin or ibuprofen or naproxen for pain if they think they're that good (but the chances this will happen are slim to none and, really, slim just left town).

LIFESTYLE CHANGES

Heart healthy = joint healthy. Almost anything that reduces the risk of heart disease appears to prevent or reduce the progression of OA, too. Never forget this please.

Exercise more. Aerobics, resistance training, tai chi—they all help to reduce stress on the joints by strengthening the muscles around them and by helping you lose weight. The goal is to keep moving so your muscles stay strong; if they get weak, the joints take all the pressure. If you have more severe types of OA, you should work with your physician.

Apply heat or cold? Cold reduces inflammation and swelling, and it reduces pain better than heat, but it can also cause temporary stiffening. Heat relaxes muscles and tendons and encourages circulation to the area, so I think it's a better choice for increasing mobility. Here's a good tip: Apply heat to a specific joint before physical activity, and use a cold pack afterward.

Drop pounds. Excess weight is your number one modifiable risk factor for OA. (Google the ADAPT, or Arthritis, Diet, and Activity Promotion Trial.) Wow! Losing just a little weight or a few inches from your waist (if you are overweight) can take pressure off some joints and reduce pain. Research bears this out time and time again. It's just a no-brainer (or should I say, "no-jointer").

Take a salt bath. Using Epsom salt (magnesium sulfate) in the tub can be very effective for reducing joint or muscle pain. Magnesium penetrates skin and helps fight inflammation and relieve pain along with hot water. Just make sure that the water completely covers or surrounds the sore area for at least 10 to 15 minutes.

Eat more gelatin. Gelatin is a cheap home remedy for joint pain that is very popular and safe, but it's also untested. It comes from the collagen inside an animal's (cattle, pigs, and horses) skin and bones. When you ingest it, it may reach the joint and provide some protection or lubrication. There are gelatin substitutes available—such as liquid fruit pectin or konjak (another gelatinous fiber)—that have similar gel-forming features and may work the same way. Some people think gelatin is no more than a placebo, but it's safe, so why not try it? (If I had a dime for all the folks who told me it helps, I would have a house full of dimes and a wife who would be upset with me for leaving dimes all over the house.)

WHAT ELSE DO I NEED TO KNOW?

- Topical rubs that heat the skin, such as Bengay, can help with joint and muscle aches. They work as counterirritants, producing a mild and localized inflammation that crowds out pain messages from nearby muscles and joints (for all its intricacies, your brain is very focused and can generally process only one primary pain signal at a time). It's kind of like creating white noise for your brain so it doesn't recognize what's coming from the joint.

- My favorite over-the-counter pain reliever is naproxen because the dosage you need is so low and it may carry less cardiovascular toxicity than other over-the-counter NSAIDs. And you can use it with many OA supplements.

Osteoporosis

Dr. Moyad Secret Osteoporosis drugs in the United States are widely overprescribed, and this is bad for a few reasons. First, studies are now showing that lifestyle changes *alone* can profoundly increase bone mineral density and reduce fracture risk. Second, most osteoporosis drugs have incredibly long half-lives (longer than most other drugs!). They are the gift that keeps on giving, which is good because they work well when needed, but it is also bad because this could lead to overexposure, thus increasing the risk of side effects. I encourage patients to ask their doctors about taking a "drug holiday" after being on one of these drugs for 3 to 5 years. Thanks to two important trials of alendronate (Fosamax), it is now known that taking a break won't increase fracture risk significantly, even if users do lose some bone. (If there is serious bone loss in the hip or spine after stopping the drug, it should be started again ASAP.)

Now let's talk about those side effects. There are some nasty yet rare problems that can occur over time after being on osteoporosis drugs, including atrial fibrillation, potentially irreversible and incurable bone loss in the jawbone because of an infection (osteonecrosis), bone and muscle pain, damage to the esophagus and esophageal cancer, and bizarre upper leg fractures (known as atypical femur fractures) after minimal trauma. Again, these side effects are extremely rare, and the drugs have been a miracle for many people, but patients should always be thinking of how to minimize exposure to the drugs while still preserving bone mineral density. One last thing to keep in mind: Almost every successful trial of both new and old osteoporosis drugs also used moderate intakes of calcium or vitamin D (or both) to increase the effectiveness of the medication.

WHAT IS IT?

Osteoporosis is thinning of the bones, which causes them to become weak and break. It's the most common bone disease, and it affects women two to three times more often than men. However, men have a higher risk of dying from an initial fracture, so it really is an equal opportunity problem.

Most osteoporosis-related fractures occur in the hip, spine, or wrist, which are the areas evaluated during a bone mineral density (BMD) test. Dual-energy x-ray absorptiometry, or DEXA, is the most widely used bone density exam (it delivers just 10 percent of the radiation of a normal x-ray). There are other detection methods, including a quantitative CT scan (QCT) and a heel ultrasound (HUS), but my favorite is DEXA, mainly because it is safe and low cost, has been well studied in relation to fractures, and looks directly at the most common fracture sites.

BMD results come in the form of a T-score for the hip, spine, and wrist, which is essentially a comparison between your BMD and that of an average 25- to 30-year-old who has no bone loss. A T-score of -2.5 or lower (measured in standard deviations from what is seen in a younger person) means osteoporosis (significant or severe bone loss). So, a T-score of -1 to -2.5 is indicative of osteopenia (moderate bone loss), and greater than -1 is considered minimal bone loss. It's not unusual to have osteoporosis of the lower spine, osteopenia of the hip, and normal wrist BMD, or some other combination. You should also receive a Z-score, which compares your BMD to the average of someone your age so you can see what is "normal" for your age group. Doctors use these scores along with other data to determine treatment.

WHAT WORKS

1. (tie) Calcium 1,000 to 1,200 milligrams a day and vitamin D 800 to 1,000 IU a day or the amount needed to normalize the 25-OH vitamin D test

I'm lumping these together because taking calcium without vitamin D doesn't make much sense—vitamin D improves the absorption of calcium, and both help increase bone density and muscle coordi-

nation. Before you roll your eyes and think, *Well I heard recently that calcium and vitamin D do* not *prevent fractures*, I want to make sure you have the full story. First, keep in mind that calcium and vitamin D have been a part of almost every successful osteoporosis drug clinical trial.

Both nutrients together have been shown to reduce bone fractures in *compliant* users. In the largest clinical trial of these supplements to prevent bone loss and fractures ever completed (the Women's Health Initiative, or WHI study), women who took calcium (1,000 milligrams) and vitamin D (400 IU) daily—or at least most days of the week—for 7 years had a 29 percent reduction in hip fractures compared to a placebo. Almost 5 years after the study ended, the women still reported fewer vertebral (spine) fractures, which are the most common osteoporotic break, but no significant difference in hip fractures. In statistical terms, this basically means that for every 10,000 women taking supplements every year, there would be four fewer vertebral fractures. Not amazing, but no other supplement has ever been shown in a major clinical trial to have this impact on fractures.

In addition, both supplements reduce parathyroid hormone, which can cause bone loss when levels are high, and they may improve coordination, which can lower the risk of falls.

The current Recommended Dietary Allowance for calcium is 1,000 to 1,200 milligrams per day, ideally from food sources (cereal, veggies, fish, dairy, or fortified milk)

CALCIUM PROS AND CONS

FORM OF CALCIUM SUPPLEMENT	PROS	CONS
Calcium carbonate	The most tested and cheapest supplement for bone loss/fracture prevention; most concentrated calcium source; easy to take	Should take with meals for better absorption; increased risk of kidney stones and constipation
Calcium citrate	Can take with or without food; may reduce the risk of kidney stones (ideal for those with a history of stones); some data on prevention of bone loss and fractures	Not a highly concentrated source of calcium, so more pills are needed; tends to be more expensive; increased risk of constipation
Calcium phosphate	Almost as concentrated as calcium carbonate, so fewer pills are needed; same type of calcium found in milk, so there is a history of bone benefit	Need more research to compete with calcium carbonate or citrate; may increase risk of stones; should take with food for better absorption
Calcium gluconate and others (glycerophosphate and lactate)		No good research on fracture prevention

Note: Bone meal, oyster shell, and dolomite calcium products primarily contain calcium carbonate, but they could contain detectable quantities of lead in rare cases. They should not be used during pregnancy, if at all. Coral calcium and many other ocean-based calcium products are really just calcium carbonate supplements in disguise, so opt for the less expensive calcium carbonate products and save your money.

that may work as well as or even better than taking supplements because food provides small quantities of calcium over the day with other nutrients (versus just taking a supplement in the morning), which improves absorption and incorporation into the bone. Taking too much calcium can increase the risk of kidney stones though, and some researchers believe it may also increase the risk of calcification of the arteries and heart attacks. No one knows yet if this is true, but I recommend erring on the side of moderation. (To figure out which form of calcium to take, see the table above.)

In the WHI trial, hip fractures were nonsignificantly lower in women with vitamin D blood levels that were approaching normal, which is 30 to 40 ng/mL on a 25-OH vitamin D test in my world. This is another example of where supplementing may not help much if you're not substantially low in D. However, I believe—and studies support this—that normal doses of vitamin D (and raising your D levels naturally through weight loss and exercise) really help to prevent falls, especially in the elderly and frail. Receptors for this vitamin are found in most tissues and cells, including muscle tissue. By improving the ability of the muscles to finely coordinate activity, you lower the risk of slipping and falling. The current National Institutes of Health recommendation is 600 IU per day for people 70 or younger and 800 IU for those 71 and older. (I think dosage should be either 1,000 IU or based on blood testing and lifestyle factors.)

There are two primary types of vitamin D supplements: vitamin D_2, which comes from a plant source, and vitamin D_3, which usually comes from sheep lanolin (there's also a new plant source that is just hitting the market). Most major clinical trials for bone loss prevention have used D_3, but many studies suggest D_2 is equally as or just slightly less effective than D_3. I like both of them, but once it's easier to get vitamin D_3 from plants, I will probably recommend that one more often. A new form of vitamin D known as 25-OH vitamin D_3, similar to what is measured in the blood, may be available soon, and it may have even greater ability to raise blood levels.

Finally, let me reiterate here what I have emphasized throughout this book: You can get sufficient calcium and vitamin D for bone loss and fracture prevention almost exclusively from lifestyle changes and diet. If you can't consume enough that way, then and *only* then should you make up the deficit with supplements. The food world is loaded with calcium (almond milk has about 450 milligrams per 8 ounces), and now many foods are fortified with vitamin D. Recent major clinical studies (the WHI, for example) have shown that most people are getting *plenty* of calcium and vitamin D from their diets; the need to supplement, especially calcium, is decreasing.

WHAT'S WORTHLESS

Note: Almost every time a supplement claims it can beat calcium, vitamin D, and exercise for bone health, it loses. These products may be able to slow bone loss, but they don't lower the risk of fractures. And much of their bone health data was derived from studies on foods that contain these nutrients, not the supplements themselves, which isn't comparable.

Strontium citrate. Found in bone, strontium is similar to calcium in structure. In fact, the human body absorbs it as if it were calcium. You can find it in seawater, wheat bran, root veggies, meat, and dairy products. Not much is known about the side effects of the supplement, strontium citrate. However, we know more about the prescription drug, strontium ranelate. Strontium ranelate is a good osteoporosis prescription medication that has been approved in many countries around the world, but not yet in the United States. It appears to work as well in men with osteoporosis as in postmenopausal women with osteoporosis, and it has been shown to reduce the risk of vertebral and nonvertebral bone fractures. It doesn't just stop bone loss; it also strengthens existing bone and may promote bone growth. Strontium ranelate has a long track record of success in the drug world (up to 10 years), and overall it appeared to have similar side effects to a placebo.

Recently, however, there has been a concern about its potential to have cardiovascular toxicity, especially in people who are at high risk. I was going to make strontium ranelate an honorable mention, but because of this new heart-health data, I had to move it to this section. With the new drug concerns, I can't recommend the supplement form right now either.

Vitamins K_1 (phylloquinone) and K_2 (menaquinone). These have been touted to prevent bone loss primarily based on dietary studies (eating foods that contain them), but well-done clinical trials have not shown a consistent increase in bone density at major skeletal sites. Advocates argue that vitamin K_2 (and even K_1) might reduce the risk of bone fractures, although studies have not addressed this well and results have been inconsistent. I remain skeptical until someone can show a true consistent benefit here. (I hope they can.)

Soy isoflavone These supplements do not work better than a placebo at preventing bone loss in women who are already getting 1,000 to 1,200 milligrams of calcium and vitamin D daily and who are within 5 years of menopause (perimenopausal or early menopausal). It's women who have vitamin D levels below 20 ng/ mL who seem to be getting some small benefit from soy supplements. If you're concerned about bone loss, you need to address any vitamin D deficiency before you consider doing anything else.

Boron, omega-3s, and the "latest and greatest" bone health supplements. Manufacturers continue to advertise that boron, omega-3s, and whatever is the supplement du jour are bone healthy, but the reality is they have weak data. You can easily get many of these so-called bone-support nutrients from even a moderately unhealthy diet (the pizza-with-flaxseed-and-beer diet).

LIFESTYLE CHANGES

Heart healthy = bone healthy? You bet! People with heart disease have a higher risk of fractures, which I believe shows a link between bone loss and heart disease. Individuals who are active and do aerobic (weight-bearing) and resistance-training exercise, maintain normal to low cholesterol, and do other things to reduce their risk of heart disease appear to have a lower risk of bone fractures. I cannot emphasize enough how your bones and muscles follow the "use it or lose it" philosophy. Daily cardio workouts (walking, jogging, or group exercise classes) and twice-weekly strength sessions should be a part of almost everyone's weekly routine to help prevent bone loss. New research from Australia suggests daily moderate and intense exercise may work as well as calcium and vitamin D and some medications for improving BMD. And, of course, quit using tobacco!

Moderate your alcohol intake. Too much increases bone loss, but drinking in moderation (one a day for women and one or two for men) might slightly help bones by acting as a weak estrogen, which is needed for bone formation and to prevent loss. However, it's not a reason to start drinking if you don't currently imbibe. Did you know that beer contains silicon, which helps maintain bones? Just another reason I will never give up drinking it!

Get calcium and vitamin D in your diet. Five or 10 years ago it was difficult to get calcium from food and beverages, but today it's easy. Dairy products, almond milk, mushrooms, egg yolks, kale, and fatty fish are better than pills any day.

Cover up. Yes, your body makes vitamin D from sunlight, but telling people to get more sun is one of the dumbest recommendations out there (second only to telling someone to use a tanning bed). Ultraviolet light is a carcinogen and accelerates aging. Vitamin D is so inexpensive and easy to purchase, and it doesn't increase your risk of dying young.

Eat more C. This vitamin is essential for creating collagen, improving bone repair, and strengthening bones. I have tested it in the past and it appeared to improve some bone markers. It's best to get it from food sources, which is really just another way of saying, "Eat a heart-healthy diet."

Cut out sodas. The more soda you drink, the less room you have for foods that contain real nutrients, like calcium (it's a phenomenon called milk displacement). Plus, the phosphoric acid in large amounts of soda might increase bone loss.

Maintain a healthy weight. Being underweight (body mass index below 18.5) increases the risk of bone loss.

Review your medications. Some drugs, such as acid reflux medications, can increase the risk of osteoporosis or fractures.

Practice fall prevention. Educate yourself on all the ways to reduce falls and fractures, including wearing shoes with good traction, installing grab bars in the tub or shower, improving lighting, tossing out throw rugs, getting your vision checked, using a nonslip rubber mat in the bath, and improving your balance and coordination through exercise.

WHAT ELSE DO I NEED TO KNOW?

- The World Health Organization (WHO?—sorry, nerd joke) created an incredible tool called FRAX that can predict your 10-year fracture risk. It's a breeze to complete—there are 12 simple questions—but you will need results from your DEXA or some other type of bone test as well. When evaluated together by your doctor, the information helps give a clearer picture of your real-world risk of suffering a fracture in the next decade. It's similar to how your cholesterol level by itself can predict your odds of having a heart attack, but

TO VIBRATE OR NOT TO VIBRATE?

Whole-body vibration machines, such as the Power Plate, were all the rage a few years back, and some are still claiming that they can improve bone density. These machines look promising for individuals with limited to no mobility (you can stand or sit on them and the vibration is supposed to stimulate bone). However, they haven't really improved bone density in healthy postmenopausal women any better than getting 1,200 milligrams of calcium and 1,000 IU of vitamin D daily (as shown in studies), so opt for those simple lifestyle changes if you're healthy with normal mobility.

adding lifestyle, family history, blood pressure, and blood sugar information can more precisely define your risk.

- Many patients ask me about hormone replacement therapy drugs for bone loss (estrogen or progesterone). And this works well as long as you're willing to accept the risk, which is a higher incidence of breast cancer, cardiovascular disease, and dementia. If you're going to use it, you should be on the lowest possible dose of hormones and should also normalize your calcium and vitamin D intake.

- Since cholesterol-lowering drugs might also reduce bone loss by blocking cells that break down bone, I wish someone would do a study of red yeast rice extract (see the High Cholesterol section, page 234) to prevent bone loss. I bet you it would yield some positive results.

Parkinson's Disease

P

Dr. Moyad Secret Conventional medicine's track record in fighting Parkinson's is awful. After hundreds of millions—if not billions—of dollars in research, there are simply no medications available that can dramatically slow the progression of this devastating disease. However, there are many medications and some supplements to treat the symptoms associated with it. If someone in my family had this disease, I would not hesitate to try one of the supplements recommended in this section to at least reduce the risks or complications associated with it, such as dementia, depression, or bone loss. Several major clinical trials of supplements for Parkinson's are being conducted, which reflects the desperate need for effective treatments.

WHAT IS IT?

Parkinson's disease (PD) is a progressive neurodegenerative disorder with a variety of potential symptoms, including slowness of movement, rigidity (movements are not smooth), tremors usually during rest, difficulty walking (gait abnormalities), loss of muscle mass and strength, and an increase in muscle and joint pain. Dementia, depression, and other mental health issues are also common with this disease (see the Alzheimer's Disease, Dementia, and Mild Cognitive Impairment section, page 65, and the Depression section, page 166). In fact, it's now the second leading cause of dementia.

Although experts aren't sure what causes it, people with PD do have an abnormally low number of neurons in a part of the brain known as the substantia nigra pars compacta (as well as differences in other supportive brain structures). The loss of neurons, which are the primary providers of dopamine to other parts of the brain, can lead to some of the physical problems of PD. This is why the main treatment for PD, which has been the primary treatment since I was a baby (that is a long time, folks), is using drugs that increase dopamine levels in the brain.

WHAT WORKS

1. (tie) Inosine (inosine monophosphate) 500 to 3,000 milligrams a day, depending on uric acid levels

If the research on this supplement continues to be positive, it will take the top spot soon, although it does come with

359

risks (more information on that in a moment). Inosine plays a role in energy production in the body, which has intrigued athletic-performance researchers for years (so far to no avail). But inosine has other roles, and here's what's really fascinating about this compound: It can dramatically raise uric acid, which naturally blocks certain compounds that increase inflammation in parts of the body, including the brain. Parkinson's patients often have lower uric acid (or urate) levels than people without the disease. In some cases, PD sufferers with higher urate levels appear to have a slower progression of the disease. Researchers are currently studying inosine for relapsing-remitting multiple sclerosis and Parkinson's disease specifically for this reason (see the Multiple Sclerosis section, page 331). The complete outcome is still unknown, but it appears to be helping some patients with multiple sclerosis, and I have had families of PD patients swear by it.

The Michael J. Fox Foundation for Parkinson's Research and other groups helped finance the latest inosine study, called SURE-PD (Safety of Urate Elevation in Parkinson's Disease). Researchers studied doses of 500 to 3,000 milligrams of inosine per day (versus placebo) in early-stage PD patients with urate levels less than 6 mg/dL at baseline. The preliminary results came in as I was finishing this book: Not only was inosine as safe as a placebo overall (no significant differences in side effects except for three cases of kidney stones in the inosine group of 51 patients

over 24 months), but it also significantly raised uric acid levels in the cerebrospinal fluid and blood and there's some hint that it could be slowing the progression of the disease. The SURE-PD researchers announced that inosine should move to a Phase 3–like trial ASAP. Based on these results, it's time to talk about this option with your doctor today.

Inosine increases the risk of kidney stones, so if you have a history of gout or kidney issues, you should avoid it or work closely with your doctor to make sure your uric acid levels are not going too high.

1. (tie) Creatine monohydrate
20 grams for 5 days and then 4 to 10 grams a day

Creatine is well known in athletic circles for providing a minimal to moderate exercise boost. Small studies have shown significant improvement in muscle strength and reduction in muscle fatigue with 5 grams per day (after a loading, or "ramp up," dose of 20 grams daily for the first 5 days). Studies with PD patients have shown that creatine monohydrate, along with resistance exercise, may improve muscle weakness, fatigue, muscle loss, and mood and may allow some people to reduce their dose of conventional dopaminergic drugs. Researchers have studied daily doses as low as 4 grams, and they appear to be as safe as a placebo (except for some weight gain).

The results with creatine are so compelling—not only as an energy source for muscle tissue but also as a neuroprotectant—

that it is moving to a major government-funded Phase 3–like trial with PD patients (the FDA requires Phase 3 trials for pharmaceuticals before approving them). The National Institute of Neurological Disorders and Stroke Exploratory Trials in Parkinson's Disease network is conducting a study, called LS-1, that will track 1,700 PD patients over 5 years to see if creatine monohydrate (10 grams daily) slows clinical decline better than placebo. It's the largest trial ever of early-stage PD!

The biggest concern over creatine is whether these dosages might negatively impact kidney function in older patients, but this hasn't been an issue so far in clinical studies. This side effect is overhyped by people who don't have much knowledge in the area of supplements or PD. Weight gain and (rarely) gastrointestinal upset are more of an issue.

2. Vitamin D₃ 1,200 IU a day or enough to raise blood levels to approximately 40 ng/mL

If you read all the other sections in this book, you'll know that I rarely recommend vitamin D supplementation and testing. It's simply overhyped these days. But I *am* recommending it for Parkinson's patients! Vitamin D reduces the risk of falls in older people, and PD patients have a higher risk of falls and hip fractures (plus, they tend to be low in D). In a 12-month randomized trial with 114 Parkinson's patients in Tokyo, vitamin D₃ appeared to reduce the progression of the disease, which may simply be a result of increasing muscle strength and balance (most tissues and cells have receptors for this vitamin, including muscle tissue, and improving the ability of the muscles to finely coordinate activity improves balance). Patients in this trial started with a vitamin D level of 22 ng/mL, which increased to 42 ng/mL after taking 1,200 IU per day (side effects were similar to the placebo). This study suggests low vitamin D levels could increase disease progression because there was little to no progression in the supplement group compared to the placebo group.

3. Caffeine pills 50 to 200 milligrams twice daily maximum or 1 to 2 cups of coffee

Some of the largest epidemiologic studies to address the impact of caffeine on disease prevention have essentially found that just two to four cups of coffee a day—about 300 milligrams—could reduce the risk of Parkinson's. And they have discovered that caffeine may improve some of the symptoms of PD as well. Caffeine works by blocking receptors of a substance called A2A adenosine that may play a role in Parkinson's symptoms. The equivalent of 1 to 2 cups of coffee per day may reduce involuntary movements (such as tremors) and may increase the ability to perform voluntary movements. It can also help with fatigue, which is a problem in PD patients, so I'm a fan regardless. Most clinical trials have used between 100 to 200 milligrams in pill form twice a day, but I've seen 50 milligrams work, too (an 8-ounce cup of coffee contains about 100 milligrams), and studies have shown that caffeine in beverages may work just as well. In the CALM-PD trial, subjects who consumed more than 12 ounces of coffee a day reduced their risk of developing dyskinesia, which is difficulty performing voluntary movements, a common side effect of Levodopa treatment for Parkinson's. (You can also get caffeine in guarana, an Amazonian plant, and in yerba mate, but look for the tea or drink forms because pills with these ingredients lack good research up against the beverage sources in the area of PD.)

HONORABLE MENTION

Omega-3 fatty acids (at just 1,000 to 2,000 milligrams per day) may have a slight impact on depression in people without PD, but more research on this is needed. A well-done smaller, older trial with PD patients from Brazil found that taking fish oil with or without regular antidepressants appeared to further reduce depressive symptoms when compared to a placebo. And other studies in elderly patients without PD suggest omega-3 fatty acids might help maintain

and increase muscle. There is no question that omega-3s from marine sources are overhyped, but this is a situation where there is at least some rational reason for testing it.

WHAT'S WORTHLESS

High doses of CoQ10 and vitamin E. Preliminary studies suggested that large doses of these two supplements could slow the progression of PD, but it looks like a bust. The National Institute of Neurological Disorders and Stroke stopped a large Phase 3 trial (known as the QE3 study, administered by the Parkinson Study Group) in progress because these dietary supplements in large doses were *not* helping early-stage PD patients.

LIFESTYLE CHANGES

Heart healthy = brain and body healthy. Lowering cholesterol may decrease the risk of PD because it could have an anti-inflammatory effect and improve bloodflow in the brain. Moderate to vigorous exercise (30 to 60 minutes) on most days of the week is also associated with a lower risk, again, perhaps due to improved bloodflow. Interestingly, smoking/nicotine use may *reduce* the risk of PD.

Control your blood sugar. Diabetes may increase the risk of brain cell damage as well as PD. Reducing glucose to normal levels could help slow the progression of the disease.

Peripheral Artery Disease
(Intermittent Claudication)

THE JURY'S STILL OUT

Dr. Moyad Secret Be careful when trying any supplement for peripheral artery disease (PAD) because conventional medicine is so much better and every time "experts" say there's a better supplement, it has either failed or made PAD worse! So the goal here is to not take supplements unless a compelling case is made for why any should be added to proven limb- and life-saving conventional treatments.

PAD impacts about 5 to 15 percent of people between the ages of 50 and 80, and it leads to a higher risk of leg amputation and premature death. A common symptom is leg pain while walking because of clogged arteries in the legs. Risk factors for PAD should sound familiar (and remind you of heart disease risk factors) and include: reduced exercise, tobacco use, alcohol abuse, obesity, excessive caloric intake, hypertension, insulin resistance, high cholesterol, heart disease, increased inflammation, and family history. (Heart healthy = blood vessel healthy!) Statins could be beneficial enough to save a limb, especially in the advanced stages of PAD, and if you have trouble taking them, be sure to check out the High Cholesterol section, page 234, for alternatives.

Some of the supplements that you should *not* use for PAD include: omega-3s, high doses of vitamin D, ginkgo biloba, and L-arginine. For omega-3s, we're still waiting on results from clinical studies, such as the omega-PAD trial; high doses of vitamin D simply have no evidence right now. After 14 trials were evaluated, ginkgo biloba still hasn't been shown to be effective, and L-arginine at 3 grams per day performed significantly worse compared to placebo in the Stanford University NO-PAIN trial (Nitric Oxide in Peripheral Arterial Insufficiency study).

Peripheral Neuropathy

Dr. Moyad Secret If you've ever had your leg, foot, arm, or hand fall asleep after sitting in an awkward position for too long, you've had a tiny glimpse at what people with peripheral neuropathy experience 24/7. Patients have actually stopped their cancer treatments because they can't take the neuropathy! There are so many different drugs being thrown at PN in an effort to find something—anything—that helps alleviate or control the pain. This includes antidepressants, anticonvulsants, and opioids—expensive drugs that come with their own challenging side effects, such as dizziness and drowsiness. More than 70 Americans die per day—and more than 27,000 per year—from unintentional prescription drug overdose, so this is an epidemic problem! Anything that can be done to prevent or reduce the progression of this disease is welcome.

WHAT IS IT?

Peripheral neuropathy (PN) is caused by injury or damage to the nerves and the blood vessels surrounding them, usually as a result of trauma, infection, diabetes, chemotherapy, and other drugs. Symptoms include aching, burning, itching, numbness, and pain, and they make something as mundane as buttoning a shirt or even walking around the block difficult (see "How Neuropathy Feels" [page 365] for more symptoms). Those with diabetes are at especially high risk for neuropathies because high blood sugar levels damage the vessels and nerves.

More than 100 types of peripheral neuropathies have been identified, but physicians tend to focus on three general categories: motor, sensory, and autonomic. Motor nerves send commands from the brain to the muscles, and they manage movements that are under conscious control, like talking, walking, and grasping things. Sensory nerves transmit information about sensory experiences, such as a light touch or pain from a paper cut, from the periphery (outside your body) to the brain. Autonomic nerves regulate all those things that you don't consciously control, such as breathing, digesting food, and the pumping of your heart. Most people experience one or two types of neuropathies. Those with diabetes, however, can have all three types if it's not aggressively controlled. The most common form in those with type 1 and 2 diabetes is known as diabetic sensorimotor polyneuropathy. It occurs in 10 percent of people with diabetes within the first year of diagnosis and in up to 50 percent of patients after 25 years of living with the disease. Most treatments recommended here are

HOW NEUROPATHY FEELS

- Aching
- Burning
- Electric shock–like sensations
- Heaviness in hands and feet
- Increased sensitivity to cold
- Itching
- Loss of reflexes (especially at the ankle and knee)
- Numbness
- Pain
- Pins and needles, as if part of the body is falling asleep (this is known as paresthesia)
- Prickling
- Reduced sensation
- Stabbing
- Tenderness
- Throbbing
- Tingling
- Weakness

for neuropathies related to sensory nerve tissue, especially diabetic peripheral neuropathy, but supplements that help with one type of neuropathy appear to help other types as well.

WHAT WORKS

1. (tie) Alpha-lipoic acid (ALA)
600 milligrams a day in divided doses

Alpha-lipoic acid is involved with countless functions in every human cell. And ALA is the number one dietary supplement for peripheral neuropathy in terms of the amount of human research that's been done on it. Part of the reason it has received so much attention is that it's used as a prescription oral and IV drug in many parts of the world. There have been more than 15 randomized trials looking at the benefit of giving 300 to 600 milligrams of ALA per day for 2 to 4 weeks to patients with PN. It was found to improve nerve conduction and reduce neuropathic symptoms, and it has a great safety record. It is generally the only therapy that can both help prevent and treat PN, along with heart-healthy lifestyle changes and controlling blood sugars.

Patients in the clinical trials experienced reduced neuropathy within as little as 2 weeks, but you should stay on it for at least 2 months to give it a chance to build up and see if it's working. Daily doses as high as 1,800 milligrams have been used, but that amount can rarely cause nausea, vomiting, headache, vertigo, and itching, and the 600-milligram daily dose seems just as effective. ALA should be taken on an empty stomach (30 to 60 minutes before or 2 hours after a meal) for better absorption, and the dose can be divided if any side effects are experienced. (*Warning:* ALA can make your urine smell the same way it does after you eat asparagus; it's harmless.) Many doctors will combine this supplement with other conventional drug treatments, but the vast majority of the research on ALA for neuropathy is as a monotherapy (by itself). The R-form of ALA appears to be better absorbed than the S-form, so look for a supplement that contains the R-form or at least racemic ALA (a 50/50 mix of R and S).

In humans, ALA is produced by the liver and several other tissues, and it can be obtained from plant and animal sources, such as organ meats. Spinach, broccoli, tomato, Brussels sprouts, garden peas, and rice bran are good sources of the R-form of ALA. Yet, the amount in our diets can never come close to the therapeutic levels that were tested and worked in clinical trials. Plus, as we age, our ability to produce ALA drops (similar to many other compounds in the body).

I don't think people have heard enough (if anything) about ALA for the treatment of PN. I think we'll be seeing exciting research about this supplement in the future.

1. (tie) Capsaicin cream (0.075 percent) applied up to four times a day

The active ingredient in chile peppers, capsaicin works by reducing levels of a compound in the body called substance P, which is released when there's pain. Capsaicin pills are starting to be researched, but I have no faith that they'll show any benefit for peripheral neuropathy anytime soon; they're just too irritating for the GI tract. The topical cream is where the research is, and it's especially effective for more superficial pain, like neuropathies. The American Association of Neuromuscular and Electrodiagnostic Medicine, the American Academy of Neurology, and the American Academy of Physical Medicine and Rehabilitation all agree that capsaicin cream at 0.075 percent is probably effective and should be considered for treatment of diabetic peripheral neuropathy. Always apply it with gloves or a cotton swab, though; if you get capsaicin on your fingers and then into your eye, the burning sensation can be quite painful and potentially harmful. There's also a new patch on the market, which makes application easy.

Higher concentrations (up to 8 percent) are going through clinical trials, but you have to obtain these through a prescription and they usually come in patch form (Qutenza). Side effects are generally minimal, but the prescription can cause a rapid change in blood pressure when it's first applied (that is a lot of concentrated capsaicin, folks!). Keep in mind that capsaicin should *not* be combined with anything else that can heat the skin, such as a heating pad, because it can burn the skin.

I'm bullish on capsaicin because it provides quick (albeit temporary) relief for PN and can be combined with ALA. I recommend it for arthritis pain, too (many people experience both arthritis and PN).

2. B vitamins only as directed by your doctor

Vitamin B$_1$ (thiamin) deficiency is a common cause of neuropathy in alcoholics and people who've had weight loss (bariatric) surgery, and recent research suggests people with diabetes may also lack B$_1$ or other vitamins. An alternate form of B$_1$ (a drug called benfotiamine) has been tested with some success at higher daily doses (25 to 100 milligrams), so there are some experts who believe supplements can be beneficial for people with low levels of vitamin B$_1$. Low levels of vitamin B$_6$ and especially B$_{12}$ have also been associated with neuropathies; these vitamins play a role in nerve health, function, and transmission. Here's what's really important, though: Numerous common medications, such as metformin for diabetes and proton pump inhibitors for gastroesophageal reflux disease or ulcers, can reduce blood levels of some B vitamins, so these could be contributing to neuropathy in some people.

I have seen very little neuropathy-relieving benefit from any supplements beyond alpha-lipoic acid and capsaicin, but when it comes to B-vitamin deficiencies, it's worth the blood test. It provides a quick answer and can save you tons of time and money wasted chasing down other causes. So, if nobody can explain why you're experiencing neuropathy, ask for a B-vitamin blood panel.

WHAT'S WORTHLESS

Acetyl-L-carnitine. Experts have been recommending acetyl-L-carnitine for years for treating PN, but it actually made symptoms significantly worse in a major study of breast cancer patients taking it to reduce the risk of neuropathy from chemotherapy. While this study only looked at chemo, I believe the results suggest this supplement could make PN worse no matter what the cause, so I'd avoid it. Major medical "oops" here, folks!

High doses of vitamin B$_6$. Some people take high doses of B$_6$ (300 milligrams or more) to increase energy, reduce the risk of kidney stones, or simply get more B vitamins because they were told to. Although supplementing at certain doses may help PN, more is not better. Such high doses over several weeks to months can actually *cause* sensory neuropathy.

Vitamin E. "Experts" often recommend large doses of vitamin E for PN because it's supposed to absorb free radicals that can cause neuropathy. But at higher doses it can create free radicals, lead to toxicity, and perhaps block the effect of some conventional drugs to treat

PN. I recommend it only in a few special cases in this book, such as for nonalcoholic fatty liver disease, age-related macular degeneration, and Alzheimer's (see those sections, pages 338, 311, and 65, respectively).

LIFESTYLE CHANGES

Heart healthy = nerve healthy. My theory is that anything that reduces your risk of heart disease potentially reduces the risk or occurrence of peripheral neuropathy. This means keeping your cholesterol, blood pressure, and glucose levels within normal ranges, exercising, and avoiding smoking.

Be aware of your surroundings. Since PN can reduce mobility and the ability to sense pain, it is necessary to pay close attention to situations and objects that can be dangerous. Wear gloves and warm socks in the winter, use pot holders, have a family member test the water temperature, remove throw rugs, install a shower chair, and use handrails on stairs.

Try alternative therapies. There's only a small amount of positive research regarding acupuncture and PN so far, but I think acupuncture is always promising for chronic pain, especially if it can reduce the amount of hard-core pain medication being taken.

Get magnetized. A fairly large and well-done study found that magnetic shoe insoles with a strength of 450 G (Gauss) reduced burning, numbness, and tingling, as well as exercise-induced foot pain after 3 to 4 months. It hasn't been replicated, and so far minimal to no benefit has been seen for general pain from magnet therapy itself (or being exposed to pulsed electromagnetic fields for brief periods of time), so try it at your own risk. It may just be a great placebo, but who cares? I like anything that can stop the cycle of frequent, high-dose drug use for PN.

WHAT ELSE DO I NEED TO KNOW?

Heavy metals—such as arsenic, mercury, and lead—in supplements can make neuropathies worse. These are found naturally in the earth, and they inevitably end up in supplements, especially if the manufacturer does not have good quality control and testing standards. This is just another reason to do your research and know whom you're buying from. Always look for an NSF, NPA, or USP label on the packaging, which indicates the product meets certain safety and quality standards. And if you're taking a ton of supplements, be aware that you could be getting unnecessarily high doses of these toxic heavy metals.

Peyronie's Disease

P

Dr. Moyad Secret No, this condition was not named after an Italian beer! (Not a month goes by where I don't hear someone at a party talking about Peroni beer and mispronouncing it as *pay-ROH-nee*, as in Peyronie's disease.)

Here's another situation where the research has finally convinced doctors that some dietary supplements work! In fact, now most physicians want their patients to take some form of dietary supplementation along with the conventional treatment for Peyronie's disease. However, keep in mind that supplements are most effective for the early stages of Peyronie's disease (acute or early chronic). As a final thought, ask your doctor about the newly approved drug Xiaflex.

WHAT IS IT?

Peyronie's disease is a deformity of the penis that impacts 5 to 10 percent of men. It's most common among 55- to 65-year-olds, but it has been reported in younger men as well. It's caused by fibrous lesions that form inside the penis near the surface (they can sometimes be felt and even seen). Researchers aren't sure why some men are more susceptible to this condition than others, but some experts consider it to be a wound-healing disorder. When the penis is partially or fully erect during intercourse, it can cause subtle microtears to the tissue inside the penis, resulting in bleeding below the skin and formation of a clot or clots. In some people, the subsequent immune response to clean up the damage (an otherwise natural process) leads to excess collagen being laid down at the site and plaque formation. Peyronie's

disease has been associated with erectile dysfunction and several other conditions, including diabetes (30 percent of patients), high blood pressure or cholesterol, obesity, smoking, pelvic surgery, and low testosterone levels.

Men with Peyronie's generally have three primary complaints:

- Painful erections that can interfere with sex (about 50 percent of sufferers experience this)

- Palpable plaque formations on the penis; they can be soft, tender, or really hard

- Curvature of the penis (seen in about 80 percent of patients)

Peyronie's has two phases: acute and chronic. The acute phase includes pain and curvature of the penis and the formation of one or more nodules, or plaques, that can be felt and sometimes even seen. The pain

369

and discomfort comes and goes and can resolve with treatment over 6 to 18 months. In the chronic phase, there is usually little to no pain, nodule size generally stays the same, and there is some degree of deformity of the penis. The standard treatment for Peyronie's, usually in the acute or early chronic phase, includes injections, prescription medication, or corrective surgery.

WHAT WORKS

1. L-arginine 2,000 milligrams a day in divided doses or L-citrulline 1,000 to 1,500 milligrams a day in divided doses

L-arginine increases nitric oxide in the blood, which boosts bloodflow to the penis; it may also have an antifibrotic effect, reducing the development of scars and improving wound healing. (Laboratory studies have suggested that it can prevent inflammation and fibrosis in the liver, kidneys, lungs, and cardiovascular system.) Research is still ongoing in regard to Peyronie's, but researchers from Rush University Medical Center in Chicago are seeing reduced fibrosis and scarring from taking 1,000 milligrams of L-arginine twice a day along with conventional treatment, including drugs or injections. Perhaps the primary benefit for Peyronie's is that L-arginine helps improve erectile dysfunction, which can be a symptom of this disease. (See the Erectile Dysfunction section, page 186.) While L-arginine has significant research, I believe L-citrulline, a precursor to L-arginine, is far better and safer. I recommend taking 1,500 milligrams per day of L-citrulline, but see which one works for you.

2. CoQ10 300 milligrams a day

CoQ10 (coenzyme Q10) appears to have anti-inflammatory effects and may also improve bloodflow to different parts of the body, from the heart to the penis. Recently, researchers have been studying its ability to reduce production of a compound called TGFB1 (or transforming growth factor, beta 1), which may contribute to the abnormal inflammatory response, and subsequent scarring, seen in Peyronie's. In studies, 300 milligrams of CoQ10 per day for 6 months worked better than a placebo to reduce plaque size, penile curvature, and pain; improve sexual function; and slow the progression of the disease in 85 percent of subjects with early chronic Peyronie's. CoQ10 is a fat-soluble supplement, so it should be taken with food. It can interfere with blood thinners, so check with your doctor before taking it.

3. Carnitine 2,000 milligrams a day

Carnitine, which comes in various forms, may be able to lower calcium levels inside endothelial cells, which line the inside of the penis, leading to a reduction in the risk of plaque formations or fibrosis. Research has shown that after 3 months of supplementation with acetyl-L-carnitine (1,000 milligrams twice a day), men with Peyronie's who were also on conventional prescription treatment saw less pain and curvature of the penis but no significant change in plaque size (although it did help a little). Another clinical trial with 2,000 milligrams per day of propionyl-L-carnitine along with conventional medicine (10 milligrams of intralesional verapamil weekly for 10 weeks) showed significantly reduced penile curvature, disease progression, and plaque size compared to verapamil without carnitine. This supplement isn't widely accepted yet among physicians because it needs more research. Just an FYI: There is no good research on drug interactions with these carnitine supplements, so check with your doctor first. I have seen minimal drug interactions in patients, and most doctors will allow some sort of dietary supplementation with conventional treatments for Peyronie's.

WHAT'S WORTHLESS

Vitamin E. This vitamin (400 to 800 IU daily or more) used to be one of the most common nonsurgical treatments for Peyronie's, but recent research suggests high doses of vitamin E supplements may be dangerous for the heart and prostate and could cause internal bleeding. As little as 400 IU daily increases risk for prostate cancer and bleeding. I only recommend vitamin E (or other potentially dangerous supplements) when there are no other good options for a disease and it can make a dramatic difference (for example, in individuals with fatty liver disease or moderate to advanced stages of the dry form of macular degeneration; see those sections, pages 338 and 311, respectively, if you're curious). *However*, using vitamin E cream

directly on the penis appears to be less dangerous; it's a good potential compromise, so ask your doctor about it.

Vitamin C. This supplement is capable of increasing the production of collagen in the body, which is exactly what you do *not* want while receiving conventional treatment for acute Peyronie's. Plus, there is no research that says vitamin C helps.

Propolis. Honeybees extract propolis from the saps or buds of trees and other plants and use it as a protectant for the hive from wind, rain, cold, other insects, and even disease. It appears to have antioxidant and anti-inflammatory properties and blocks the production of certain compounds (interleukins) that could make the inflammatory response worse. It sure sounds like it would be helpful for Peyronie's, but research hasn't shown it to be beneficial.

Blueberry extract. Blueberries have strong antioxidant properties and may even have an antifibrotic effect, but again, the research on the extract hasn't panned out.

LIFESTYLE CHANGES

Heart healthy = penis healthy. This means that maintaining a healthy weight and normal cholesterol, blood pressure, and blood sugars have been associated with a lower risk of Peyronie's.

WHAT ELSE DO I NEED TO KNOW?

Without treatment, about half of men get worse and the other half get better or stay the same. In many instances, the pain or

371

OLDIE BUT A GOODIE

I remember this moment like it was yesterday. One day when I was 9 or 10, my dad, who's a doctor (he's 80 years old and still practicing because he simply loves his job; he's the best urologist on the planet!), wore a T-shirt that said something like, "Keep straight with Potaba." We didn't have Google or Bing back then so I had no idea what the T-shirt meant, but now I do and I wish I had that shirt!

Researchers aren't quite sure exactly how Potaba (potassium para-aminobenzoate) works, but the theory is that it decreases the production of collagen, which leads to a reduction in fibrosis (the effective dose is 3 grams daily for a year). Recent research shows that it may reduce plaque size but not pain or curvature of the penis. No research has been done with para-aminobenzoic acid, the supplement form of Potaba, but it should be tested. It's easy to find and inexpensive.

curvature of the penis is the deciding factor on when to get treatment. In other words, it comes down to quality of life (and sex!). This is why a specialist is needed. Some studies of potential interventions look at pain improvement, but pain can decrease over time even without treatment. Other studies look at a reduction in the size of the plaque on the penis, but this does not always improve curvature. Thus, many urologic experts believe the best way to judge a potential treatment for Peyronie's is whether it can reduce any deformity (narrowing, shortening, or curvature). But only a specialist can help you decide if the treatment might be worse than the disease itself. Getting surgery or injections is not fun.

Surgery is considered the gold standard to fix the deformity associated with Peyronie's, but it should only be used in men whose condition has stabilized for 3 to 6 months (in other words, it's not getting worse or better). The best candidates are men who have a painless deformity, cannot engage in sexual activity because of the deformity, have hardness issues, or have plaque formations that cannot be corrected with nonsurgical options. Surgery gives the fastest and best result, on average, and most men can still have orgasms and ejaculate afterward. It can't always fully correct a curvature, and in some cases it can reduce the length or hardness of the penis or (rarely) reduce some penile sensation, so talk to your doctor.

Polycystic Ovary Syndrome (PCOS)

Dr. Moyad Secret This is the most common hormone problem and the number one cause of infertility in women of reproductive age (5 to 10 percent of reproductive-age females with polycystic ovary syndrome, or PCOS, have difficulty becoming pregnant). The supplement NAC (N-acetylcysteine) at 1,200 milligrams per day appears to work well along with conventional treatment for inducing ovulation in preliminary research. It may actually improve ovulation and pregnancy rates! Talk to your doctor, who should check the medical literature because this is a cheap supplement with a great safety profile.

PCOS is a common hormonal disorder characterized by an irregular menstrual cycle, high levels of male hormones (androgens), and polycystic ovaries; insulin resistance impacts more than half of PCOS patients. Many women do not have ovarian cysts, however, which is why the National Institutes of Health concluded that the name is confusing and blocks progress to research and better care. In truth, it's a complex mix of metabolic, hypothalamic, pituitary, ovarian, and adrenal interactions or abnormalities, and it causes hormonal changes that affect women in multiple ways. The cause is unknown, but experts suspect a combination of genetics and environment. Symptoms include acne, excess hair growth on the body and face, irregular menstrual periods, ovarian cysts, thinning scalp hair, weight gain, chronic pelvic pain, bloating and fluid retention, depression, and migraines. Long term, PCOS may increase the risk for some cancers, such as uterine (endometrial) cancer.

Because there is insulin resistance and an increased risk of type 2 diabetes in PCOS, high insulin levels are the primary problem. There is also usually an increase in blood pressure and cholesterol and fat in the abdomen. Taking 1 to 1.5 grams of fish oil per day can reduce triglycerides and increase HDL (good cholesterol) and may even improve blood sugar levels. (See the High Cholesterol section, page 234.)

Although half of women with PCOS are of normal weight, if you're obese or carrying extra pounds, losing weight can spur a profound improvement in symptoms and fertility. Statins (prescription cholesterol-lowering drugs) may be able to reduce androgen levels, and if that's the case, red yeast rice supplements might be a good option to try because they function like some statins. In some women with PCOS, high-dose statins could make insulin resistance worse, though, so work with your doctor carefully on this to see if you qualify for a statin or red yeast rice.

Pregnancy

Dr. Moyad Secret Approximately 50 percent of pregnancies are unplanned, and by the time a woman finds out, she's usually well into her first trimester. That's why I always recommend women (and even men) who are of childbearing age take a multivitamin with folic acid daily. Better folic acid intake (either in the many fortified foods that are now available or via supplement) is one of the greatest public health success stories of my lifetime because it reduces the risk of disabling or fatal neural tube defects (NTDs). Now, there's new preliminary research suggesting this B vitamin may even reduce the risk of autism, but this needs more research. Regardless, it's encouraging that during one of the most delicate and critical moments in life—pregnancy—supplements can be life saving and life changing.

WHAT WORKS FOR . . .

Note: Before taking any drugs or supplements during your pregnancy, please check with your OB-GYN.

Preventing neural tube defects. Healthy women who are of reproductive age with no history of NTDs should take 400 to 800 micrograms of folic acid (vitamin B_9) or another form of folate (such as L-methylfolate) daily, usually in a prenatal vitamin. Pregnant women at high risk of a neural tube defect should take 4 milligrams. (In a study of 1,800 high-risk women, the Medical Research Council Vitamin Study Research Group found that folic acid supplementation led to a *72 percent reduction* in risk of NTDs.) This B vitamin helps with red blood cell development and cell replication and division, and it is known conclusively to help pre-

vent neural tube defects, such as spina bifida (66 percent of NTDs) and anencephaly (33 percent of NTDs). In spina bifida, the spinal column doesn't close to protect the spinal cord. Nerves get damaged, leading to lifelong paralysis of the lower body and bladder and bowel problems in the majority of cases. In anencephaly, most or all of the brain fails to develop. The baby typically dies in utero or after birth. That's why prenatal vitamins with folic acid or another form of folate are so critical.

Certain medications can alter how much folic acid you need, so ask your doctor about the correct dosage if you're taking medication for epilepsy, type 2 diabetes, rheumatoid arthritis, lupus, psoriasis, asthma, inflammatory bowel disease, kidney disease, liver disease, sickle cell disease, or celiac disease. If you consume more than one alcoholic drink a day, also talk to your doctor about how much to take. Breastfeeding women need 500 micrograms of folic acid per day.

Some women may benefit from taking a specific form of folate known as L-5-methyl-THF (it's in a commercial product called Metafolin, also known as L-methylfolate). It's somewhat similar to folic acid but generally costs more (it's considered a medical food, so it's best to work with your doctor when taking it, but you don't need a prescription). A small percentage of women have a genetic risk factor for neural tube defects and may be put on Metafolin if they test positive for this genetic mutation (the MTHFR gene). (Hispanics have the highest risk of this and African Americans the lowest.)

Why a vitamin versus just eating more folate, you ask? Folate in food is only 50 to 80 percent as available to the body as the folic acid in supplements. All of the major clinical studies that showed benefits against NTDs were primarily with folic acid supplements.

Now, since autism is a neurodevelopmental disorder that may occur during early pregnancy—especially in the first month when folate is known to be essential—taking folic acid before conception is critical. (Some children with autism spectrum disorder or autistic symptoms have a deficiency of brain levels of folate, which could be due to autoantibodies blocking the folate receptor. Extra folate may help overcome some of these issues in children.) More research on this is still needed, but women of reproductive age

MOYAD TIP: Iron is critical in a prenatal vitamin, as is vitamin C because it improves the absorption of iron. Ask your doctor how much you may need.

should be taking folate anyway, so there's no risk here. (See the Autism Spectrum Disorders section, page 85, for more information.)

Acid reflux/heartburn. If you need to supplement your dietary calcium intake to get to the daily Recommended Dietary Allowance or you occasionally experience acid reflux symptoms or heartburn, of which there's a higher risk in pregnancy, use calcium carbonate. Some of the best-selling over-the-counter acid reflux meds—from Tums to Rolaids—are primarily composed of calcium carbonate. One potential bonus: There is some research suggesting calcium may help reduce the risk of hypertension during pregnancy.

Bone health. There is preliminary evidence that a mother's calcium and vitamin D status during pregnancy can impact the bone health of her child. Ask your doctor whether you should have a vitamin D blood test to determine if you need extra doses of D (600 IU is the standard recommendation during pregnancy and breastfeeding for women with normal D levels). Normal calcium intake should be from 1,000 (19 years or older) to 1,300 milligrams per day (14 to 18 years of age), and you can get most of it from diet. Bottom line: It's important to address calcium and vitamin D needs during pregnancy. I consider a vitamin D blood level of 30 to 40 ng/mL (on a 25-OH vitamin D test) to be completely normal, and megadosing to get beyond this level makes no sense. Please refer to the Osteoporosis section, page 352, for more information on bone health.

Constipation. Fiber is your friend! Getting fiber from food—such as vegetables, cereal, and bread—can keep you regular during pregnancy. And staying hydrated is just as important as using a fiber product. If this isn't doing the job, talk to your doctor about taking a fiber powder supplement (5 to 10 milligrams a day of psyllium, for example). Keep in mind that using iron supplements during pregnancy and having a history of constipation before pregnancy are two of the best predictors of whether you'll be constipated during pregnancy. (Overusing calcium supplements can also cause constipation.)

Depression. Postpartum depression and depression in pregnancy are serious issues, and you should discuss them with your doctor if you're concerned. See the Depression section, page 166, for lifestyle tips that can help; the research with supplements just isn't great for postpartum depression, I'm afraid. (There is some research to suggest low vitamin D levels may be linked with a higher risk of postpartum depression, though.)

Leg cramps. Taking 300 to 900 milligrams of magnesium sulfate per day may reduce pregnancy-related leg cramps, but there have only been a small number of studies and diarrhea is one of the most common side effects of magnesium supplements.

Nausea. About half of women experience nausea and vomiting early in their pregnancies, and another 25 percent have just nausea. Even though this is known as morning sickness, it should really be called anytime-day-or-night sickness. In a small percentage of women, the nausea and vomiting can become so severe that it leads to weight loss, electrolyte imbalances, and dehydration (and requires treatment).

Pregnancy triggers nausea and vomiting due to rising levels of the hormone hCG (the same hormone used in testing kits to indicate pregnancy). It stimulates estrogen production from the ovaries, and the estrogen increases the risk of nausea and vomiting.

There's a theory that B-vitamin deficiency may increase the risk of nausea because multivitamins or prenatals with B vitamins can reduce nausea. Taking vitamin B_6 (10 to 25 milligrams) every 8 hours can help. (Research shows that taking a multivitamin even around the time of conception can reduce the severity of nausea and vomiting during pregnancy.)

Taking ginger supplements (125 to 250 milligrams four times a day or 350 to 500 milligrams three times a day) for 4 days to 3 weeks has shown success for nausea and vomiting in the first trimester of pregnancy. Most of the past successful clinical trials have used between 500 to 1,500 *total* milligrams per day (taken in divided doses). Never go above this because excessive ginger consumption can cause uterine stimulation, increased heartburn, and other problems. Past clinical trials of ginger in pregnancy saw no greater rate of birth defects, miscarriages, or deformities compared to pregnant women who weren't taking ginger.

Note: Ginger is one of the only *herbal* supplements, apart from cranberry supplements for urinary tract infections, that I recommend for use during pregnancy and *only* after talking with your doctor. Other supplements might help, but the risk could exceed the benefit due to contaminants found in some herbal products.

Keep your eye on protein powder supplements because they're being tested to reduce nausea. Protein is not only the most satiating macronutrient, it could have some impact on reducing bowel stimulation and preventing the triggering of nausea centers in the brain (it just needs more research).

Preeclampsia. This medical condition, which can occur in pregnancy or right after, results in high blood pressure and excess protein in the urine, which can endanger the health of both mother and baby. If left untreated, it can progress to eclampsia (life-threatening seizures) during pregnancy. Recent large studies have used the supplement L-arginine along with other vitamins and minerals in women who are at higher risk of preeclampsia, and researchers achieved large preliminary reductions in risk. It appears L-arginine was responsible for the real benefit in these studies (versus the other vitamins and minerals).

L-arginine can improve bloodflow to various organs of the body by increasing blood levels of nitric oxide, which dilates vessels, but it could also have some blood-thinning effects, so more safety studies are needed (see the Hypertension section, page 251). If L-arginine becomes an option in the future, researchers should also test L-citrulline, which appears to work just as well but at half the dosage. This is an ongoing and exciting area of research, and if you're at risk of preeclampsia, you should discuss it with your doctor. I will not recommend dosages here because this is a conversation to have with your OB-GYN.

Additionally, the US Preventive Services Task Force recently recommended taking low-dose aspirin for women at high risk of preeclampsia. It may also reduce the risk of preterm birth and intrauterine growth restrictions. While aspirin was originally derived from willow bark, I don't recommending taking this supplement. But taking a low-dose aspirin is certainly worth discussing with your doctor if you are at high risk for preeclampsia.

Urinary tract infections. See the Urinary Tract Infection section, page 435, for details on how to choose the right cranberry supplement to prevent recurrent UTIs.

Varicose veins and hemorrhoids. Please refer to the Varicose Veins and Chronic Venous Insufficiency section, page 442, and the Hemorrhoids section, page 226, for the research on horse chestnut seed extract and diosmin. Again, I would be very careful about using them, especially during the first trimester, because they have received little to no research in pregnancy.

WHAT'S WORTHLESS

The Moyad mantra in pregnancy (and for kids): *When in doubt, cut it out!* Of course, I'm not talking about prenatal vitamins here. I'm talking about the long list of supplements that are supposed to "improve the health of mom and baby"; this is just too delicate a time to be playing guinea pig. For example, researchers are touting lots of probiotics, but there is still not enough evidence. Plus, normalizing fiber intake acts like a perfect prebiotic, which allows the best probiotics to naturally set up shop in your colon without having to take more pills!

Fish oil. Some of the best studies to date have shown minimal to zero benefit with fish oil for reducing postpartum depression or improving the mental health of children whose mothers used this supplement during pregnancy. Still, there are multiple other randomized trials that suggest there might be a benefit. I have seen a lot of sales pitches by supplement companies and doctors who get paid by these companies, but it would be nice to see more consistent research. This is what I call a flip-of-the-coin supplement in terms of research. If you and your doctor think you need it, do not take the pills (they can exacerbate reflux and heartburn); opt for a children's flavored liquid instead. Or add low-mercury, high omega-3 fish to your diet.

LIFESTYLE CHANGES

Heart healthy = pregnancy healthy. Exercising and being a healthy weight when trying to become pregnant can reduce complications. Conversely, reduced physical activity during pregnancy can cause excessive weight gain, thus increasing the risk for gestational diabetes, hypertension, preeclampsia, delivery by caesarean section, and stillbirth. Ask your doctor about calorie intake, exercise type and amount, and other lifestyle questions.

WHAT ELSE DO I NEED TO KNOW?

Never let one tiny section in a massive book cause you to not follow your doctor's advice during pregnancy. This section, like this entire book, is intended to facilitate more discussion between you and your doctor.

Premature Ejaculation

P

Dr. Moyad Secret Remember back when PE used to mean gym class? Now that more and more physical education programs are being dropped in schools, it won't be long before PE will only refer to premature ejaculation! The nongym PE is actually the most common male sexual dysfunction (erectile dysfunction, or ED, runs a close second). The primary method of treating it is delaying ejaculation by decreasing stimulation and sexual function. Some of the most commonly used drugs for PE are either numbing topical agents (a.k.a. anesthetics, such as lidocaine or over-the-counter sprays) or a class of antidepressants known as SSRIs (selective serotonin reuptake inhibitors), which cause delayed ejaculation as a side effect. So it makes sense that supplements that work for PE either have anesthetic or antidepressant properties.

WHAT IS IT?

Premature ejaculation is ejaculation with minimal stimulation and earlier than desired, usually before or soon after penetration. The man has little or no voluntary control over it, and the situation usually (but not always) causes distress, sometimes to the point where sexual intimacy is avoided altogether. Unlike erectile dysfunction, PE is not age-related and the drugs that work for ED generally don't work for PE. Unfortunately, most men with PE never seek help; I'm hoping this section will change that.

The causes of PE are unknown. Experts have speculated that it's due to anxiety, a hypersensitive penis, or even a neurotransmitter/chemical imbalance, but there's little data to support these theories.

Most men know they have a problem, but for those who are unsure, there are questionnaires online, such as the Premature Ejaculation Diagnostic Tool. The higher the score, the likelier the problem is PE.

WHAT WORKS

1. Topical anesthetic (desensitization) creams/sprays
dosage varies

As mentioned earlier, these products work by blunting exterior sensations. Really the only topical supplement product that's been studied and has decent evidence so far is Severance Secret-Cream (also known as SS-cream), a combination of nine herbs that is produced by a Korean company (Cheil Jedan Corporation). You apply 0.2 grams

(200 milligrams) to the head of the penis 30 to 60 minutes before sexual activity and wash it off immediately after sex. The problem is, it's hard to get outside of Korea, but you can contact the company or look for it on Amazon (it's hit and miss there). It had very impressive (almost difficult to believe) results in one double-blind trial. The average ejaculatory time went from 1.4 minutes to 10.9 minutes, and the cream was 27 times more effective than the placebo in terms of increasing sexual satisfaction! Twenty percent of the SS-cream users reported mild localized irritation, including burning and pain (the partners didn't report any side effects), and some participants complained about the color and odor. Although the European Association of Urology now recommends SS-cream in its clinical treatment guidelines, I doubt this cream will be widely available outside of Korea anytime soon (my colleagues in Korea have not heard of any push to bring it to the United States or other areas). One thing you can always count on though in the supplement field is copycats (companies that copy the original formula or even sell anesthetic sprays).

The nine herbs in this product are:

- Ginseng Radix Alba
- Angelicae Gigantic Radix
- Cistanchis Herba
- Zanthoxylli Fructus
- Torlidis Semen
- Asiasari Radix
- Caryophylli Flos
- Cinnamomi Cortex
- Bufonis Veneum

2. (tie) St. John's wort 300 to 450 milligrams a day

Note: Both of the silver medalists here (St. John's wort and 5-HTP) have not been heavily researched; rather, they have similar mechanisms of action to some of the most commonly used prescription drugs for PE. I'm breaking my research rules here because of my experience with patients and doctors around the world who have used these successfully for PE.

Both St. John's wort and 5-HTP (opposite) increase serotonin, much the same way that selective serotonin reuptake inhibitor antidepressants, or SSRIs, do (see the Depression section, page 166). Researchers are still trying to figure out exactly how St. John's wort works, but it seems to block serotonin uptake (meaning the chemical hangs around longer) and alter levels of multiple brain neurotransmitters, including dopamine, norepinephrine, and GABA (gamma-aminobutyric acid). Increased levels of serotonin inhibit the ejaculatory reflex, and delayed ejaculation is one of the common side effects of antidepressants, which is why doctors frequently prescribe them for PE. While there is preliminary research showing it may help some men with PE, I'd like to see more evidence. One of the active ingredients in St. John's wort, a compound called hyperforin, has been getting some research, but it's still only in the lab; in other words, it hasn't been tested for PE in real people.

St. John's wort has been effective for *depression* at doses of 500 to 1,200 milligrams per day (in two or three divided doses) over 4 to 12 weeks. (Always look for an extract that is standardized to contain 0.3 percent hypericin.) But clinical trials for PE will use a dosage that is much lower (probably one-third to one-half of what has been used for depression). Just keep in mind that St. John's wort can reduce the efficacy of almost half of all prescription drugs in the United States, including birth control pills. (That might slow down the excitement process right there!) And never take St. John's wort if you're already on a prescription antidepressant, including SSRIs, tricyclics, or monoamine oxidase (MAO) inhibitors. You should also avoid it if you're taking immunosuppressants, antiretrovirals, blood thinners (like warfarin), or chemotherapy drugs. Side effects of high dosages of St. John's wort include insomnia, vivid dreams, anxiety, dizziness, and sun sensitivity.

Is it worth the risk? I think some of the potential drug interaction concerns are overblown, but that's something to ask your physician about. Since the number one prescription treatment for PE is SSRI-type drugs and because St. John's wort works like these drugs, it's easy to recommend this supplement for PE. If it's not effective after 1 or 2 weeks, try something else.

2. (tie) 5-HTP 50 to 300 milligrams a day

While St. John's wort keeps serotonin from being reabsorbed by cells, 5-HTP essentially helps cells create more serotonin (either way you end up with more of it). Again, there are no studies with PE yet, but it has a mechanism of action that's similar to conventional drugs for PE. As with St. John's wort, the letters and comments I've received over the years in terms of efficacy of 5-HTP have been encouraging. Most studies of this supplement for depression used 200 to 300 milligrams, but you can start as low as 50 milligrams. Keep in mind, higher doses (above 300 milligrams) are not better; they can cause nightmares, vivid dreams, and dizziness (nausea, diarrhea, and drowsiness have also been reported). Talk with your doctor about what dosage might be good for you. Most important, do not combine 5-HTP with any other medications that also impact serotonin levels, such as antidepressants, without first speaking with your doctor. I believe it can increase the risk of serotonin syndrome (which can cause diarrhea, fever, seizures, and even death) and possibly deplete other neurotransmitters.

3. L-citrulline 1,500 milligrams a day

Again, my recommendation here is based on experience, not a major clinical trial. This is a potential exception to the rule that what works for ED generally won't work for PE (ED drugs usually don't have any anesthetic effect or impact on the ejaculatory reflex). L-citrulline improves erectile function and hardness in some men (see the Erectile Dysfunction section, page 186) by increasing levels of nitric oxide in the blood, which helps improve bloodflow. There is recent evidence in the prescription drug world that low nitric oxide levels may increase the risk of PE by increasing sensitivity or stimulating the ejaculatory reflex. Therefore, despite a lack of published evidence with L-citrulline so far, I had to make it my third choice. Nothing else has a better benefit-to-risk ratio when it comes to PE (after my first two choices, of course).

Keep in mind that ED supplements (and drugs) seem to improve confidence, the perception of ejaculatory control, and overall sexual satisfaction, while reducing anxiety and the amount of time needed to get a second erection. Some studies have observed a better result for PE when combining an ED pill with an antidepressant.

WHAT'S WORTHLESS

Note: In general, prescription drugs for ED have shown minimal impact on PE and they are not approved for this condition. Most dietary supplements for ED, with the exception of L-citrulline, haven't helped either, so you see where I'm headed with this section.

Panax ginseng. This product needs more research. There are some compounds in the ginseng plant (specific ginsenosides) that might hold some promise, though, so I'm keeping my eye on it. It is an ingredient in SS-cream (my #1 pick on page 379), but only as a small percentage.

Maca. There's simply no evidence to suggest maca can help individuals with PE.

Folic acid. There's some preliminary evidence that large doses of this B vitamin (1 milligram or more) can help reduce PE because folic acid can enhance brain neurotransmitters (the primary conventional drugs used for PE impact brain chemicals), but the evidence is weak and the safety of taking so much is questionable. Plus, there is a concern that using megadoses of folic acid over long periods can enhance the growth of male cancers, like prostate cancer.

LIFESTYLE CHANGES

This is one health issue where lifestyle has a minimal impact (so I'll save you the "heart healthy" spiel). Similarly, research has not found a relationship between PE and obesity, but you can *never* go wrong by making healthy changes to your lifestyle!

Refine your technique. Here are a few ways to avoid premature ejaculation (a sex therapist or urologist who specializes in sexual dysfunction can give you more tips).

- The stop-start method is just like it sounds. It involves taking periodic breaks from sexual activity to essentially train the penis to hold off. For example, you or your partner stimulates the penis until you're close to orgasm, then stop for a bit. Repeating this over time has helped some men with PE overcome the quick urge or need to ejaculate.

- The squeeze technique has several versions, but it mainly involves squeezing the head of the penis with your thumb and forefinger when the sensation of ejaculation begins. Focus the pressure on the urethra, which is the tube running along the underside of the penis. This method pushes blood out of the penis and temporarily reduces sexual tension and the ejaculatory response.

- Masturbating before intercourse is a common technique used by younger men. (You can call this the *There's Something about Mary* technique, for all you moviephiles out there.)

- Kegel exercises tighten the pubococcygeal muscles of the pelvic floor. These muscles get activated when you cut off the flow of urine midstream. You can strengthen them by doing exactly that (starting and stopping several times when you urinate), but people may start to wonder why you're taking so long in the bathroom! You can easily mimic the same sensations anywhere without anyone knowing what you're doing. Performing several sets of 10 throughout the day can strengthen the muscles and improve ejaculatory control. In the same vein, core exercises (like plank moves or exercises on a stability ball) strengthen the pelvic floor, too.

- The most sensitive nerve endings of the vagina are in the first third of the vaginal entrance, so small, shallow movements can help you last longer than simply thrusting vigorously, and this might satisfy your partner as well.

- Sensate techniques involve setting aside time to slowly explore, touch, and kiss each other without an immediate need for intercourse or even genital touching. It helps you both get comfortable with each other, with the ultimate goal of also treating PE. Other methods include masturbating in front of each other and using massage oils and lubricants.

Get poked. In a large Turkish study, researchers compared acupuncture to the PE prescription drug paroxetine. It didn't perform as well as the drug, but it did work significantly better than a placebo. In this study, patients received acupuncture twice a week for 4 weeks. There's also some promising preliminary clinical research regarding combining yoga with prescription medication for PE.

Premenstrual Syndrome and Primary Dysmenorrhea

Dr. Moyad Secret Dietary supplement companies need to step it up when it comes to research for premenstrual syndrome (PMS). They should follow the lead of pharmaceutical companies, which look for other ancillary benefits of effective drugs that are already on the market, such as prescription antidepressants. Some of these are now FDA-approved for PMS, but they also come with many side effects, including nausea, sexual dysfunction, and decreased energy. I'd start by studying supplements that have shown benefits for depression (SAM-e, 5-HTP), fatigue (American ginseng), headaches (vitamin B_2, butterbur, magnesium), nausea (ginger, B_6), stress and anxiety (theanine, GABA), and pain (SAM-e, again). I just divulged the golden road map for success! The conventional drugs in this area of medicine are not better or smarter than supplements; the makers are just more strategic, business savvy, and sensitive to the distressing effects of moderate to severe PMS. Come on, supplement companies! Get off your gluteus maximus; you will obviously be well rewarded!

WHAT IS IT?

About 80 percent of women report experiencing some form of behavioral, psychological, or physical changes during the 2 weeks before menstruation. Most of the time PMS causes mild to moderate symptoms, but in premenstrual dysphoric disorder (PMDD), a severe form of PMS, women experience more acute symptoms that dramatically interfere with day-to-day life, including relationships, social interactions, and work.

Postovulation hormonal changes trigger PMS, and some women's bodies are more sensitive to these shifts than others. That's why birth control pills can be so effective for PMS; they reduce the chances of ovulation occurring and keep hormones steady throughout the month. In addition, there are at least two neurotransmitters that have been implicated in PMS: GABA (gamma-aminobutyric acid) and serotonin. Drugs that increase serotonin, like antidepressants, have proven very helpful for many women. Twin studies have shown that genetics/family history also increases the risk of experiencing PMS or PMDD.

Primary dysmenorrhea—pain during menstruation—is the most common gynecologic condition experienced by menstruating women. It involves recurrent lower abdominal cramps just before or during menses but with no underlying explanation or cause (i.e., a pelvic examination is normal). (Secondary dysmenor-

COMMON PMS SYMPTOMS

Some of the physical symptoms include:

- Abdominal bloating
- Abdominal cramps and pain
- Body aches
- Breast fullness or tenderness
- Fatigue
- Headaches
- Nausea
- Swelling of the legs, feet, arms, or hands
- Weight gain

Some of the behavioral and psychological symptoms include:

- Anger or irritability
- Anxiety
- Appetite changes (food cravings or overeating)
- Changes in sex drive (libido)
- Decreased concentration
- Depressed mood
- Feeling out of control
- Mood swings
- Poor sleep or an increased need for sleep
- Tension
- Withdrawal from everyday activities

rhea, on the other hand, is caused by a distinct pathological condition, such as endometriosis, pelvic inflammatory disease, or interstitial cystitis.) Pain may radiate to the lower back and thighs as well. Researchers believe dysmenorrhea is due to an imbalance of compounds—prostaglandins, vasopressin, and others—that can cause uterine contractions, cramping, and even nausea and vomiting. Risk factors include age (younger than 30), anxiety and stress, obesity or being underweight, depression (especially if it's associated with an eating disorder), family history, smoking, early age at first menses, heavy menstrual periods, premenstrual symptoms, bleeding in between menstrual

MOYAD FACT: Women who experience severe PMS on a regular basis are at higher risk of having more severe menopausal symptoms as well, such as hot flashes, reduced sex drive, poor sleep, and depressed mood.

periods, and never having given birth (nulliparity), among others.

WHAT WORKS

1. Calcium carbonate
1,200 milligrams a day in two divided doses

Several randomized trials have found positive benefits for PMS with calcium carbonate dietary supplements (1,000 to 1,200 milligrams per day in two divided doses). Yet, it was a large US multicenter trial (the PMS Study Group at 12 US sites) that brought the most attention to it. A total of 466 participants took 1,200 milligrams of calcium carbonate or a placebo daily for three treatment cycles. By the third treatment cycle those taking calcium carbonate had a 48 percent reduction in total PMS symptom scores compared to 30 percent in the placebo group. Pain was reduced by 54 percent with calcium carbonate versus a 15 percent *increase* with the placebo. Negative mood aspects (swings, depression, tension, anxiety, anger, crying spells) were reduced by 45 percent with calcium carbonate and 28 percent with the placebo. Food cravings were reduced by 54 percent versus 35 percent with the placebo, and water retention was reduced by 36 percent versus 24 percent. The beneficial impact of calcium carbonate began to be significant in the last two cycles, which means you have to give it a couple of months.

The tolerable upper limit or maximum for calcium for women (ages 12 to 50 years) is 2,500 to 3,000 milligrams per day; the average dietary intake is 600 to 800 milligrams, so taking extra calcium in the form of a supplement appears safe for PMS. However, postmenopausal women should be careful about getting too much calcium because it could slightly increase their risk of kidney stones. Overall, calcium carbonate is the most tested supplement for PMS; it's safe for women who may become pregnant and also very inexpensive, which makes it the perfect Moyad product to recommend!

Rare side effects with calcium supplementation include constipation, nausea, loss of appetite, headaches, and nonspecific pain. And calcium carbonate can potentially interfere with some prescription medications, especially tetracycline drugs and thyroid hormone pills (thyroxine). You can still use these drugs; just take the calcium at least 2 to 4 hours before or after the drug because it can reduce absorption.

Many studies of calcium suggest that vitamin D may play a role in reducing PMS as well. If you're experiencing problematic symptoms, ask your doctor about a blood test for vitamin D. (Other calcium supplements, such as calcium citrate, have not been researched in the area of PMS, so I'm not recommending them.)

2. Vitamin B$_6$ (pyridoxine) 50 to 100 milligrams a day

In general, B vitamin supplements don't have consistent research for PMS, with the exception of vitamin B$_6$. An analysis of at least nine randomized trials showed that daily doses of vitamin B$_6$ ranging from 50 to 600 milligrams reduced PMS symptoms. However, I'm not a fan of taking large doses because it can cause sensory neuropathy or nerve damage (especially at levels above 300 milligrams per day). Plus, the clinical studies using 100 milligrams per day of vitamin B$_6$ looked as impressive as the higher-dosage studies, so stick with my suggested range. This vitamin is also commonly used to reduce nausea—a common symptom of PMS—in the first trimester of pregnancy with good success (see the Nausea and Vomiting section, page 333).

3. Chasteberry (*Vitex agnus-castus*)
20 milligrams a day on average

This herbal contains casticin, an ingredient that decreases levels of the hormone prolactin by occupying specialized cellular receptors in the body known as dopamine (D2) receptors. Higher levels of prolactin may cause more severe PMS symptoms in some individuals. The best trial with chasteberry—published in *BMJ* (*formerly known as the British Medical Journal*)—used an extract known as Ze 440 (which contains a standardized amount of casticin). Fifty-two percent of the women who took the extract (there were 170 subjects total) reported at least a 50 percent reduction in their PMS symptoms, versus 24 percent of those who took the placebo. They reported a significant improvement in a variety of symptoms, including head-

ache, irritability, mood changes, and breast symptoms, and the side effects were no different than a placebo. This is the trial that most likely launched this herb into commercial success. Another study that was not double-blind found a 42 percent reduction in PMS symptom scores, with the largest improvements in pain, behavior changes, negative feelings, and fluid retention. When compared to a commonly used prescription antidepressant (fluoxetine), both worked equally well.

A more recent study from Germany that compared doses of 8, 20, and 30 milligrams of Ze 440 with a placebo found that the 30-milligram dose worked no better than the 20-milligram dose, but the 20-milligram dose worked significantly better than the 8-milligram and placebo groups.

Chasteberry is arguably the most commonly recommended herbal product for PMS by alternative medicine experts, and although I agree that it has some efficacy, it also has quality-control issues. Research with this supplement has focused on two extracts, Ze 440 (one 20-milligram tablet) and BNO 1095 (one 4-milligram tablet), both of which can be hard to find in the United States. Once you venture away from these, all bets about effectiveness are off, so buyer beware. If it weren't for this, I would have ranked chasteberry higher.

Uncommon side effects include nausea, headache, and skin rashes. There isn't good information about major drug interactions, but ask your doctor if you're using any type of hormonal contraceptive (which usually can help alleviate PMS anyway) or taking drugs that affect prolactin or dopamine (several antipsychotic drugs rely on dopamine); chasteberry shouldn't be used with them. The biggest general concern is that this herb could reduce the effectiveness of oral contraceptives, and I wouldn't recommend it if you're planning to become pregnant or are pregnant.

HONORABLE MENTION

Omega-3s, 1,200 milligrams daily of the active ingredients EPA and DHA, can help reduce pain during PMS, according to one study. Another trial with 2,000 milligrams daily found they significantly reduced depression, anxiety, and bloating, especially after 2 to 3 months of use.

Magnesium (200 milligrams per day of magnesium oxide) has preliminary evidence for reducing water retention, breast tenderness, and mood symptoms.

WHAT'S WORTHLESS

Saffron. In one study, taking 15 milligrams twice a day for two menstrual cycles reduced symptom severity by half in 19 out of 50 patients. However, as with most PMS dietary supplements, this study has not been replicated—or improved upon—to see if it really works better than a placebo.

Evening primrose oil. It contains the omega-6 GLA (gamma-linolenic acid), which alleviates breast pain and abdominal cramping by being metabolized into prostaglandin E1, which is a natural anti-inflammatory in the body. The problem is, rigorous studies of evening primrose oil have shown no benefit over a placebo. Adolescents with epilepsy should avoid it because there have been reports that it may lower the seizure threshold.

Black currant oil and borage seed oil are somewhat similar to evening primrose oil in that they have a high GLA content—even higher than evening primrose oil. Yet, there is no adequate human research to suggest these work for PMS either.

Black cohosh. Recent research suggests it has minimal to no impact in this area, but it may have a role in treating menopausal symptoms because of its apparent impact on neurotransmitters (see the Hot Flashes section, page 245).

Wild yam root. Wild yams contain the compound diosgenin, which some supplement manufacturers claim gets converted into progesterone in the body, reducing PMS (and even menopausal symptoms). Unfortunately, this conversion has not yet been proven.

Dong quai. This herb is widely used in Chinese medicine for gynecological problems, including PMS. Yet, there is no adequate research in the area of PMS.

Soy, vitamin E, or ginkgo biloba. These individual supplements don't yet have enough clinical research to determine if they work better than a placebo.

St. John's wort. By itself, St. John's wort has not worked much better than a placebo in PMS studies. But when researchers start pairing it with other supplements that have been shown to be effective for PMS, I feel more confident that it may help reduce symptoms.

LIFESTYLE CHANGES

Heart healthy = menstrual cycle healthy? Maybe. Doctors generally recommend increasing exercise and reducing caffeine, salt, and refined or simple sugars when dealing with PMS, but there's very little research to support these recommendations. In fact, there's very little research being done at all in regard to lifestyle choices and PMS. But if you look at many of the symptoms that can occur with PMS and PMDD (fatigue, anxiety, poor focus), there is plenty of research outside of PMS to suggest that exercise and healthy lifestyle changes can make a difference.

Most of the dietary and supplement research over the past 25 years in the area of PMS has revolved around addressing deficiencies during the menstrual cycle, whether it's calcium, vitamin D, omega-3s, B vitamins, or whatever. The heart-healthy Moyad diet outlined in the beginning of this book addresses these deficiencies as well. So, as a result, I do believe that being heart healthy can make your menstrual cycle healthier. A well-known older study from Virginia Commonwealth University found that obese women had a nearly threefold increased risk of PMS compared to nonobese women. Another study from Basel, Switzerland, of more than 3,500 women found that PMS was associated with an increased risk of poor physical health and psychological distress. The question remains whether the poor health and distress leads to PMS or vice versa.

Eat more Bs. Researchers working on the large Nurses' Healthy Study 2 (one of the largest and longest studies to evaluate the impact of lifestyle habits on overall health) found a lower risk of PMS in women who had higher intakes of vitamins B_1 and B_2 from food sources. Foods that are high in these vitamins include organ meats, pork, brewer's yeast, fortified cereals, beans, wheat germ, bran, wild rice, mushrooms, milk, soybeans, eggs, broccoli, and spinach (mostly heart-healthy foods). In one well-done randomized trial with 556 young women (ages 12 to 21), 100 milligrams daily of vitamin B_1 (thiamin hydrochloride) worked better than a placebo at reducing dysmenorrhea during menstruation. I'd like to see more recent research on this because 87 percent of the participants had their pain eliminated in this older study!

Try acupressure. This is getting a lot of preliminary positive research for primary dysmenorrhea. Massaging two points—just above the ankle bone and a few inches below the knee—on the inside of the lower leg (called Spleen 6 and Spleen 8) has helped reduce pain.

389

Pressure Ulcers/Wound Healing

Dr. Moyad Secret Pressure ulcers are also known as bedsores; they're caused by constant pressure on an area, which restricts bloodflow. They're very common in nursing homes and challenging to treat. There have been many studies showing protein supplements can improve wound healing, and they have been as short as a week and as long as almost a year. One protein supplement does not stand out over others, but I would suggest talking with your medical team about taking a highly concentrated protein powder with nutrients.

   L-arginine. Lower dosages (4,500 milligrams per day or less) continue to show some promise for improving healing times. Arginine can stimulate insulin release and improve the transport of amino acids to body tissues that are in need of repair. This needs a major clinical trial and perhaps should be combined with other nutrients, including L-citrulline, which is even more efficient than L-arginine and at lower doses.

Prostate Cancer

Dr. Moyad Secret The list of dietary supplements that, when taken in large dosages, can *increase* the risk of prostate cancer, especially more aggressive forms of the disease, is downright scary! The SELECT trial showed vitamin E supplements at 400 IU and selenium supplements at 200 micrograms per day increased the risk, and taking more than one multivitamin per day, high-dose zinc supplements, and even high-dose folic acid (1 milligram or higher) may also increase risk after many years of use. In fact, in the most recent update from the SELECT trial, men with normal to high intakes of dietary selenium appeared to have a significantly increased risk of aggressive prostate cancer when taking selenium supplements. Whether you believe the research or not, these supplements are certainly *not* lowering the risk of prostate cancer.

I like to use the acronym SAM to remind me of drugs and potential supplement equivalents that are beginning to garner enough research to suggest they *could* help prevent prostate cancer and reduce the risk of dying from this disease. SAM stands for **s**tatin drugs, **a**spirin, and **m**etformin, which are all primarily generic drugs originally derived from natural sources. Statins came from a fungus (red yeast rice), aspirin from willow bark, and metformin from the French lilac. I find it incredible that three low-cost, heart-healthy drugs, used to prevent cardiovascular disease and diabetes, have become some of the best ways to potentially prevent prostate cancer and could be used with conventional treatment to slow the progression of this disease. Who qualifies to take them? People who need any of these three drugs due to their cardiovascular disease or diabetes risk and who may want the additional benefit of lowering their prostate cancer risk. What am I trying to say? Heart healthy = prostate healthy!

Almost all heart-healthy lifestyle changes—maintaining a healthy weight, adopting a good diet that includes fiber, and exercising—could reduce the risk of prostate cancer. (Heart-healthy diets, such as the Ornish diet and others, have preliminary evidence that they prevent or slow the progression of nonaggressive prostate cancer.)

In general, I don't believe there's a single supplement right now that should be used to prevent or treat prostate cancer, but since statins may lower the risk of aggressive prostate cancer by lowering the amount of cholesterol utilized in the prostate, there's a chance red yeast rice (see the High Cholesterol section, page 234) will work because it acts like a low-dose statin. And there is some preliminary evidence that it may discourage prostate cancer growth.

Although I indicated aspirin is beginning to get research for potentially lowering the risk of dying from prostate cancer, please do not pop an aspirin a day if you're only worried about prostate cancer because the harm could exceed the benefit if your cardiovascular risk is low. Go to reynoldsriskscore. org (women can use it, too) to determine your risk of heart disease, and discuss the results with your doctor. If your risk is high, you may be a candidate for baby aspirin, but if it's low, the side effects (ulcers, bleeding into the brain, and so on) may not be worth it. I get so tired of "experts" pushing aspirin on everyone because they think it's a miracle drug, which it can be for the people who qualify for it, but for those who don't, it could be a life-threatening disaster.

See the Hot Flashes section, page 245, and the Low Energy and Chronic Fatigue section, page 293, for information on addressing side effects from cancer treatment.

Flaxseed. There's a silly myth floating around the Internet that flaxseed can increase the risk of prostate cancer based on the observation in some studies that higher levels of plant omega-3s were found in some prostate cancer patients. What few folks realize is in one of the largest and best dietary clinical trials ever done in prostate cancer, published in the journal *Cancer Epidemiology, Biomarkers & Prevention*, flaxseed was shown to be both heart and prostate healthy—and it costs pennies a day! Taking 30 grams a day of flaxseed powder before surgery to remove the prostate appeared to work as well as if not better than a low-fat diet, based on an incredibly well-done study from Duke University.

Capsaicin. Preliminary research from the University of Toronto on capsaicin pills appears to show some activity against prostate cancer in the laboratory, but this needs a clinical trial.

WHAT'S WORTHLESS

Pomegranate (and others): I do not believe the juice or the pills work any better than placebo (I hope I'm proven wrong). I have seen countless "natural products" like these come and go during my lifetime—lycopene, shark cartilage, green tea supplements, saw palmetto, zinc, and others—but these have not proven themselves to be prostate- or heart-healthy, so they've never made my final cut.

Psoriasis

P

Dr. Moyad Secret Heart healthy = skin healthy! Psoriasis is a chronic inflammatory autoimmune skin disease that can also impact the joints and is associated with an increased risk of cardiovascular disease (CVD). Obesity, which is an inflammatory condition as well, and weight gain can make psoriasis worse. Researchers in a recent 16-week randomized trial had overweight patients with psoriasis follow a low-calorie diet (800 to 1,000 calories daily for 8 weeks and then 1,200 calories per day for another 8 weeks) or a standard healthy (not calorie-restricted) diet with no effort to lose weight. Skin-related issues and symptom severity decreased in the weight loss group. Other studies have found that the response to conventional psoriasis medicine is greater when overweight patients lost weight. Better yet, in other clinical studies, exercise appeared to further improve symptoms. Now researchers are studying the effects of lowering cholesterol on psoriasis.

Miscellaneous. Topical honey and aloe vera may slightly improve plaque psoriasis, the most common type of psoriasis, which occurs in raised patches, but the placebo response rate was high in these clinical studies. Topical vitamin D is approved by the FDA for treatment of psoriasis, but it can cause skin irritation. Since some studies suggest patients with active psoriasis have low levels of B_{12}, there is some preliminary positive data that supplementing with topical and oral vitamin B_{12} can be beneficial. And high-dose inositol may also play a role in psoriasis treatment, but the dosages in small studies (6 grams per day) are unrealistic; smaller dosages should be evaluated. Finally, there are several ongoing clinical trials looking at how marine omega-3s can be used with conventional psoriasis therapies.

Sunlight. Sun exposure or ultraviolet light–based therapies can help treat psoriasis because they have an immunosuppressive effect. This is an important lesson for people without psoriasis, though: Sun exposure *suppresses* the immune system!

WHAT'S WORTHLESS

Selenium, taurine, zinc, and kukui oil from Hawaii have failed to do anything.

Pulmonary Hypertension

THE JURY'S STILL OUT

Dr. Moyad Secret Normal, or systemic, hypertension occurs when the blood vessels that run from the left ventricle of the heart out to the rest of the body narrow, harden, and become inflexible, which increases the pressure in them. Pulmonary hypertension occurs when the blood vessels that run from the heart to the lungs do these same things, which puts added stress on the right ventricle, the chamber of the heart that pumps blood to the lungs. Similar to systemic hypertension (see page 251), the only supplements that are worth considering are those that could improve bloodflow, which explains why erectile dysfunction supplements, such as L-arginine and L-citrulline, are being researched for this disease. The improved bloodflow and reduced pressure in the lungs decreases hypertension.

Not surprisingly then, Viagra-like drugs are being used because they improve respiratory circulation. In fact, sildenafil, which is the generic form of Viagra, is prescribed as Revatio, an FDA-approved drug for adults with PAH (pulmonary arterial hypertension), but long-term therapy may increase the risk of death in children, according to the FDA. So that brings us back to L-arginine and L-citrulline. In some pulmonary diseases, L-arginine levels are metabolized and rendered ineffective at a much quicker pace than normal, so supplementation is crucial. There's preliminary research showing L-citrulline malate, at 1,000 milligrams three times a day, can improve walking distance and quality of life and reduce average arterial pulmonary hypertension numbers. This is exciting stuff, but more research is needed.

Raynaud's Phenomenon

THE JURY'S STILL OUT

Dr. Moyad Secret Since there are no FDA-approved medications for this condition, there is a lot of room for improvement. Most of the drugs being used are off-label (calcium-channel blockers and Viagra-like drugs to improve blood-flow and open blood vessels), and many are expensive and carry significant side effects. So any supplements that can slightly mimic a Viagra-like effect (such as L-arginine and L-citrulline) have the most promise here because they increase bloodflow.

In Raynaud's phenomenon, the arteries that carry blood to the fingers, toes, and uncommonly the nose and ears begin to spasm when they're exposed to cold or stress, which results in poor circulation to these areas. Warming helps relieve the problem. There are two classes of Raynaud's: primary Raynaud's, where the cause is unknown, and secondary Raynaud's, where the symptoms are a result of other diseases (such as scleroderma, lupus, or similar connective tissue diseases).

L-arginine. Taking 1,000 to 2,000 milligrams twice a day when symptoms begin could increase the amount of nitric oxide in the hands and toes, which increases blood vessel size and blood circulation. L-citrulline, which works as well as L-arginine to improve nitric oxide levels but at half the dose, needs a clinical trial now.

Fish oil. An older study found using 6 to 7 grams daily improved the symptoms of primary Raynaud's. Yikes! Who wants to take this much fish oil?

Restless Leg Syndrome

Dr. Moyad Secret What researchers are now learning from some of the largest studies of people with restless leg syndrome (RLS) is that it runs in families and could be associated with other conditions, such as heart disease, kidney problems, pregnancy, neuropathy, depression, and many other medical issues. (This is a good reason to reduce your heart disease risk.)

Up to one in 10 adults has RLS, and most—about 70 percent—are misdiagnosed with things like poor circulation, back problems, arthritis, depression, and varicose veins. Some medications—such as those for high blood pressure, depression, colds, and allergies—can make it worse, so talk with your doctor about this. Alcohol, caffeine, and smoking can also make RLS worse. While the cause is still unknown, many researchers theorize it's due to lower levels of the neurotransmitter dopamine or a deficiency of iron. (Doctors often use dopamine agonist drugs or iron supplementation to treat RLS). New research from Harvard University with more than 50,000 men and women suggests obesity and/or high cholesterol may be associated with an increased risk of RLS. So heart healthy = leg healthy? Looks like it!

RLS has four key features: An intense urge to move the legs, usually accompanied by a "creepy crawly" feeling, aching, or uncomfortable sensations; symptoms begin or worsen during rest or inactivity; symptoms are relieved to some degree by walking or stretching; and symptoms are worse or only occur in the evening or at night.

Iron. RLS can be a symptom of iron-deficiency anemia, so you should have your iron levels (especially ferritin) tested. A ferritin level less than 50 ng/mL has been associated with RLS. If levels are low, work with your doctor to determine the correct supplement dosage.

Rheumatoid Arthritis

R

Dr. Moyad Secret Rheumatoid arthritis (RA) is a terrible disease that can lead to joint destruction. What needs more attention in those with RA, however, is the high risk of cardiovascular disease (CVD), probably due to the high rate of inflammation. Recent studies suggest a 50 to 60 percent increased risk of death from CVD in RA patients, primarily from heart disease and stroke. So people with RA need to reduce their risk of CVD to as close to zero as possible. A supplement that could help reduce RA symptoms *and* CVD risk would be ideal!

Rheumatoid arthritis is an autoimmune disease characterized by chronic inflammation of the joints. It impacts 1 percent of the population and can affect any peripheral joint—such as those in the feet, knees, and hands—and it can be very painful and debilitating. The cause and triggers of RA are unknown, but one strong theory is that an infection or trauma causes an initial inflammatory response in the affected joint(s), which gets out of control. Healthy joints don't normally contain white blood cells (leukocytes), but in RA a variety of them are seen. As the disease progresses, the cells of the lining in the joint increase and release a variety of compounds, causing a loss of cartilage, bone destruction, and a large reduction in function. The best RA drugs are ones that can reduce this immune response.

Fish oil. In studies, krill oil (from tiny crustaceans found in the ocean) at 300 milligrams per day resulted in less pain and stiffness after about 2 weeks. And an analysis of more than 20 randomized trials found that dosages of fish oil ranging from 2,700 to 6,000 milligrams per day for a minimum of 3 months could slightly reduce the progression of RA as well as reduce the need for NSAIDs (nonsteroidal anti-inflammatory drugs) or pain medication in some RA patients. More recent data suggests heavier individuals may get more benefit compared to thinner individuals. Regardless, many of these clinical trials were using omega-3 supplements along with conventional medicine.

Red yeast rice. Cholesterol-lowering statin drugs may not only reduce the risk of CVD in RA, they may also slow the progression of the disease. This is why red yeast rice supplements, which are like taking a low-dose statin, should also be tested!

Rosacea

Dr. Moyad Secret Perhaps the most important thing to know about this disorder is that a good dermatologist can change your life. And here's how you know you have a doc who's truly looking out for your best interests: She doesn't jump to write you a prescription for antibiotics. She prefers to try other solutions first, like prescription topical medications or supplements. So many rosacea patients are overprescribed antibiotics, which can help in the short term but come with risks, including intestinal infection; death of good bacteria; stomach upset; skin sensitivity to light; headaches; ringing in the ears; and, of course, antibiotic resistance. According to the Centers for Disease Control and Prevention, antibiotic resistance is becoming "one of the world's most pressing public health threats." Dermatologists in the United States write up to 4 million topical antibiotic and up to 9 million oral antibiotic prescriptions per year for inflammatory and infectious diseases (most are tetracycline antibiotics). But rosacea can be effectively treated without antibiotics.

WHAT IS IT?

Rosacea is a common, chronic inflammatory skin problem that affects the face primarily. It's characterized by facial flushing, redness and bumps in a symmetrical distribution, and acnelike breakouts in some of the flushed areas. People also complain of extreme sensitivity to environmental triggers, such as sun, wind, hot liquids, spicy foods, and facial cleansers and soaps. Women get it more than men, but men will often progress to more advanced stages, perhaps because they are less likely to seek treatment.

There are four subtypes of rosacea: acne rosacea (papulopustular), which is acne along with rosacea; vascular rosa- cea (erythematotelangiectatic), which is characterized by enlarged small blood vessels in the facial skin that may appear to be broken (also called telangiectasias); ocular rosacea, which impacts the eyes leading to dryness, redness, and swelling; and phymatous rosacea, a severe form that causes visible thickening of the skin, especially around the nose, enlarged pores, and oily skin.

Experts aren't sure what causes rosacea, but it may be genetic, some kind of sensitivity to environmental triggers, a bacteria—or some combination of all three. (Some researchers believe that *Helicobacter pylori*, the bacterium that's been linked to ulcers and cancer in the gastrointestinal tract, may also increase the risk of rosacea, but this is very controversial and hasn't been proven.) Unfortunately, there are no specific laboratory tests for rosacea; your doctor will diagnose it based on an exam and your complaints.

WHAT WORKS

Note: Before using any topical ingredient always do a spot test on a small area of the face first so you don't exacerbate the problem if you're sensitive to it.

1. Niacinamide (vitamin B₃ or nicotinamide) combination see
dosage information below

Vitamin B_3 can take two forms: niacinamide or niacin (also known as nicotinic acid). However, only niacinamide has anti-inflammatory properties that may help several dermatologic conditions, including rosacea and acne (see the Acne section, page 47). Make sure you don't get them confused when you're perusing store shelves. In a trial known as NICOS (the Nicomide Improvement in Clinical Outcomes Study), a dietary supplement formula containing niacinamide (750 milligrams), zinc (25 milligrams), copper (1.5 milligrams), and folic acid (500 micrograms) reduced the severity of rosacea (and also acne) and improved facial appearance after 4 and 8 weeks of daily use. In fact, it appeared to work as well as antibiotics! (Some people may experience nausea and stomachache, so take it during or right after a meal.)

The NICOS trial was groundbreaking for rosacea because for many years there was skepticism about how well it could be treated without antibiotics. I've seen this supplement combination work with patients, and it can even be used with conventional topical treatments (like azelaic acid), so by all means, start with this before going the antibiotic route. I've had patients see reduced redness and faster skin healing with a 2 percent niacinamide facial moisturizer as well.

The exact product used in the NICOS trial, called Nicomide, is available, but you have to ask your doctor about it, or you can make your own version, which is pretty inexpensive to do. There is also a prescription dietary supplement known as NicAzel that contains nicotinamide, azelaic acid, zinc, B_6, copper, and folic acid. It reduces acne and scarring and accelerates healing, based on the NICOS results (look for a product called NicAzel Forte).

2. Azelaic acid topical cream
3 to 10 percent concentration

Prescription-strength (15 to 20 percent) azelaic acid, an anti-inflammatory, has a long, successful track record for rosacea, but the jury is still out on over-the-counter formulas (3 to 10 percent concentrations). I've seen this lower-dose plant-based supplement—which is found naturally in wheat, rye, and barley—work, and it's a good option for people who find the higher concentration to be a little too harsh. There just needs to be more extensive testing. Plants use azelaic acid as a warning signal when they're invaded or infected. It triggers the release of salicylic acid and other defense compounds to attack the pathogen, and scientists think it may work similarly in humans; it's essentially an antimicrobial. Apply it every 6 to 8 hours (no more than three times a day) until the redness begins to fade.

3. Omega-3 fatty acids and omega-6 fatty acids dosage varies by type

Researchers now know that omega-3 and omega-6 supplements may be effective for treating dry eye (see the Dry Eye section, page 181). The ocular form of rosacea causes dry eye problems along with inflammation, and although these supplements haven't been studied for ocular rosacea, they work well for related conditions, so in this case the benefit exceeds the risk. (It's also worth asking your dermatologist if you can try omega-3s or omega-6s for facial redness and dryness.)

Omega-3s: Flaxseed oil can be taken as a dietary supplement softgel, but you would need to take six or seven a day to get the 3,300-milligram-per-day dose that has shown anti-inflammatory benefits for the eyes in studies. It's much easier to just take 1 or 2 tablespoons daily of flaxseed oil (my favorite is Omega Swirl from Barlean's). Alternatively, you could take 800 to 1,500 milligrams (one or two pills daily) of the active ingredients in marine or fish oil (EPA and DHA omega-3 fatty acids); Omega Swirl also has an incredible-tasting fish oil option.

Omega-6s: If you are allergic to marine products, prefer not to take them, or aren't seeing enough benefit from omega-3s, you can take 200 to 300 milligrams of gamma-linolenic acid (GLA), which is an anti-inflammatory omega-6, and 100 to 200 milligrams of linoleic acid (LA), another omega-6, in the form of evening primrose oil, black currant oil, or even borage oil. That's the equivalent of one or two softgels a day from most companies. We're often told that omega-6 fatty acids are bad for us because they *create* inflammation, but this is a gross generalization. Some omega-6 compounds have anti-inflammatory effects when used in the moderate dosages recommended in this section, which is why they are potentially effective for the treatment of ocular rosacea.

I recommend combining omega-3 and omega-6 supplements only if your rosacea does not improve in 3 months of taking either type on its own. The benefit in combining them is that they fight inflammation in different ways, so it's possible for someone who's not responding to omega-3 supplements to get a better response from omega-6s and vice versa; and some people do better with both. It's like taking aspirin or ibuprofen: Both reduce inflammation and pain, but in some individuals one works better than the other or the combination works better than either one alone. Regardless, many sources of omega-3s (like flaxseed) also contain some omega-6s and vice versa, but larger doses are often needed to really see a benefit. If you want to combine them, try taking either 750 to 1,000 milligrams of fish oil or 1,000 milligrams of flaxseed oil *plus* up to 100 milligrams of GLA or 150 milligrams of LA.

WHAT'S WORTHLESS

Niacin. If I had a dime for every call I've gotten from someone who thought they had rosacea, only to discover this person was taking niacin, I would be so rich I could buy an island. This is a popular supplement for managing cholesterol, although recent evidence has begun to question whether it's truly beneficial. Regardless, niacin causes facial flushing in doses as low as 50 milligrams, and this can give the appearance of rosacea or temporarily make it look worse.

Zinc. In a recent clinical trial, individuals with rosacea took 220 milligrams of zinc sulfate twice daily for 90 days, and researchers found that it worked no better than a placebo. Although an earlier study of zinc sulfate (100 milligrams three times daily) appeared to help rosacea, this recent research, along with the potential for side effects (such as nausea) at these larger dosages, makes this difficult to recommend.

Curcumin and capsaicin. Because these supplements have anti-inflammatory properties, some people are taking them for rosacea, but more research is needed, plus they can cause gastrointestinal problems, like stomachache. Remember, when there is no research, my rule is first do no harm. (I got that little tidbit from some dude named Hippocrates, who also said "Let food be thy medicine.") Also, keep in mind that capsaicin is the active ingredient in hot chile peppers, and heat-generating compounds can only make the redness of rosacea worse.

LIFESTYLE CHANGES

Try limiting carbs. Recent studies linking low-carbohydrate diets with a reduction in duration, frequency, and severity of acne have come as a surprise, and I suspect researchers would potentially find similar benefits with rosacea. Here's a soapbox moment: With everything that's known about rosacea being an inflammatory disorder with numerous environmental triggers, you would think there'd be a plethora (my SAT teacher would be proud of me for using that word) of studies exploring the connection to diet and lifestyle, but there aren't. So if any of you readers are planning on going into dermatology, initiate a diet-and-rosacea study and you will be famous.

Go retro with sunscreen. You definitely want to protect your skin from the sun if you have rosacea, but the newer sunscreen formulas with chemical blocking agents (avobenzone, oxybenzone, etc.) can be irritating to skin, so stick with "older" products that have physical blockers that aren't absorbed as easily, such as zinc oxide and titanium dioxide. This is one area that has seen extensive research, and it's striking how many sunscreens cause sensitivity and irritation in those with rosacea.

401

Identify your triggers—and avoid them. There are all sorts of things that can cause rosacea, including emotional stress, sun, hot or cold weather, wind, hot liquids, spicy foods, facial cleansers and soaps, heavy exercise, and alcohol (the National Rosacea Society has found that red wine may be a greater trigger than other alcohols).

Up your fiber intake. There is a small amount of evidence suggesting that the faster food moves through the gut, the less chance there is for it to cause facial flushing or irritation. Fiber (25 to 30 grams per day) can help speed up transit time through the intestinal tract. Look at it this way: Even if it doesn't improve symptoms, it can help reduce inflammation in general. Fiber also functions as a prebiotic, so it helps improve healthy bacteria colonization in the gut. I have seen many rosacea patients get better after increasing fiber intake.

Slather on oats. Colloidal oatmeal has historically been used to treat itching and skin irritation because it soothes inflammation. It's available over the counter and there's minimal risk to trying it.

Shingles

THE JURY'S STILL OUT

Dr. Moyad Secret Shingles (a.k.a. herpes zoster) is caused by the same virus that causes chickenpox. It's a rash that usually occurs as a strip on one side of the face or body and eventually turns into blisters. Please get the shingles vaccine (Zostavax) if you've had chickenpox. Even if you've already had a shingles outbreak, ask your doctor if you can still have the vaccine for further protection, especially since new research has come out indicating stroke risk may be increased after a shingles outbreak (so getting the vaccine could be a heart-healthy strategy!). It not only dramatically reduces the risk of shingles, it also reduces the severity. The nerve pain (postherpetic neuralgia) associated with shingles can be awful.

Capsaicin cream. This topical supplement could improve quality of life and sleep and reduce the significant pain and fatigue associated with a shingles outbreak (see the Peripheral Neuropathy section, page 364). While I recommend a cream at 0.075 percent concentration, there are stronger prescription versions (up to 8 percent) available to help with more severe pain.

S

Sickle Cell Anemia

Dr. Moyad Secret Sickle cell anemia is a potentially fatal hereditary blood disorder in which the blood cells are misshapen, leading to problems in many different organ systems and areas of the body. It impacts people around the world, but I can count the number of good dietary supplement studies that have been completed for it on one hand. It is known that low levels of L-arginine are associated in some cases with worse outcomes, so why not test L-arginine or L-citrulline supplements to improve bloodflow or vasodilation in more studies? NAC (N-acetylcysteine) at 1,200 to 2,400 milligrams per day needs a large trial to look at its ability to reduce painful crisis (these are essentially serious flare-ups requiring immediate treatment that are caused by blood cells getting stuck in vessels around the body) based on its history of increasing cell antioxidant levels (glutathione).

On the other hand, high doses of vitamin C (1,400 milligrams) and vitamin E (800 IU) may have made the condition worse in a preliminary 180-day trial in Brazil, but there isn't enough research on negative effects of supplements either. Vitamin A or D supplementation could help based on very preliminary research, but there hasn't been any follow-up. More research here is needed now!

Omega-3 fatty acids. Children with sickle cell disease in the Sudan received omega-3 fatty acids (278 milligrams of DHA and 39 milligrams of EPA) versus a placebo for a year. The researchers found that the omega-3 group had a reduced rate of vaso-occlusive events (painful episodes where the red blood cells get stuck), blood transfusion, and white blood cell count and were less likely to miss school because of illness.

Folic acid and other B vitamins. Many sickle cell anemia patients are put on 1 milligram of folic acid daily by their doctors to improve red blood cell production, which makes sense. However, also talk to your doctor about being tested for vitamin B_{12} deficiency because it is not uncommon with this disease.

Skin Cancer and Skin Aging

THE JURY'S STILL OUT

Dr. Moyad Secret Research from Queensland, Australia, which arguably has the highest rate of skin cancer deaths in the world, has remarkably changed the course of this disease through promoting greater awareness of sunscreen use and other sun-protective measures (such as seeking shade and the use of wide-brim hats, sunglasses, and long-sleeve shirts and pants). Look up the Australian "Slip, Slop, Slap" campaign. And the advice is working better than any pill for prevention will ever work!

WHAT'S WORTHLESS

Selenium. Selenium at 200 micrograms per day can increase the risk of skin cancer recurrence (especially squamous and basal cell carcinomas), according to the Nutritional Prevention of Cancer clinical trial.

Heliocare. This dietary supplement pill comes from a fern extract. Some people take it for UV protection, but experts estimate it only offers the equivalent of an SPF 3 product. It's similar to beta-carotene supplements, which, when used long term, provide an SPF of about 4. However, this supplement has *never* been shown to prevent skin cancer. In fact, in a 12-year randomized trial with 22,000 participants called the Physicians' Health Study, beta-carotene supplementation had no impact on skin cancer. I would be more inclined to use a broad-spectrum (UVA and UVB) sunscreen of SPF 15 or more or a traditional sunscreen, such as zinc oxide or titanium dioxide.

Skin Health

Dr. Moyad Secret Okay, let's talk skin antiaging for a second. The smartest thing you can do is reduce your exposure to UV light, either from the sun or tanning booths. That's a good start, but healthy skin is also about skin hydration, and there is plenty of preliminary data that supplements can really help here.

Flaxseed oil. Researchers conducted a 12-week randomized study with women where one group took about 2,200 milligrams of flaxseed oil versus safflower seed oil capsules daily. The flaxseed oil group reported significant reductions in skin sensitivity, skin water loss, roughness, and scaling and increased skin smoothness and hydration. This was a small study, but the results were impressive enough and flaxseed oil is safe enough that I recommend trying it, especially in the wintertime for people who struggle with dry, scaly skin. After I analyzed this study, even I began to take flaxseed oil for my skin. Another reason I'm willing to believe the results of this study is because some recent studies have shown that taking omega-3 supplements (one fish oil pill plus 1,000 milligrams of flaxseed oil) for 3 months or less may also reduce the risk and symptoms of dry eyes. Not bad for such a low-cost product. (Nutrients that are healthy for the eye are healthy for the skin because the tissues are similar.) I recommend using a teaspoon or two (up to a tablespoon) of flaxseed oil itself versus pills. Otherwise, the sheer number of pills you'd have to take to equal this amount of omega-3s from plants would be huge.

Lutein and zeaxanthin. These two compounds (10 milligrams of lutein and 0.6 milligram of zeaxanthin) can improve skin health based on a preliminary clinical trial. Again, this is not a surprise because they also protect eye health.

Miscellaneous. Green tea supplements and French maritime pine bark (Pycnogenol) have initial data for skin health, but more research is needed. Vitamin C from foods has been associated with a lower rate of skin aging, but whether the supplement can do the same thing (by potentially improving collagen production) is unknown. Vitamin C is an ingredient in a lot of effective topical medicines, though.

WHAT'S WORTHLESS

Vitamin A. High doses (beyond 10,000 IU) can really dry out the skin.

Smoking Cessation
(And Other Addictions)

THE JURY'S STILL OUT

Dr. Moyad Secret Lets face it: Quitting nicotine sucks, and that's why relapse rates are so high. Most conventional drugs for smoking cessation don't work much better than a placebo overall, and they don't work much better than going cold turkey. Plus, they're costly and come with side effects, such as hostility, depression, and agitation.

Smoking is the number one cause of preventable death and disability. Stress, weight gain, and withdrawal symptoms make it difficult to quit. In fact, weight gain and increased appetite are one of the most common complaints from "quitters." If you're kicking the habit, have a diet and exercise program prepared.

NAC (N-acetylcysteine). NAC may discourage the craving and reward sensations of certain addictions. A small preliminary randomized study suggested that taking 3,600 milligrams per day of NAC caused less rewarding feelings when restarting cigarettes about 4 days later compared to a placebo. It deserves more attention because NAC has shown some preliminary potential for other addictions, too. A very well-done randomized trial in adolescents (ages 15 to 21) found that those taking 1,200 milligrams per day of NAC over 8 weeks were twice as likely to have a *negative* cannabis urine test. The side effects are similar to a placebo, so this is a great option along with conventional treatments.

NOT PROVEN BUT YOU NEVER KNOW . . .

Antidepressant supplements. have been tested for addiction without success, which is not surprising to me because antidepressant drugs haven't been successful. I think antianxiety supplements might be promising, though. For many people who've quit smoking, including my daughter, I recommended L-theanine and GABA (gamma-aminobutyric acid). If the anxiety of withdrawal is extreme, take one GABA pill (100 to 150 milligrams per day), and if the withdrawal is minimal, take one L-theanine pill (100 to 200 milligrams) once or a few times a day. If you've tried everything to no avail, ask your doctor about Snus, a smokeless tobacco product that has a lower concentration of carcinogens. Research shows a reduction in lung cancer risk versus smoking with this product.

S Statin-Induced Myalgia

Dr. Moyad Secret Statins (HMG-CoA-reductase inhibitors) are the most widely prescribed cholesterol-lowering drugs in the world. And they get a lot of attention, both good and bad. Some of it is deserved and some of it is ridiculous (kind of like celebrity gossip). The next time you read an exposé and start thinking statins are overrated or part of some conspiracy to pad the pockets of "big pharma," come over to my house (well, not really). I'll tell you about how many coronary artery bypass surgeons and cardiologists are looking for extra work and how many cardiovascular procedures are no longer done (saving billions of dollars annually), all because these drugs are keeping most of your circulatory system free of cholesterol. And most statins are now available as generics, so many of them cost less than dietary supplements! I (as well as many other researchers) have been investigating the benefits of lowering cholesterol and am convinced statins and low cholesterol prevent many other conditions from occurring as we age, from brain diseases to sexual dysfunction to some aggressive cancers.

One of the side effects of statin use is muscle pain, and this condition is called statin-induced myalgia (SIM). Supplements are a very good option for SIM but not the best one because there are so many contributing factors. The best option (besides finding the specific cause) is to exercise more and make dietary changes to reduce cholesterol. Time and time again, I have seen patients make moderate changes to their lifestyles that dropped their statin dosage down to almost nothing or that allowed them to stop taking the drug altogether. The second-best option for SIM is to lower your current statin dose or switch to one of the newer prescriptions—such as rosuvastatin (my favorite), atorvastatin, pitavastatin, or even ezetimibe (it blocks cholesterol absorption from food and you take it in addition to your statin)—which you may be able to take once or twice a week instead of daily. The third option is to either switch to a red yeast rice supplement to lower cholesterol or take a dietary supplement to reduce the side effects of statins (such as CoQ10 and others).

WHAT IS IT?

Myalgia is muscle ache, pain, or weakness *without* any obvious underlying cause, such as muscular disease or damage, in which case you would see elevated creatine kinase (CK) in the blood. At least 10 to 20 percent of statin users complain of muscle problems, and it's the primary reason people quit taking them. Of course, as we get older, we tend to get more muscle aches and pains anyway, which can confuse the situation, but statin-induced myalgia will usually start within 6 months of taking a statin. Research suggests that taking half the recommended dose (and making up the difference with better diet and exercise habits) appears to dramatically reduce or completely eliminate the risk of muscle problems for many people. Even if you're not experiencing muscle pain, the higher your dose, the greater the risk of experiencing other side effects, such as reduced libido, memory loss, type 2 diabetes, and liver damage. So the goal should always be to take the smallest dose that will work.

Just a quick note about myositis, which is muscle pain accompanied by increased levels of CK, indicating there is injury or breakdown of the tissues: This is rare but can occur with statins, especially at higher doses. It's also a medical emergency, so if you're having muscle pain and you're on a statin, ask your doctor for a CK test. If it's high, a urine myoglobin test (to detect muscle-breakdown by-products in the urine) might also be ordered, or even a muscle biopsy in really rare cases.

You should never just deal with the pain or take a supplement to solve it first. Work with your doctor to figure out the true cause and try to resolve it without taking more pills. While statins can trigger pain, often it's because of another underlying factor, and this is what frequently gets missed with SIM. Here's the latest evidence-based list of factors that can increase the risk of SIM.

- Age (older than 70)
- Alcohol abuse
- Carnitine deficiency syndromes
- Diabetes
- Exercise (excessive exercise can raise CK levels way above normal)
- Female
- Genetics
- Grapefruit/grapefruit juice (It and perhaps even pomegranate juice has the ability to reduce the metabolism or breakdown of statins, leading to higher blood levels over time, almost as if you had taken a higher dose, as well as cause muscle pain and liver damage. Grapefruit impacts atorvastatin, lovastatin, and simvastatin the most and does not appear to affect fluvastatin, pitavastatin, pravastatin, and rosuvastatin.)
- Hereditary muscle problems
- High blood potassium levels
- High statin dose
- High triglycerides
- Hypertension (Some medications can increase risk, such as amiodarone, verapamil, or diltiazem; you may need to switch to another drug.)
- Infection
- Kidney problems (low glomerular filtration rate or high creatinine levels)
- Liver problems (fatty liver, hepatitis, high liver enzymes)

- Low thyroid levels (untreated hypothyroidism)
- Low vitamin B_{12}
- Low vitamin D
- McArdle's disease
- Muscle pain when taking statins previously
- Other cholesterol medications (It's not uncommon to take two different types of cholesterol medications. However, some nonstatin meds, such as gemfibrozil, can increase the amount of statin active ingredients in your bloodstream, leading to toxicity.)
- Small body frame or low body mass index
- Substance abuse (amphetamines, cocaine, heroin)
- Surgery

WHAT WORKS

Note: Again, these supplements are only for myalgia *without* elevated CK levels. Also, always consult your doctor when altering your statin dose.

1. Red yeast rice 600 to 2,400 milligrams divided into two daily doses either in place of a prescription statin or with a lower-dose statin

The first prescription statin drugs may have been isolated from red yeast rice, which is a mixture of yeast and rice. The active cholesterol-lowering ingredient in red yeast rice (RYR) is known as monacolin K, a compound that blocks the same cholesterol-synthesizing enzyme in the liver that prescription statins do. (See the High Cholesterol section, page 234, for more detailed information on red yeast rice.)

In studies, RYR has been found to lower LDL (bad cholesterol) by 10 to 30 percent at dosages as low as 600 milligrams (1 pill) and as high as 1,800 to 2,400 milligrams. (Monacolin K has a similar structure to the drug lovastatin, so take RYR with food and avoid all forms of grapefruit and pomegranate when taking this supplement.) RYR has consistently been shown to help people lower their cholesterol without increasing the risk of SIM. RYR may have fewer muscle pain side effects because its active ingredient is more diluted than the active ingredient in statins, or it may be due to other compounds in RYR that haven't yet been researched. Regardless, RYR has become a wonderful option for people with SIM who don't want to continue on a prescription statin or who want to lower their dose.

Here's the frustrating thing about RYR: Dietary supplement companies are *not* supposed to standardize it, meaning they can't guarantee the amount of monacolin K in each product. Because RYR works too much like prescription statins, the companies can get in trouble for selling an over-the-counter product that acts too much like a drug. This is one of the dumbest penalties against dietary supplement companies that I have ever witnessed. Either the supplement should be banned entirely from the United States or companies should be able to standardize the monacolin K amount in red yeast rice! The bottom line: You have to test different brands to see which ones have enough of the active ingredient to make a difference in your cholesterol levels. Also, since RYR is a natural statin that works somewhat similar to synthetic drugs, it can also cause liver and muscle side effects in rare cases, so your doctor still needs to monitor you as if you were on a prescription statin.

2. CoQ10 (ubiquinone) 100 to 600 milligrams a day

This fat-soluble antioxidant is used in every cell of the human body. One of the building blocks of CoQ10 is created in the liver as part of the cholesterol-production process. Statins block the ability of the liver to make cholesterol, so when you take them, the amount of CoQ10 produced by the body drops! Atorvastatin (Lipitor), for example, can cause a 50 percent reduction in CoQ10 levels in the blood in just 30 days. Since the mitochondria in every cell need CoQ10 to produce energy, a lack of it can impact muscle tissue, leading to pain. Even the drug companies realize it has some potential benefit; some of them tried to obtain a patent on it for reducing SIM. CoQ10 has, by far, the most human research of any dietary supplement for lowering the risk of muscle problems with statins. But the results are mixed, with about half the studies showing some ben-

efit and the other half showing no benefit. Again, since there are so many underlying causes that can increase the risk of SIM, there is no dietary supplement or drug that will ever prevent or reduce this condition in everyone.

That said, most studies have participants taking 100 to 600 milligrams of CoQ10 daily to prevent or reduce myalgia, with higher dosages showing more efficacy. One of the biggest side effects of CoQ10, however, is the cost! If it's not working within 4 weeks, increase the dose, and if it's not working at the maximum dosage (600 milligrams per day), then it's time to give up. (Or you can continue to use it for its many other benefits, such as increasing muscle performance during exercise, boosting strength, or reducing muscle fatigue in statin users.)

Side effects are rare with CoQ10, but GI problems and allergic rash have been reported. Weirdly, it has both antiplatelet (blood-thinning) and *pro*clotting effects, depending on what medications you're taking it with, so always check with your doctor. Ideally, you should take CoQ10 with a meal that has some fat in it for better absorption (save your money and don't buy brands that say they have better absorption; they're not worth it, and most studies tested the cheaper ones). Let your doctor know you're taking CoQ10 as she may want to monitor blood levels.

3. Four-way tie! There are so many effective supplements that I couldn't just pick three.

Creatine monohydrate powder
5 grams a day

Inside muscle tissue, creatine helps produce energy. In fact, many people take it to boost their workouts, especially weight lifters (it's one of my recommended supplements for athletic enhancement; see page 77). Some individuals experience a decrease in creatine when taking a statin or other drugs, which can lead to muscle pain. Preliminary research published in the *Annals of Internal Medicine* indicates taking 5 to 10 grams of this powdered dietary supplement daily (with water) can reduce myalgia. But here's how you have to do it: Take a "loading dose" of 10 grams for the first 5 days with no statin drug and then 5 grams a day after that with reintroduction of the statin. It can help some individuals reduce or eliminate myalgia after 2 to 3 months. (Use creatine powder please, not the pills; otherwise, you have to take too many.)

Carnitine 1,000 to 2,000 milligrams a day

Some people, whether they're taking statins or not, have a difficult time metabolizing carnitine, an amino acid that is crucial for energy production. Researchers are not certain why this is, but it's not uncommon for people with carnitine-metabolizing abnormalities to suffer from SIM. Dosages of 1,000 to 2,000 milligrams per day (with or without food) of a type of carnitine called L-carnitine (acetyl-L-carnitine, for example) should help. The research on this is just getting started, but

in my experience—and based on the high number of carnitine problems in people with SIM—it's smart to give this a try, especially since the benefit outweighs the risk; just work with your doctor.

Vitamin D at least 1,000 IU a day

Vitamin D has many functions within muscles, including reducing inflammation, preventing injury, and simply improving function. Being deficient in D (less than or equal to 20 ng/mL on the 25-OH vitamin D blood test) can cause pain. Your doctor will look at your blood levels to determine how much D you need to correct an insufficiency. Some doctors want to correct these big deficiencies right away and will give something like 50,000 IU of vitamin D as a prescription twice a week for 3 weeks and then continue or discontinue it based on the lab results, eventually introducing the statin again. I'm concerned that radically normalizing any deficiency with megadoses comes with its own toxicity, especially since vitamin D acts more like a hormone than a vitamin.

Phytosterols (plant sterols and stanols) 2,000 milligrams a day

Phytosterols block the uptake of cholesterol from dietary and bile sources in the intestinal tract. They reduce "bad" (LDL) cholesterol but don't really impact HDL (good cholesterol) and triglycerides. Phytosterol supplements are really just less potent copycats of the drug ezetimibe (Zetia), which can reduce LDLs by approximately 20 percent (at a 10-milligram dose). These supplements can help reduce your statin dose, which can help minimize SIM. At 2,000 milligrams per day, they've been shown to lower LDL by an average of 10 to 11 percent. Phytosterols may also reduce the absorption of some fat-soluble vitamins, so you need to take a multivitamin daily as well. Finally, always take this supplement before every meal (or just before large meals with lots of cholesterol) to block cholesterol absorption. (Phytosterols are now FDA approved to be used in food products, such as margarine and orange juice; I like the margarine option best.)

WHAT'S WORTHLESS?

Omega-3 fatty acids. Taking omega-3s to reduce cholesterol levels is perhaps one of the biggest mistakes people make. Fish oil can *increase* LDL cholesterol as you increase the dosage! Some experts discount the rise and say it's not a big deal, but it *is* a big deal! Fish oil (or the active ingredients EPA and DHA) is FDA approved to lower triglycerides, not LDL! Do not take fish oil to lower LDL cholesterol or for SIM. (See the High Cholesterol section, page 234.)

Niacin or no-flush niacin. Niacin dietary supplements, which cause facial flushing, can only add to the toxicity of a statin by increasing the risk of liver injury. The no-flush niacin (inositol hexaniacinate), so named because it doesn't cause the telltale flushing that regular niacin does, also doesn't work to lower cholesterol levels or for SIM. No flush = no work!

Vitamin E and selenium. Experts used to believe these popular antioxidants reduced SIM by preventing muscle injury, but neither of them reduced SIM in clinical studies with people taking statins.

LIFESTYLE CHANGES

Change your diet. Low-fat diets have a profound impact on reducing LDL, and low-carbohydrate diets have a profound impact on reducing triglycerides *and* LDL. Research has also shown that higher daily intakes of plant sterols (1,000 to 2,000 milligrams), soy protein (11 to 15 grams), soluble fiber (5 to 10 grams), nuts and seeds, and veggies and lower intakes of beef, poultry, fish, and eggs reduced LDL by 10 to 15 percent on average. The better your diet, the less you have to rely on a statin.

Add fiber. Reduce your statin dose slightly and add 5 to 15 grams of psyllium fiber powder or another soluble fiber product to your diet. An older study from the Robert Wood Johnson Medical School in New Jersey found that 10 milligrams of simvastatin along with 15 grams of fiber lowered LDL just as much as taking 20 milligrams of simvastatin with no fiber! Nice! Fiber blocks the absorption of cholesterol and helps bacteria in the intestines create compounds that lower the production of cholesterol.

Stress and Anxiety

S

Dr. Moyad Secret Want proof that stress and anxiety can negatively impact your health almost immediately? Just look at the millions of people around the world who have "white coat hypertension": Their blood pressure rises, sometimes to dangerous levels, only in a doctor's office; the rest of the time it's normal. If short-lived stress or anxiety can spike blood pressure, imagine what feeling like this day in and day out can do to the body!

Stress is both psychological and physiological. But one secret to treating it lies in your brain. Stress and anxiety supplements (at least the ones I'm going to talk about here) work by altering your brain waves, as seen on an electroencephalogram (EEG). There are four basic waves that researchers look at on an EEG: delta, theta, alpha, and beta; the latter two are especially important in clinical studies of these supplements. Your brain emits alpha waves during periods of relaxed and effortless alertness and beta waves during highly stressful periods when it's difficult to focus. Having more alpha and fewer beta waves is a marker of being relaxed, awake and aware, and better able to concentrate (i.e., lower stress). And the supplements in this section can increase alpha and decrease beta waves. Pretty cool stuff!

WHAT IS IT?

Stress and anxiety trigger extreme internal changes that can negatively impact physical and mental health as well as quality of life. Whether the stressor is internal (worry about job loss) or external (being chased by a dog), the body's reaction is the same, resulting in profound physiological changes. Common triggers include work, relationships, money, childhood trauma, drugs or alcohol, illness, lack of sleep or exercise (as well as too much exercise), and even genetics.

Stress and anxiety are like house-guests. When they show up every once in a while, they don't really cause a problem; when they stay too long, it makes you crazy. A certain amount of stress can improve alertness and be beneficial (exercise is a "good" type of stress, in moderation). When you're stressed day in and day out, it impacts your quality of life and starts to negatively affect your body. Common symptoms of stress and anxiety include feeling weak or tired; sweating or trembling; increased heart and breathing rate; feeling powerless; a sense of panic, danger, or doom; increases in blood pressure, heart rate, breathing, and blood sugar; palpitations; muscle tension (sometimes leading to headaches); trouble sleeping; depression; and a weakened immune system.

When you're stressed, the adrenal glands release excessive amounts of fight-or-flight hormones, including norepinephrine, epinephrine, and cortisol. These can increase your heart rate, blood pressure, and blood sugar, which, over time, can cause cardiovascular problems. Stress and anxiety can weaken your immune system by causing a reduction in specific immune cells that fight infections. They can also impair your memory, focus, and concentration and make it difficult to get adequate sleep or rest, causing both mental and physical fatigue. Stress can even reduce the amount of healthy bacteria found in your gastrointestinal tract and cause digestive problems (ever heard of nervous stomach?). Stress also reduces compounds in the body that can help you fight stress, so it's a vicious circle.

There are different types of stress and anxiety (for example, generalized anxiety disorder, panic disorder, and post-traumatic stress disorder), and most of the research with supplements and anxiety has been for generalized anxiety, but researchers have also studied supplements for situational anxiety (such as taking a test). Keep in mind: If stress and anxiety are interfering with day-to-day living, it's important to seek treatment from a professional.

WHAT WORKS

Note: Taking an antistress supplement along with prescription medications for stress, anxiety, or depression may cause potentially dangerous drug interactions, so always check with your doctor or pharmacist. Also, sudden withdrawal from any supplement or drug that reduces stress or anxiety as well as your blood pressure, such as beta blockers, may be dangerous because it can cause a dramatic increase in blood pressure or heart rate; always taper off gradually over several weeks.

1. GABA (gamma-aminobutyric acid) 50 to 200 milligrams a day

This amino acid is prescribed as a drug in many parts of the world, but in the United States it's considered a dietary supplement. GABA is a naturally occurring brain neurotransmitter, but it's also found elsewhere in the body. GABA dietary supplements increase alpha-wave activity and decrease beta-wave activity—which is proof that it works to promote relaxation but maintain concentration—and may reduce levels of the stress hormone cortisol. In preliminary studies, daily doses of only 50 to 200 milligrams have been shown to be effective (taken with or without food). Once I had an A-list friend (no name dropping here) call me before a big speech in New York City. It was one of the most important events of his career, and he was understandably nervous. He didn't want to take a prescription drug because it would make him too relaxed and drowsy, reducing his ability to focus. I told him about GABA (and theanine, the next supplement) and he took it. I found out later it was the best speech of the night!

Researchers haven't documented the side effects, including drug interactions, of this supplement very well because the studies haven't been long term. I'm always concerned about drug interaction and dependency with antistress products, so check with your local pharmacist about any new concerns. Although GABA does help promote a sense of calm alertness, it also could lead to drowsiness in some people.

2. L-theanine 100 to 250 milligrams a day in a single or divided dose

This is a fascinating amino acid found in green and black tea (there are about 20 milligrams in a cup of black tea), and it actually counteracts the stimulatory effects of caffeine—an excellent example of nature balancing itself. Regardless, L-theanine has a fabulous record and has been used as an additive in candy, foods, and beverages in Japan for decades. (Some

people even use it to calm their children down, although I'm not condoning this!) Scientists first isolated it in tea in 1949 and then in mushrooms in the early 1950s. It has worked in studies by increasing GABA and other brain neurotransmitters, such as dopamine and serotonin; blocking the uptake of the neurotransmitter glutamate in the nervous system, which helps with learning and memory; encouraging the release of glycine, an inhibitory neurotransmitter; and even providing some protection for nerve cells of the brain. All of these have a relaxing or calming effect.

Because it has such a good safety record so far, L-theanine is my favorite antistress supplement when used at a dosage of 100 to 250 milligrams per day (200 to 250 has shown more consistent impact). I did not rank it number one only because GABA is more effective. Like GABA, it increases alpha waves in the brain, but it's a milder effect, and I believe its ability to profoundly reduce stress and anxiety is limited. That's not really a disadvantage, though; in fact, it's another reason why it's so safe. The patented form of theanine, known as Suntheanine, has the most research. (The FDA has considered it a Generally Recognized as Safe, or GRAS, product since 2007.) In studies, at 200 milligrams it improved both subjective and objective feelings of stress, such as heart rate, alpha-wave activity, and immune response (GABA does this also, of course). Take it with or without food and either as one daily dose or divided in half.

Unfortunately, some supplement companies are combining L-theanine with numerous other ingredients in order to create a unique blend, however, there's no research on these combinations. The most effective clinical trials were with L-theanine by itself.

3. (tie) *Rhodiola rosea* (look for the extract called SHR-5) 100 to 300 milligrams a day in divided doses (half in the morning and afternoon)

This supplement is also known as roseroot or rosenroot. It appears to favorably impact neurotransmitters in the brain, counteract the impact of adrenaline (a fight-or-flight hormone) on the body, and block cortisol release. It would have ranked higher, but most of the positive research with it was on a standardized proprietary extract from the root called SHR-5, and many of the trials had some methodological issues. Yet, there's too much clinical evidence to ignore it. Researchers are now testing higher daily doses of SHR-5 extract (576 milligrams) and getting positive preliminary results for stress-related fatigue. (It's also getting good attention as an antidepressant; see the Depression section, page 166.) It's not always easy to find SHR-5, but with a little footwork, you can track down several companies that use the extract (for example, Swedish Herbal Institute's Original Arctic Root).

Small studies with *Rhodiola rosea* have shown that 170 milligrams twice daily can reduce generalized anxiety disorder, but the more impressive clinical trials overall were with SHR-5; it reduced stress-related fatigue and improved mental performance.

Researchers are studying several active ingredients from this plant, including rhodioloside, salidroside, triandrin, tyrosol, and rosavin. The extracts used in some studies have also been standardized to what is believed to be the two more active ingredients, rosavins (3 percent) and salidroside (0.8 percent). (The naturally occurring ratio of these compounds in the root is 3:1, but I would just look for the SHR-5 extract.) Studies do not consistently indicate whether to take it with or without food, but you should divide the dose (take half in the morning and half in the late afternoon or evening).

The only problem I have with this herb in the stress and anxiety trials is that there has not been enough safety information published on it. Most studies have reported no side effects beyond a placebo. Mild side effects—such as irritability, allergic reaction fatigue, and insomnia—have been reported in rare cases, especially with higher doses.

3. (tie) *Bacopa monnieri* (Brahmi or bacopa) 200 to 450 milligrams a day in divided doses

This is an alternative Ayurvedic medicine that in preliminary clinical trials reduced stress and anxiety better than a placebo. Although this plant has been used in India and Pakistan for various ailments, the real focus lately has been on its potential for memory enhancement (see the Memory

417

Loss section, page 318, and the Alzheimer's Disease, Dementia, and Mild Cognitive Impairment section, page 65) and reducing anxiety.

Many of the components of bacopa were isolated years ago and include alkaloids, saponins, sterols, bacopa saponins, and bacosides. The bacosides appear to be involved in nerve cell repair, production, and signaling, and they also appear to have some antioxidant benefit in different areas of the brain, including the hippocampus, frontal cortex, and striatum. The specific compounds garnering attention and research for their effect on the brain are bacosides A and B.

In one 12-week trial, a 300-milligram daily dose (with 55 percent combined bacosides, meaning a combo of A and B) resulted in a significant improvement in memory, learning, and speed of information processing. In addition, some participants reported less anxiety early in the study, and it's this finding, along with other studies reporting similar effects, that has people excited about bacopa as an antianxiety herbal. Lab studies with 25 percent bacoside A have shown an ability to reduce anxiety that's similar to some prescription drugs, but without the temporary memory issues. A 1-month trial of bacopa syrup (30 milliliters daily in two divided doses) in individuals with anxiety demonstrated a significant reduction in anxiety and mental fatigue, an increase in memory, and a decrease in blood pressure. A clinical trial with healthy individuals that compared 450 milligrams of bacopa

extract with a placebo (over 12 weeks) did not find any profound effects *except* for a trend toward less anxiety with bacopa.

Based on these studies, I recommend using 200 to 450 milligrams (divided during the day) for a minimum of 12 weeks to see if it works (it should be standardized to a minimum of 25 percent bacoside A or 50 percent total bacosides). The most common side effect is mild gastrointestinal upset, such as abdominal cramps, increased stool frequency, and nausea.

WHAT'S WORTHLESS

Kava or kava-kava. This herbal supplement has the most positive research for reducing anxiety, but I cannot recommend it because safety has to come first (see the Insomnia and Jet Lag section, page 266). Otherwise, it would be my number one supplement choice for anxiety.

Kava is an extract from the roots of a Polynesian plant (*Piper methysticum*), and it's used in the South Pacific (Polynesia, Melanesia, and Micronesia) to calm, relax, and promote well-being. It is even used as an aphrodisiac. And many people in the United States use it as a substitute for Xanax or Valium. It contains several active ingredients, including kawain, dihydrokawain, and methysticin, but the most interesting ones are the kava pyrones (better known as kavalactones); as many as 15 of them exist.

Side effects overall have been low (1 to 5 percent in most studies), but the problem is that it's getting the reputation as a liver

418

killer. Regulators in the UK pulled it off shelves after reports of users needing liver transplants and complaints of other liver problems. However, some researchers are arguing that this was not justified and that it's time to let kava regain popularity. More than a decade ago, the FDA issued a warning about an increased risk of liver toxicity with kava, but it's still legal in the United States (so they can't be that concerned, right?).

Every time I'm ready to recommend kava again something makes me nervous. For example, the National Toxicology Program is a well-known laboratory study group that tests supplements, especially if they're popular (their research with Panax ginseng made me more comfortable recommending it). They usually conduct 2-week, 3-month, and 2-year toxicity and carcinogenic studies in rats and mice. When they examined kava, there was some hint of liver problems when combining this supplement with other drugs or supplements. In other words, the risk exceeds the benefit for now.

Fish oil. It's touted for everything these days, and while it does deserve some of the accolades, stress and anxiety is an area where fish oil is overhyped. In some people it can slightly reduce blood pressure and heart rate, but this hasn't resulted in a consistent reduction in stress or anxiety.

Valerian. Valerian is not a good anti-stress or antianxiety supplement because it's a good sleep aid. People who are stressed and anxious usually need to func-tion during the day at work or at school. Being knocked out and unable to focus will just lead to more problems. Take valerian to sleep, not for stress.

Miscellaneous. There are many popular (but unproven) sleep supplements that are also supposed to be good for decreasing stress and anxiety, including passionflower, hops, wild lettuce, Jamaican dogwood, California poppy, chamomile, lemon balm, skullcap, and *Patrinia* root. But they're not worth the money. As with valerian, using any of them just doesn't make sense; it's like taking an Ambien for stress. Plus, I can count the number of good studies that have been done with these supplements on one hand—whether for sleep *or* stress. (See the Insomnia and Jet Lag section, page 266.)

LIFESTYLE CHANGES

Heart healthy = less stress. Anything that throws the body into physiological stress—being overweight or having high blood pressure, blood sugar, or cholesterol—can increase mental stress and anxiety. So any diet or activity that reduces these and improves overall heart health can help.

Experiment with different stress-busting strategies. There are many ways to combat stress and anxiety, including joining a support group, journaling, art therapy, guided imagery, hypnosis, music therapy, horticultural therapy, yoga, meditation, tai chi, and more. Many of these are even *free* (check your local community recreation center). Pick a method that suits your personality (some people would rather de-stress by boxing than meditating), and if that doesn't work, keep trying until you find something that does. (I'll let you in on a secret: Stress happens when you feel like a situation is out of your control. The reason many of these activities work is because they help you gain control over your situation and even your own bodily reactions. As a result, blood pressure, heart rate, stress, and anxiety go down.)

Avoid self-medicating. If you're prone to anxiety, self-medicating with alcohol, tobacco, or caffeine can create a roller-coaster ride of dependency and make anxiety worse. Your body develops resistance to them, so you need higher doses to get your "fix," potentially leading to huge swings in blood pressure and heart rate. Keep your alcohol intake to moderate levels (one or two drinks a day) and eliminate tobacco products. Similarly, it's good to limit your intake of caffeine to one or two cups a day.

Work out more. Exercise is one of the best ways to reduce stress and anxiety. It lowers heart rate, blood pressure, and blood sugar levels and releases "feel-good" endorphins. It also reduces sympathetic nervous system overload—the fight-or-flight response—which is a massive problem as we age (the internal mechanism that keeps this response under control doesn't function like it did when you were 20). You don't have to go for a run or take up boxing to feel better, either. Yoga, tai chi, and walking are perfectly good for reducing stress and anxiety.

Try alternative therapies. Meditation and massage can help with stress reduction, and I believe that acupuncture has enough positive clinical trials now in the area of stress and anxiety to warrant recommending it.

Stroke Prevention

S

Dr. Moyad Secret The five factors that in combination lower stroke risk by 80 percent are: Don't smoke, maintain a healthy weight, don't drink alcohol in excess, exercise regularly, and eat a healthy diet. Keeping blood pressure normal is the single biggest thing that prevents stroke. (See the Hypertension and Prehypertension section, page 251.) Strokes are now the fourth leading killer in the United States—almost 800,000 occur a year!

With the exception of red yeast rice, which may prevent atrial fibrillation like other statins do, I don't highly recommend any supplements for prevention since lifestyle is the key. Also you should know that vitamin E can increase the risk of hemorrhagic stroke, and ginkgo and B vitamins are worthless for prevention.

Tinnitus

Dr. Moyad Secret I have tinnitus (a.k.a. ringing in the ears) in my left ear, and it drives me crazier than Republicans and Democrats saying they want to work together. The truth is, no single conventional or alternative treatment exists for this problem, despite the fact that it's very common. There are just so many risk factors and conditions associated with the disorder. For example, antibiotics can increase the risk of tinnitus by damaging the inner ear cells that transmit sound to the auditory nerve, all the more reason to avoid taking antibiotics if you don't need them. Doctors should be open to a variety of potential supplement treatments for tinnitus because the benefit outweighs the risk in most cases. I can't promise a supplement solution, but I think it's worth being a guinea pig.

WHAT IS IT?

Tinnitus is the conscious perception of a constant or intermittent ringing, buzzing, hissing, or whistling sensation that occurs in the absence of a sound or other stimulus. It can be heard in one or both ears, or centrally within the head, although some describe an external sound source, as if it's close to the ears. In most cases, you're the only one who can hear it (subjective tinnitus), but in some rare cases, others can also hear it (objective tinnitus). In other rare cases, patients can hear a thumping sound that is sometimes in sync with their heartbeat (pulsatile tinnitus).

Tinnitus impacts approximately 10 to 15 percent of the population, and close to one in three will seek medical attention for it. (I got a hearing test, which was normal, and multiple reassurances that I was going to be okay. I also had an MRI, which was negative, because you always want to make sure there isn't a tumor growing near the auditory nerve.) It's usually caused by damage to the nerve cells in the ear. Seventy percent of cases are due to trauma (working around loud machines or going to a loud concert) or aging, but the remaining 30 percent can be traced to any of 20 different factors, from ear problems, like infection or excess wax, to temporomandibular joint disorder (TMJ), to more systemic diseases, such as rheumatoid arthritis, lupus, and diabetes. More than 200 drugs (including pain killers, antibiotics, and diuretics) can cause it as well!

Tinnitus affects men and women equally, but, as mentioned earlier, there is an increased risk with aging, especially for those between 60 and 70 years old.

Half of sufferers report tinnitus in both ears or centrally within the head, but in the other half, tinnitus is more left-sided than right for some unknown reason. Unfortunately, way too many individuals are told to "learn to live with it," which makes no sense. Although there are so many potential causes, there are also so many different treatment options, from sound therapy and dietary supplements to surgery. If tinnitus does not get better in a few months or if it is associated with dizziness or vertigo, see an otolaryngologist (also called an ENT doc).

WHAT WORKS

Note: Most supplements that are touted for tinnitus help by supposedly improving inner ear circulation. Although this sounds good and might help, many of them have not been proven to do this. Also, many supplements offer a money back guarantee within 60 days, but tinnitus can be temporary or decrease over time, so you may get better on your own (I don't recommend holding off on trying a supplement, though). The bottom line: No product for tinnitus has great research behind it and no single supplement stands out, so these are not listed in order of effectiveness. Consider them all bronze medals.

1. Melatonin 1 to 3 milligrams daily or as needed

Tinnitus can disrupt sleep, so any safe supplement that will help sufferers catch some z's is useful. While writing this book, I experienced bad tinnitus, and going to sleep or staying asleep was tough! I took 3 milligrams of melatonin about 15 to 30 minutes before bed, but some people respond well to only 1 milligram. (Higher doses are being tested.) A new review of tinnitus clinical trials now suggests melatonin may actually reduce tinnitus and not just help you sleep better with the condition. Always start low; too much can create a cycle of dependence and make you feel groggy or fatigued the next day.

2. Pycnogenol 100 to 150 milligrams a day

A small clinical trial of Pycnogenol (an anti-inflammatory supplement derived from the bark of the French maritime pine tree) demonstrated a potential to improve circulation in the inner ear, and it may even reduce the severity of tinnitus over 1 to 2 months. It also has an excellent safety record. The problem with Pycnogenol is that the research suggests it can benefit a wide variety of conditions. When a supplement has preliminary research suggesting it's beneficial in so many areas, I get skeptical. It's hard to be a "jack of all trades" as a supplement and be really good at any one of them. However, I'm willing to make an exception in the area of tinnitus.

3. Bioflavonoids 200 to 800 milligrams a day

These are some of the most common

423

protective compounds found in plants. They're antioxidants, but are generally not absorbed well by the body. However, their anti-inflammatory, procirculatory, and cellular defense properties make them a commonly studied supplement for a variety of difficult-to-treat conditions, such as tinnitus. There is some evidence to suggest that people with otosclerosis-induced tinnitus (an inner ear bone abnormality) might benefit from a bioflavonoid supplement. For example, the bioflavonoid ipriflavone (derived from soy and also known as 7-isopropoxyisoflavone) is being studied for the treatment of osteoporosis. Some small studies using 200 milligrams four times per day for up to 6 months have found some benefit in reducing or stopping tinnitus. If you have tinnitus caused by otosclerosis, ipriflavone might stave off further problems with the small inner ear bones that could make the problem worse.

Another bioflavonoid dietary supplement called Lipo-Flavonoid Plus (follow package dosing) is perhaps the best-selling tinnitus dietary supplement in the United States, and I am often asked whether it works. (I became much more interested in answering this after I got tinnitus that didn't go away after a few weeks.) The supplement was developed specifically for people with tinnitus by an otolaryngologist at the Mayo Clinic, and it contains the following:

- Eriodictyol glycoside (an extract from lemon citrus bioflavonoid)

- Vitamins B_1, B_2, B_3, B_6, and B_{12}

- Choline, inositol, and pantothenic acid

- Vitamin C

At first glance, it appears to be a glorified multivitamin with one special ingredient from lemon citrus bioflavonoid. The research cited by the Web site and in the packaging is for a condition called Ménière's disease, an inner ear disorder that causes vertigo, tinnitus, and hearing loss. Although tinnitus is one of the primary symptoms of Ménière's, I'm not convinced it will help tinnitus sufferers who don't have it. Regardless, since it contains a bioflavonoid complex, I think it's worth a try for 3 months.

WHAT'S WORTHLESS

Ginkgo biloba. It's one of the most commonly recommended supplements for tinnitus due to its blood-thinning properties (thinner blood should improve inner ear circulation, goes the thinking), but the research is weak and good studies have shown no overall benefit. In addition, there have been quality-control issues with this supplement, so the risk exceeds the benefit

Zinc. It is supposed to improve the health and function of the auditory nerve and is often recommended for tinnitus, but I never bought into this. When researchers tested a daily 50-milligram dose of zinc sulfate for 4 months in people with tinnitus from various causes, they found it worked about as well as a placebo.

And excessive zinc (100 milligrams or more a day) has been shown to damage the sense of taste and smell. If that's the case, I wonder if it will damage hearing as well!

B vitamins. Older research suggested B vitamins might reduce tinnitus by correcting an underlying deficiency, but recent studies show they don't work better than a placebo. Regardless, some supplement manufacturers still use this deficiency-correcting argument in ads. But don't buy into it. Another marketing theory is that B vitamins can reduce stress, which can reduce tinnitus. Sorry! B vitamins have never been proven to reduce stress *or* tinnitus. If you are worried about your B_{12} status, just ask your doctor for a blood test.

WHAT ARE THE OPTIONS FOR KIDS?

When children get tinnitus, they generally appear less distressed by it than adults. There's no research regarding the impact of supplements on tinnitus in kids. I recommend following the adult suggestions above, (especially melatonin, which has been tested in kids) but at half the dosage.

LIFESTYLE CHANGES

Heart healthy = ear healthy. Say it with me: Lowering blood pressure and cholesterol, consuming less salt, exercising, reducing stress, *and* getting enough rest will help my ticker and my ears.

Protect your ears. Loud noise can lead to or worsen tinnitus, so wear earplugs at concerts or even in loud workout classes.

Reduce blood pressure–increasing products in excess. Caffeinated beverages, alcohol, and nicotine can make tinnitus worse.

Review meds with your doctor. Besides antibiotics, high doses of aspirin or ibuprofen and certain antihypertensive drugs can cause tinnitus or make it worse.

Check out magnesium. This important mineral is being tested as an otoprotectant. The Recommend Dietary Allowance for adults is 320 milligrams (women) to 420 milligrams (men). It's one of the nutrients that people tend to lack in their diets. Fish, nuts, beans, seeds, and veggies are some of the highest sources.

Consider a hearing aid. The better you hear, the less you may notice tinnitus (hearing loss can cause the brain to turn up its internal volume—like feedback from an overly sensitive microphone). A hearing aid (or in more severe cases, a cochlear implant) could lower the volume of your tinnitus.

Explore therapy. Counseling or cognitive behavioral therapy may not reduce tinnitus, but it has been shown to help with conditions that are associated with tinnitus, such as sleep problems and depression.

Travelers' Diarrhea

Dr. Moyad Secret The best way to prevent travelers' diarrhea (TD—and not the football kind) is to be prepared with a multipronged approach. For prevention, I recommend packing bismuth subsalicylate (Pepto-Bismol tablets) and a probiotic dietary supplement, such as *Lactobacillus rhamnosus* GG, and using them daily (I tell you how below). In case you're unlucky, make sure to have on hand loperamide caplets (Imodium) and the prescription antibiotic rifaximin, which has been FDA approved for travelers' diarrhea since 2004 (it's good for both treating *and* preventing TD).

WHAT IS IT?

It's been called Montezuma's revenge, the "vacation terminator," and, um, decorum does not permit me to throw in the other names. Travelers' diarrhea is the most common travel-related disease in the world: Approximately 40 to 50 percent of people who venture abroad experience an episode of diarrhea. Food and water that have been contaminated with fecal matter are the primary source of the problem.

TD usually occurs within the first week of a trip, and the longer you stay, the lower your chances of getting it (yet another reason to ask for more vacation time). Studies found that individuals who had lived abroad for a year had significantly reduced risk of TD because they had developed an acquired immunity to the microscopic invaders that cause the condition. People raised in an area with a high incidence of TD have a lower risk of getting it in the future,

while people raised in more sanitary areas have a higher risk of getting TD when traveling! This adds even more credibility to the hygiene hypothesis: Individuals who were exposed to more diverse infectious sources (animals, other kids, floors, etc.) as kids develop better lifelong immunity than people who were raised in more sterile environments. The relatively germ-free individuals may even experience an exaggerated response to an otherwise mild infection.

The average episode of TD lasts 3 to 5 days! Most cases (50 to 80 percent) are bacterial, so antibiotics could make the difference between having fun on vacation and reading *War and Peace* in the bathroom. However, viruses and protozoa cause up to one-third of cases. Regardless of the offending bug, the symptoms are pretty much the same: watery diarrhea; fever; nausea; vomiting; abdominal pain/cramps; and even nongastrointestinal complaints, such as

COMMON TRAVELERS' DIARRHEA BACTERIA

- *Aeromonas*
- *Campylobacter*
- Enterotoxigenic *Escherichia coli* and other *E. coli* strains
- *Salmonella* (nontyphoid)
- *Shigella*
- Vibrio (noncholera)

COMMON TRAVELERS' DIARRHEA PARASITES (usually longer lasting)

- *Cryptosporidium parvum* (it's a common cause of cow diarrhea)
- *Cyclospora cayetanensis*
- *Entamoeba histolytica*
- *Giardia lamblia* (called beaver fever, this usually results from drinking water from a stream or river)

COMMON TRAVELERS' DIARRHEA VIRUSES (less frequent)

- *Norovirus* (often referred to as the cruise ship virus, although it can be found anywhere; always bring a couple of good books when you go on a cruise because you could be doing a lot of reading if you get this)
- *Rotavirus*

joint and muscle pain and headache. Most people get better without serious side effects, but electrolyte deficiency can occur; if symptoms do not improve after 3 days or there is fever or bloody stools, find a doctor. The good news: If you get TD, your chances of contracting it again when traveling within the next year is lower.

WHAT WORKS

Note: Apart from over-the-counter loperamide, which is not officially a supplement (though I consider it one because it's OTC and originally derived from some natural sources), no dietary supplement should be used to *treat* TD. The current OTC and prescription treatments are just too good, and in most cases TD resolves on its own. Dietary supplements should be used for *prevention* of TD. Never use a probiotic if you are immunocompromised or taking prescription immunosuppressive medication, such as the steroid prednisone.

1. *Lactobacillus rhamnosus* GG probiotic (Culturelle) follow dosage directions on packaging for kids and adults starting 2 days before the trip and daily throughout for prevention

Lactobacillus rhamnosus strain GG can bind to intestinal cells and produce several compounds that fight bad bugs. It's been on the market longer than any other potentially effective probiotic for TD except *Saccharomyces boulardii* (see #2), but it has much more favorable research. Two studies with hundreds of travelers found a prevention rate with the GG strain between 12 and 45 percent.

This probiotic usually comes in a powder within a capsule or as a fermented milk product, does not have to be refrigerated, and lasts up to 21 months! (If you can't figure out how old your product is, just squeeze a capsule. If it's still soft and flexible, then chances are it's not expired.) In studies, there were no restrictions on taking the capsules with a meal or on an empty stomach, but the supplement container should be stored in a cool and dark place. (Side note: Probiotics claiming a benefit against TD that have to be refrigerated are a waste of your money. Trying to keep something like this refrigerated when you're traveling is unrealistic. If it's that delicate, it probably will not work.) I also like Culturelle because the adult version contains 200 milligrams of inulin, which is a low dose of fiber *and* a prebiotic, so it increases the chances of healthy bacteria coming into your gastrointestinal tract and promotes regular stool movement. I don't recommend combining GG with another probiotic supplement for prevention; how this will work is unknown, and more is not always better, even for diarrhea!

2. *Saccharomyces boulardii* probiotic 1,000 milligrams a day in two divided doses starting 5 days before a trip and daily throughout for prevention

S. boulardii (a yeast-based probiotic) has demonstrated protection in travelers going to North Africa but not to other destinations. Although, the fact that it helped in an area of the world with such a high rate of TD makes me comfortable recommending it for other parts of the globe. Again, the studies do not specify if it should be taken with or without food, so see what works for you.

3. Loperamide up to 16 milligrams a day as needed for treatment only

Loperamide (Imodium) is the most commonly used product for TD, and it's the most effective OTC treatment. There are very few drugs that can reduce diarrhea after it has started, but loperamide can. Some people consider loperamide to be a drug, but I count it as a supplement because it was potentially derived from a plant and—for all you physiology geeks out there—attaches to receptors in the intestines that normally bind other plant-derived products (opiate receptors), so your body thinks it's a plant, too!

It blocks certain receptors in the intestine to slow the movement of the gastrointestinal tract so that more water can get absorbed, reducing diarrhea. Ask your doctor whether you should take it along with an antibiotic; some say yes, others no. A word of caution about drug interactions: Loperamide is an opioid receptor agonist, so you don't want to take an opioid, such as codeine, at the same time because it can intensify the sedative side effects and cause a potentially serious drug interaction. (Don't use it if you have bloody stools or a fever either.) It is safe for kids (see "What Are the Options for Kids?" in this section).

Patients generally take an initial dose of 4 milligrams followed by 2 milligrams every 4 hours with a maximum of 16 milligrams daily. You can take loperamide for about 12 hours after normal stools begin again, but no longer than that; long-term use can alter the functioning of the GI tract. If you have trouble taking pills, liquid loperamide (usually for kids) supplies about 1 milligram of medication for each 7.5 milliliters of the liquid.

WHAT'S WORTHLESS

Antacids. I recommend avoiding calcium supplements, such as calcium carbonate, or antacids (including proton pump inhibitors and H2-blockers) while traveling because they can increase the risk of TD. Stomach acid is a critical immune barrier against GI infections, so you don't want to suppress it. If you take calcium supplements for osteoporosis, specifically calcium carbonate (the biggest-selling calcium supplements for bone loss in the world), then I suggest taking a break while on your trip. Of course, if you get heartburn or indigestion while away, then by all means take a TUMS or other antacid, but try to use it only when absolutely needed.

Lactobacillus acidophilus **probiotic.** This worked as well as or worse than a placebo in a large clinical trial of people who were going to an area with a high rate of TD. (I want to know what they put in the placebo!) *Lactobacillus* combined with other probiotics hasn't been shown to be effective either.

Prebiotics. These basically feed good bacteria in your gut, keeping them strong and healthy to fight the bad bacteria that find their way in, but the research just isn't there against TD.

"Immune-boosting" dietary supplements. Whether it's vitamin C or E or

LOW-RISK FOODS

The following generally don't harbor bacteria that can cause travelers' diarrhea.

- Bottled water with an obvious seal that has not been broken (keep in mind that infections are usually dose related, so rinsing your mouth or toothbrush with tap water is a bit safer compared to drinking the water)

- Bottled carbonated beverages, including soft drinks and beer (Yes! This makes me happy!)

- Foods that have a peel, such as oranges and bananas

- Foods with a low pH (in other words, they're acidic), such as citrus fruit

- Foods that are self-washed and self-prepared (studies show that washing and preparing your own food lowers the risk of TD, probably because you're more aware of what you're putting in your mouth)

- Foods high in natural sugar, such as honey, jam, jellies, or syrup (they act like an antimicrobial agent)

- Dry food, such as bread and rolls without butter or some other type of spread

- Any food or beverage served "steaming hot" (equal to or greater than 59°C or 138°F), such as coffee or tea

another such supplement (take your pick), they're all worthless against TD! There's no evidence they work, and I don't see researchers ever finding this evidence.

WHAT ARE THE OPTIONS FOR KIDS?

TD is more common in kids (probably because their immune systems are still developing), and they're at higher risk for dehydration and more severe illness. Bismuth subsalicylate (Pepto-Bismol) cannot be used because it's aspirin-based and can increase the risk of Reye's syndrome, a potentially deadly problem in kids that has been linked with aspirin use. Some kids older than 2 can use loperamide, but check with your child's doctor about this as well as antibiotics (some are appropriate for kids while others aren't). *L. rhamnosus* GG is an

HIGH-RISK FOODS

The following are at higher risk for containing bacteria that can cause travelers' diarrhea. Eat and drink at your own risk!

- Tap water, including ice cubes (the tap water in hotel filtration systems is often not safe!), in countries with questionable water supplies

- Fresh dairy products (they are unpasteurized)

- Raw fish and meat (even hamburgers not served hot and toppings are a major problem), oysters, and moist foods served at room temperature, including vegetables

- Food and drinks sold from mobile food stands or street vendors (I have to admit that one time when I was in the middle of Malaysia, I was starving and bought some incredible-tasting fruits and meats from some kids. I just said to heck with it and lived to write about it in this book! I live dangerously, folks!)

- Cold sauces and salsas

- Foods that are cooked and then sit at room temperature or that are reheated (Avoid the buffet and you may avoid having your head in the toilet!)

option as well (one capsule a day), but again, talk with your child's doc. Seek medical attention if your child has a persistent high fever, vomiting, dehydration, or bloody diarrhea.

Pregnant women may be at higher risk for TD because they tend to have lower levels of gastric acid and food takes longer to travel through their GI tracts. Loperamide is safe, but bismuth should be avoided; talk to your doctor.

LIFESTYLE CHANGES

Boil it, cook it, peel it, or forget it. Being vigilant about food and drink while traveling probably only prevents 10 to 20 percent of TD cases, but I think it's still worth it. Boiling water is the best way to kill all bugs. Don't get too crazy, though; studies have suggested that people who are completely obsessed with every single thing they eat or drink actually have a higher risk of getting TD (maybe the stress reduces their immune systems). Sorry, all you OCD travelers!

Bring hand sanitizer. Travel with a bottle of ethyl alcohol (62 percent alcohol or higher), and use it to wash your hands before and after every meal when you cannot trust soap and water. When I travel, I also use it to clean suspicious areas, like toilet seats and bike handles.

Bring water purification tablets. You can use potassium iodide, sodium chlorite, or other chlorine water tablets/pellets to treat suspicious water. I prefer potassium because it's faster, but taste and safety (long term) are an issue. My advice: Add some kind of flavored vitamin C, such as Emergen-C or Ester-C, to improve the taste. The safest option is just to opt for bottled water, though.

Rehydrate! If you're unlucky and get TD, be sure to replace the electrolytes and water you're losing through diarrhea and vomiting. Sports drinks, coconut water, and even kids' oral hydration products, such as Pedialyte, contain potassium, sodium, and even chloride and magnesium to get you back to normal again.

Take Pepto daily. Taking two bismuth subsalicylate (Pepto-Bismol) tablets (263 milligrams each) with meals (no more than eight a day)—or drinking 2 ounces of the liquid with meals and once at bedtime—has shown a protection rate against TD of almost 65 percent in preliminary studies. It may be helpful because it coats the GI tract, keeping bugs from taking hold (it also helps reduce bathroom trips once you have TD). The only catch is that in large quantities (more than eight tablets or 10 ounces a day) it can cause a harmless blackening of the stool and tongue, and it could even lead to a mild, temporary case of ringing in the ears.

Trichotillomania

Dr. Moyad Secret This condition is characterized by recurrent hair pulling, leading to hair loss. Mood and anxiety disorders are especially prevalent with this condition, and it can be devastating, resulting in low functioning and self-esteem. Although the title of one of the largest reviews on this subject, published in the *Cochrane Database of Systematic Reviews*, was "Pharmacotherapy for Trichotillomania," a dietary supplement (NAC; see entry below) was one of the top three recommended agents. Once again, this reflects the wide acceptance of dietary supplements throughout medicine.

NAC (N-acetylcysteine). In the *Cochrane Database of Systematic Reviews* analysis (mentioned above), which was done at the University of British Columbia in Canada, researchers found no definitive medication for treatment of trichotillomania, but two pharmaceutical medications (clomipramine, a tricyclic antidepressant, and olanzapine, an antipsychotic) and a dietary supplement (NAC) had the best preliminary evidence for treatment in adults. In addition, a small, high-quality randomized trial from the University of Minnesota Medical School compared 1,200 milligrams of NAC per day for the first 6 weeks and then 2,400 milligrams per day for 6 more weeks to a placebo. Results began to differ by 6 weeks and were statistically and clinically significant, with 56 percent of the NAC takers improved or much improved compared to 16 percent of those on a placebo. NAC is a glutamate modulator, which means it may impact impulsive or compulsive behavior (it's been used for gambling and drug addictions) and the reward centers of the brain. Case studies published recently in adult patients continue to suggest excellent benefits in reducing hair pulling and potentially improving function. A smaller Yale University study with children and adolescents (ages 8 to 17) found no benefit over a placebo with NAC at the highest dose of 2,400 milligrams per day for 12 weeks. In children, behavioral therapy is the preferred method of treatment.

Trigeminal Neuralgia

Dr. Moyad Secret Trigeminal neuralgia is a chronic pain condition named for the trigeminal nerve (the fifth cranial nerve), which is impacted in this disorder. It is more common in people older than 50 and affects women more than men. It may be caused by a blood vessel impinging on the nerve, and the resulting sharp jaw/cheek pain can last from seconds to a few minutes. The pain can be severe; it often leads to depression, anxiety, and stress. Triggers can include chewing, brushing the teeth, touching the face, or even wind or air hitting the face.

How many pain conditions can be improved with topical capsaicin? Many, including some headaches, peripheral neuropathy, osteoarthritis, and post-herpetic neuralgia. Ask your doctor if you can use a low-potency topical capsaicin (0.025 to 0.075 percent) for your pain.

Just FYI: Surgery has worked miracles for some patients with this condition.

Urinary Tract Infection

Dr. Moyad Secret A urinary tract infection (UTI) can occur over and over again, and while antibiotics work well, patients can quickly develop a resistance to them. Many health care professionals have embraced cranberry juice as a remedy to prevent the recurrence of UTIs, but the calories add up fast when you have to take it day after day for months (obesity is a clear risk factor for infections, *especially* UTIs). This is where dietary supplementation makes much more sense (and cents). Supplements have few, if any, calories and offer equal results to cranberry juice, if not better; plus, there's far better compliance (there's a 95 percent chance a patient will stick with supplements versus a less than 50 percent chance she'll continue taking cranberry juice). The key, however, is looking for the right ingredients, so keep reading!

WHAT IS IT?

The urinary tract extends from the kidneys down to the opening of the urethra.

A UTI can occur anywhere in the tract, including the kidneys, ureters (which connect the kidneys to the bladder), bladder, and urethra. A lower UTI occurs in the bladder or urethra (called cystitis), and an upper UTI occurs in the ureters or kidneys, which is known as pyelonephritis.

Approximately 85 to 90 percent of UTIs are caused by gram-negative bacteria, and about 75 to 95 percent of these bacterial infections are caused by *Escherichia coli* (from feces). Nonbacterial UTIs (usually fungal causes) are relatively rare; diabetics and people who use a catheter frequently are at higher risk of these types of infections.

Risk factors for UTIs include being female, sexual activity, certain types of birth control, diabetes, menopause, catheter use, and urinary tract obstruction (such as a stone, enlarged prostate, tumor, or narrowing of the urinary tract). Urinary tract infections are 50 times more common in adult women than in adult men, probably due to the fact that the urethra is much shorter in women, so bacteria have a short trip to reach the bladder. Also, during perimenopause and menopause a reduction in estrogen makes it more difficult for normal, "healthy" bacteria to survive, creating room for infection-causing bugs to get a foothold. Infections in men may be an early indication of a kidney stone or an enlarged prostate.

Some common symptoms of a UTI include:

- Dysuria (pain on passing urine)

- Frequency (having to go often)

- Urgency

- Pressure or pain above the pubic bone in the bladder when not urinating

- Difficulty passing urine

- Cloudy urine

- Fever

- Fatigue

- Hematuria (blood in the urine)

- Pyuria (white blood cells in the urine)

Children may not experience any symptoms, but they'll often exhibit some red flags, such as irritability, poor appetite, fever, diarrhea, and incontinence. If the infection progresses up to the kidney, it can cause nausea, vomiting, fever, and flank pain.

Many women experience recurrent bacterial infections, usually involving the same strain of bacteria that caused the first infection! The bugs survive treatment with antibiotics and lie dormant, just waiting to take advantage when there's an opportunity.

WHAT WORKS

Note: There is no supplement that has been shown to *treat* UTIs, only to *prevent* them from recurring. However, it's possible that using a supplement within the first 24 hours of an infection (along with conventional meds) may be a standard form of treatment in the future. This makes sense from a science standpoint because during the first 24 hours the bacteria are still trying to attach themselves to the lining of the urinary tract and are more vulnerable to "attack."

1. Cranberry (*Vaccinium macrocarpon*) 36 to 72 milligrams of proanthocyanidins a day in divided doses for prevention

Cranberries have been used since the early 1800s for bladder problems. While many people automatically reach for supplements made from these bitter-tasting berries at the first sign of that familiar burning feeling, they work best when taken as a preventive—just like multivitamins—especially for people vulnerable to UTIs. Cranberries are 90 percent water, but they also contain quinic acid, malic acid, citric acid, glucose, and fructose. In medical school, I was taught that quinic acid caused large amounts of hippuric acid to be produced and then excreted in the urine, which had an antibacterial effect, but recent studies have debunked that theory.

So how do they work? Current thinking is that fructose and proanthocyanidins (PACs)—especially type A (versus type B)—block *E. coli* from adhering to the inside of the urinary tract. This is why you want to find a supplement with very high levels of PAC-A. (Some products do list these, but most don't. You can always call or go on the Web to find the information, but I encourage people to start demanding that these companies report it; it's that critical.) Cranberry juice contains 37 percent PACs, on average, but cranberry also comes in syrup, capsules, and tablets. Unfortunately, processing into pills, syrups, or what have you can lower the amount of PACs (more on that later). Lab and clinical studies have found that taking anywhere from 36 to 72 milligrams of PACs daily (divided into two daily doses— morning and evening) reduces the risk of infection. The antiadhesion effects of PACs on bacteria decrease over the course of the day, which is why it's best to take the supplement in both the morning and evening.

The largest independent clinical review of cranberry juice or supplements and UTIs found that, compared to water or no treatment, these products did *not* significantly reduce the occurrence of UTIs in any group, including the following (stick with me here, I'm getting to the good part):

- Symptomatic UTI in general (14 percent reduction)

- Women with recurrent UTIs (26 percent reduction)

- Older people (25 percent reduction)

- Pregnant women (no reduction)

- Children with recurrent UTIs (52 percent reduction)

- Cancer patients (no reduction, but more recent research is showing benefits)

- People with neuropathic bladder or spinal injury (5 percent reduction)

However, the impact of cranberry was not significantly different than antibiotics for women with a history of recurrent UTIs (antibiotics worked slightly better) or in children (cranberry worked as well as antibiotics). In other words, they are a viable option to antibiotics—and without the antibiotic resistance. Here's how the study authors summed up the research: "The large number of dropouts or withdrawals from some of the studies indicates that cranberry products, particularly in juice form, may not be acceptable over long periods of time. Cranberry capsules or tablets may overcome some issues with compliance, but from the current evidence they do not appear to be any more effective than the juice, *although they may be as effective as antibiotics*." Read the last part of that sentence again. Wow! I agree with this finding 100 percent. Besides the taste, cranberry juice is high in sugar and calories. So here is my suggestion for Ocean Spray or another cranberry juice company: Find a way to put 36 to 72 milligrams per day of PACs in a serving of "light" (reduced-calorie) cranberry juice!

The problem with most cranberry supplement studies is that they do not report the amount of PACs in the products tested. So here's what I look for in a cranberry supplement. (I have five rules and a low or competitive price is just a given.)

1. It must have 36 to 72 milligrams of PACs per one or two pills (PAC-A should be as high as possible, too; as PACs increase, so does PAC-A). I look for a pill that contains at least 18 milligrams of PACs or higher, ensuring that two pills will provide 36 milligrams or more. The higher, the better, of course. (Again, you may have to call the company or search online for these numbers.)

2. It should come in enteric-coated capsules, which means the contents get released further down the gastrointestinal tract (past the stomach).

3. It should report the level of the compound oxalate per pill. High quantities of oxalate can increase the risk of kidney stones, especially in people at high risk for them. One of the only clinical studies of cranberry supplements and oxalate found that people who took them had significantly increased levels of oxalate (more than 40 percent higher on average). This is a big deal because as little as a 10 percent increase in urinary oxalate over the upper limit of normal can lead to stones. The average normal intake of oxalate from the diet is about 150 milligrams per day, but some cranberry pills contain more than 350 milligrams. Look for oxalate levels below 100 milligrams.

4. It should contain a little magnesium, potassium, or calcium (10+ milligrams of each) to counter absorption of the oxalates.

5. It should be protected from light and higher temperatures. PACs are light and temperature sensitive, so keep the pills in the refrigerator in a container that's either opaque or dark.

2. *Lactobacillus rhamnosus* GR-1 and *Lactobacillus reuteri* RC-14 probiotics at least one billion CFUs per capsule twice a day

As in the rest of the body, the urinary tract is loaded with good bacteria that keep the bad bacteria under control. Lactobacillus probiotics can produce hydrogen peroxide, which prevents other bacterial invaders from hanging around. If good bacteria are low or absent, *E. coli* has an easier time thriving. Lactobacillus vaginal suppositories for the prevention of UTIs have mixed research, as do the capsules. A large clinical trial published in the *Archives of Internal Medicine* (now called *JAMA Internal Medicine*) compared *Lactobacillus rhamnosus* GR-1 and *L. reuteri* RC-14 twice a day (at least 10^9 colony-forming units, or CFUs, per capsule) against a common antibiotic (TMP-SMX) in 252 postmenopausal women at high-risk for recurrent UTIs. The probiotics did not beat the antibiotic, but after a year almost 100 percent of the women who took antibiotics had developed resistance to the antibiotic, compared to *no resistance* with the probiotic. Regardless, this probiotic combination is now commercially available (look for Fem-Dophilus), so it's definitely worth a try for preventing UTIs.

3. D-mannose 2,000 milligrams a day in divided doses

D-mannose is a simple sugar that has some preliminary clinical research regarding UTIs. It appears to work by blocking the attachment of *E. coli* to the urinary tract. A large clinical trial with 2,000 milligrams of D-mannose (dissolved in 6 to 7 ounces of water) showed significant reductions in recurrent UTIs over 6 months, which was similar to antibiotics.

HONORABLE MENTION

Vitamin C may acidify the urine, making it less hospitable to certain bacteria. Now, it hasn't been able to do this consistently in studies, but is it so crazy to believe that a vitamin that can reduce the duration of the common cold in some folks might be able to promote an immune response that could deter or block a UTI? Regardless, it's inexpensive and safe in pregnancy so it's worth a try (200 to 500 milligrams per day; higher dosages can increase your risk of kidney stones). By the way, did you know that cranberries contain a large concentration of vitamin C, along with many other nutrients? One serving contains 100 to 150 percent of the Recommended Dietary Allowance. Coincidence?

WHAT'S WORTHLESS

Uva ursi. This shrub (also known as bearberry) is native to the more mountain-ous areas of North America, and the herbal supplement has been touted for UTI prevention and treatment in so many alternative medicine books that I have lost count. This is not based on evidence, though, and in my experience, it's minimally effective. Also, the leaves of the plant contain an ingredient known as arbutoside, which the gut turns into glucose and hydroquinone (long-term exposure to hydroquinone may be carcinogenic).

Avoid uva ursi if you're pregnant, breastfeeding, or have kidney problems or stomach issues. I have had so many people call me up complaining that a certain supplement they bought at a local health food store gave them stomach pain. I always ask, "Is there uva ursi in it?" And the answer has always been "yes."

Juniper. The leaves of this tree contain antimicrobial terpenoids, compounds that could be used against a UTI, but it's never really been tested for this in a good clinical trial. In very large doses ("large" has never been defined), it could be harmful to the kidneys.

Berberine. Laboratory studies have suggested that this compound—which is found naturally in a variety of plants, including goldenseal and goldthread—might prevent *E. coli* from adhering to the bladder wall. However, good research on this is lacking.

L-methionine. This amino acid can make the urine more acidic, which might reduce the risk of UTIs. The average dosage used in a few small clinical studies is 500 milligrams three times a day maximum. The catch is that L-methionine can increase the amount of a compound in the body known as homocysteine, which in the long term could be unhealthy and damage the kidneys.

WHAT ARE THE OPTIONS FOR KIDS?

In one study of kids with recurrent UTIs, those who drank 2 milliliters of cranberry juice per kilogram of body weight daily (with 37 percent PAC) had reduced risk of UTIs. That is the good news. The bad news is that 30 percent of the kids dropped out of the study because they couldn't tolerate the juice. Talk with your child's doctor about the possibility of using supplements at lower dosages.

LIFESTYLE CHANGES

Heart healthy = urinary tract healthy. This shouldn't be surprising anymore.

Eating a heart-healthy diet delivers nutrients—such as calcium, magnesium, and potassium—that may reduce the risk of kidney stones and UTIs. However, one of the smartest things you can do is maintain a healthy weight because extra pounds could increase blood sugar levels and the risk of developing insulin resistance, which creates a more favorable environment for a UTI. Recent research shows that lowering cholesterol levels may also protect the urinary tract and reduce

the risk of a UTI because the concentration of other compounds that bacteria have been known to utilize when they invade or adhere to the bladder is reduced as well.

Don't OD on juices. Fruit juices in general have too many calories, which can increase weight, blood sugar, and the long-term risk of a UTI. However, if you are convinced they work for UTIs and want to sip a few ounces a day for prevention, that's okay. Drinking just 1.5 to 2 ounces of lingonberry (*Vaccinium vitis-idaea*) concentrate with cranberry concentrate per day over 6 months showed some benefit in preventing UTIs.

Get moving. Exercise makes you thirsty, and the more you drink, the more you pee. Urination is a wonderful protective mechanism against bacterial infections because it constantly flushes out little bugs. Exercise also reduces your risk of diabetes and weight gain.

Get your five servings—and more. Eating fresh fruit can lower your risk of UTIs, and so can noshing on fermented dairy products (such as yogurt and kefir), probably because they contain probiotics. However, coffee, tea, nonfermented milk products, and soft drinks do not affect risk.

Switch birth control methods. Spermicide use (including using condoms that contain spermicide) is a very strong risk factor for UTIs, especially when used with a diaphragm. Spermicides alter the natural bacteria balance in the vagina and increase the chance that other more hostile bacteria can settle in. Just an FYI: Sexual intercourse is one of the strongest risk factors for UTIs. Reducing the frequency of intercourse or intermittent abstinence may be beneficial for some people, but that's for you to decide!

Follow good hygiene. Urinating shortly after intercourse, not delaying urination, wiping front to back with toilet paper, and avoiding douching and wearing tight underwear have not been studied against UTIs, but they just make good sense.

Topical (not oral) estrogen prevention. Postmenopausal women with a history of symptomatic UTIs should ask their doctor about topical (oral has not been effective from four studies) vaginal estrogen cream therapy. It has excellent prelim-

inary evidence from two studies that it is significantly reduces risk in those with recurrent UTIs.

WHAT ELSE DO I NEED TO KNOW

Officially this might not be a dietary supplement, but Phenazopyridine hydrochloride has a specific analgesic effect on the urinary tract. It's a dye (an "azo" dye) that coats the lining of the urinary tract and acts like an anesthetic (kind of like a toothache numbing agent for the urinary tract) to reduce UTI pain and perhaps even the burning and urgency. Some examples of products that contain this compound are AZO and URISTAT.

Varicose Veins and Chronic Venous Insufficiency

Dr. Moyad Secret Dietary supplements are now part of the standard medical treatment for varicose veins and chronic venous insufficiency (CVI). Many of them are considered prescription drugs in other areas of the world (such as Europe), which shows, once again, that the line between an effective dietary supplement and a drug is often just perception. In other words, many powerful supplements should be thought of no differently than conventional drugs (around one-third of which come from natural sources).

Research has shown that some dietary supplements can reduce leg swelling and the appearance of varicose veins and minimize the risk of getting more of them. They won't eliminate varicosities—only a qualified doctor can make that happen—so never believe a dietary supplement company that's trying to convince you otherwise.

By the way, some supplements that can reduce the impact of CVI and varicose veins can also help in the treatment of hemorrhoids (see Hemorrhoids section, page 226), and they may even be beneficial in treating conditions like lymphedema (swelling in the arms or legs as a result of fluid buildup), which is a side effect of some cancer treatments. More research is needed!

WHAT IS IT?

Veins carry deoxygenated blood to the heart, which sends it immediately back out to the lungs to get reoxygenated. In chronic venous insufficiency, the venous walls or the valves inside the veins malfunction, causing blood to stay in the veins. The leg vessels are especially vulnerable because they have to work hard against gravity to send blood up to the heart; they rely on muscles in the legs to contract and keep pushing blood upward. And with age and long periods of time spent sitting or standing or being inactive, the veins and valves get weak. High blood pressure in the veins (called venous hypertension) can damage them as well.

Symptoms of CVI include swelling in the lower legs and ankles; aching, tired, and heavy legs; dry, itchy skin; leathery-looking skin or a change in skin color; skin ulcers; and varicose veins (bulging, twisted, and swollen veins that are visible just below the surface of the skin and can cause leg pain and swelling). Think of varicose veins as a milder form of CVI. They're more likely to occur in people with a family history or who have had multiple pregnancies. Being tall or overweight can increase your risk as well. As with CVI, sitting or standing for long periods of time increases the risk of varicose veins. By the way, spider veins are simply smaller varicose veins (they're actually capillaries), so the same prevention tips and treatments apply.

WHAT WORKS

1. (tie) Horse chestnut seed extract (*Aesculus hippocastanum*) 50 to 75 milligrams of escin once or twice a day for 12 weeks

Horse chestnut seed extract has been shown to reduce leg pain and itching and ankle and calf swelling as well as compression stockings do. The active compound in horse chestnut is escin (also called complex active triterpenoid saponins or just aescin), which has been shown to block the destruction of structural components in the walls of veins.

In studies, the dosage has generally been in the range of one capsule once or twice a day, with each capsule standardized to contain 50 to 75 milligrams of escin. Again, this supplement can strengthen the veins and reduce swelling and other issues in the short term. Long-term studies (more than 12 weeks) have not been done. Still, with more than seven placebo-controlled trials, this is one of the best dietary supplements for mild to moderate CVI, and it can be used with conventional treatment options in many situations (as always, talk to a trusted doctor about this). Gastrointestinal upset and dizziness were reported in up to one-third of test subjects in about half of the studies conducted; the rest of the trials reported mild to minimal side effects. Horse chestnut has not received adequate research in the area of potential drug interactions. Regardless, do not use it if you're pregnant, breastfeeding, or taking a blood-thinning medication.

1. (tie) Diosmin 500 milligrams a day in divided doses

Diosmin is a flavonoid (a compound that may have health-protective benefits). And Daflon is the best-known product containing diosmin. In fact, it's a semisynthetic prescription drug in Europe. It's considered a micronized purified flavonoid fraction, or MPFF, because it contains a 90:10 ratio of flavonoids: 450 milligrams of diosmin (a compound found in citrus fruits) and 50 milligrams of other flavonoids, which are found in plants. *Micronized* means that the particles were reduced in size to less than 2 micrometers (that's really tiny) to improve its solubility and absorption. Although it's a drug in other countries, in the United States diosmin is a regular dietary supplement. The standard dosage is 500 milligrams a day divided into two or three doses taken every 8 hours.

Most of the studies on Daflon have lasted between 2 to 6 months, and they've shown that it can decrease inflammation in veins, help prevent damage to the lining inside veins, improve venous tone and lymph drainage, and reduce calf and ankle swelling and other symptoms of CVI. Researchers believe it can also help keep

443

more varicosities from forming. I recommend you take it for at least 12 weeks.

There is also some preliminary evidence to suggest Daflon can be used with conventional treatments for CVI, which generally involve vein removal or shrinkage procedures. Do not use it if you're pregnant or breastfeeding. There hasn't been any good research in the area of drug interactions, so ask your doctor about it. However, I would be careful about combining diosmin with aspirin or other anticoagulants because it may increase blood thinning.

2. Rutosides (O-beta-hydroxyethyl-rutosides, a.k.a. rutin or oxerutin)
1,000 to 2,000 milligrams a day

Rutosides appear to protect blood vessel walls from damage and discourage other cells from adhering to the vessel walls so they can continue to function normally. Tests with products containing rutosides have shown a reduction in some CVI symptoms, including cramping, pain, feelings of heaviness in the legs, and swelling. One of the most commonly tested rutoside products has been Venoruton (from Novartis), a prescription drug in Europe. There's also a gel or cream form that can be used topically in addition to taking the supplement.

It's hard to find a product with the same exact ingredients that were tested in the trial mentioned earlier outside of Europe, but you can look for rutin at your local health food store. It's close in molecular structure to the rutosides that have been used in studies, and I believe it works about as well as they do, plus it's cheaper! (Rutin is also found in asparagus and buckwheat and in the rinds of limes, lemons, grapefruits, oranges, and apples, for example.)

The side effects of rutosides or rutin are rare and include gastrointestinal upset (nausea, heartburn, and diarrhea), rash, itching, headache, and hot flashes. You can purchase gel and pill forms online, such as on Amazon. There are also some rutinlike copycats out there, such as red vine leaf (*Folia vitis viniferae*) extract. It shares similar properties with rutosides and rutins, and when it was tested at 360 and 720 milligrams once daily for 12 weeks in people with stage I and II CVI, both dosages reduced lower leg swelling and size to a similar degree as compression stockings. I recommend taking it for 8 weeks.

3. Pycnogenol 150 to 360 milligrams a day

A standardized extract from the bark of the French maritime pine, Pycnogenol contains polyphenols, especially proanthocyanidins (PCOs), which appear to be the active ingredient with protective properties. You can now find Pycnogenol supplements that contain 95 percent proanthocyanidins. Studies with Pycnogenol have found it reduced leg cramps, pain, heavy feelings, and swelling. In one 8-week trial, Pycnogenol (150 to 300 milligrams daily) improved CVI symptoms faster and better than Daflon (at 1,000 milligrams daily). (This was a small study with some bias, but it's interesting nonetheless.) A 4-week study with 360 milligrams of Pycnogenol compared to 600 milligrams of horse chestnut seed extract found that Pycnogenol reduced lower leg swelling better. Now, the active ingredient in Pycnogenol—PCOs—is not cheap, but you can find it in peanuts and grape seed extract, which are less expensive. Grape seed extract is a fairly well-known supplement, but there's no adequate research with varicose veins.

WHAT'S WORTHLESS

Buckwheat or buckwheat herbal tea. This common plant (which is not a true wheat product) is supposedly high in rutin, but due to poor quality control, you just don't know if you're actually getting any rutin in the product. Regardless, clinical trials are lacking for this herb. Buckwheat itself is a common food allergen, though, so beware. I currently only recommend buckwheat for coughs: In a head-to-head study, buckwheat honey reduced coughing as well as the best-selling over-the-counter cough suppressant, dextromethorphan (see the Common Cold and Flu section, page 141).

Gotu kola. This well-known tropical medicinal plant contains a variety of extracts that researchers were excited about when I was a kid, but nothing ever came of it. Very little CVI-related research

has been done recently with this herb, while the others that I've discussed in "What Works" continue to garner good research.

Butcher's broom. This one is sure to upset some experts. This herb has anti-inflammatory properties and the *potential* to be useful for CVI problems because it has an active ingredient—called ruscogenin—that may block the enzyme elastase, which contributes to the breakdown of blood vessels. Here is the problem, though: Due to poorly designed studies, an effective dosage is unknown, and studies with products that contain butcher's broom as one of several ingredients haven't performed better than a placebo. Also, it can cause contact dermatitis or allergic reaction in rare cases, as well as swelling, nausea, and other gastrointestinal side effects. And tyramine, another compound in butcher's broom, can negatively interact with prescription medicines, such as MAO (monoamine oxidase) inhibitors (a type of antidepressant).

I'm not saying it's worthless; I just don't think it's worth it. (I love the name butcher's broom, though; it sounds scary and hygienic at the same time. Apparently, it arose from the fact that the herb has stiff twigs that butchers used to bind together and use to clean their cutting boards.) If studies can prove it's safe and pinpoint how much is effective, then I'll be swept off my feet (get it) and endorse it. Until then, this is one broom that you should take out of the closet and put in the trash.

LIFESTYLE CHANGES

Heart healthy = vein healthy. Can you believe that some experts don't think we know whether diet affects CVI and varicose veins? Granted, there's little to no research proving this, but come on! It is already known that heart-healthy diets reduce the risk of damage to blood vessels and that weight gain puts unnecessary pressure on blood vessels, so it's really a no-brainer.

Exercise regularly. Working out (even walking the dog) makes leg muscles contract, which improves circulation and sends stagnant blood up to the heart and lungs.

Quit smoking. Tobacco thickens the blood, reduces circulation, increases blood pressure, and creates inflammation and damage throughout the circulatory system, all of which set the stage for CVI.

Try vibrating. Many patients claim standing on a vibration platform, such as the Power Plate, can help reduce leg swelling. The rapid, tiny vibrations force the lower leg muscles to contract (while shaking you like a martini). While I don't buy into using them for general muscle or bone strengthening, it makes sense for CVI and is certainly worth a try.

Avoid long periods of sitting or standing. If you have a desk job, get up and walk around for a few minutes every hour. If you have to be on your feet, then sit down every few hours. (People who sit most of the day have a greater chance of gaining weight and having poor circulation, though.) When you're sitting, avoid crossing your legs because it puts pressure on veins.

Loosen up your wardrobe. Constrictive clothing, like a tight belt or girdle, can restrict bloodflow in both directions. That said, compression stockings, which are worn on the lower legs, can be beneficial for CVI. They come in different compressions (8 to 10 mm Hg up to 40 to 50 mm Hg) based on the severity of the condition, but a prescription is generally needed for stockings with more than 20 mm Hg compression. Check with your doctor.

Kick up your heels. Elevating your legs for at least 30 minutes a day can help reduce any ankle or foot swelling by making it easier for blood and lymph to circulate back to the upper body. While you're seated, point and flex your feet 10 to 15 times. This employs the muscles around the lower legs, which helps squeeze blood back up through the veins, preventing pooling and excessive pressure on the lower legs and feet.

Vertigo

Dr. Moyad Secret Vertigo is a common condition similar to seasickness without the sea; people feel like the world is spinning around them, and it can lead to nausea, vomiting, headaches, and other problems. One of the most common types of vertigo is benign paroxysmal positional vertigo (BPPV), which occurs increasingly with age. BPPV can usually be treated with simple head movements performed in a doctor's office or at home. (The Epley Maneuver involves moving your head through a series of positions to move calcium deposits in the inner ear, which are the root of the problem.) This is far better than any supplement and will save you a fortune! Another common vertigo cause is vestibular neuritis, an infection of the inner ear probably caused by a cold virus.

Ménière's disease is when the inner ear swells up intermittently, and these attacks can cause terrible vertigo along with many other symptoms. The initial treatment is a low-sodium diet and a diuretic blood pressure pill (see the Tinnitus section, page 422). Sudden vertigo along with speech, vision, and balance problems can be a sign of something else, like a stroke.

Weight Loss

Dr. Moyad Secret The major problem with weight loss supplements and prescription medications (and the reason most of them have been yanked from store shelves—think fen-phen, sibutramine, and ephedra) is heart-related side effects. They can increase heart rate, blood pressure, cholesterol, and blood sugars, and they can even increase feelings of stress and depression. And since cardiovascular disease (CVD) is the number one killer of men and women, any pill that helps with weight loss but *increases* the risk of CVD is just not worth it! So is it possible to find a supplement that controls appetite, ramps up metabolism, or potentially reduces the risk of certain diseases *while* helping you lose weight? Yes! (Along with diet and exercise, of course.)

WHAT IS IT?

Obesity has just overtaken smoking as the top preventable cause of illness and premature death in the United States. Approximately 70 percent of the population is now overweight or obese, and obesity in children has tripled over the past 30 years—it's what I call a super epidemic. Just as smoking increases the risk for a variety of diseases, the health impact of obesity is staggering. Here is just a partial list of conditions that obesity can lead to or worsen.

- Acid reflux
- Atrial fibrillation
- Blood clots
- Breathlessness
- Cancer (including breast, colon, endometrial, esophageal, kidney, liver, ovarian, and prostate; and it may increase the risk of getting a more aggressive form of the cancer, as well)
- Complications from surgical procedures
- Diabetes
- Eye diseases
- Fetal defects (from maternal obesity)
- Gallbladder disease
- Gout (high uric acid levels)
- Heart disease
- Heart failure
- Hiatal hernia
- High blood pressure
- High cholesterol
- Hot flashes

- Immobility

- Incontinence

- Infertility (men and women)

- Low back pain

- Low testosterone

- NAFLD/NASH (a.k.a. fatty liver disease)

- Osteoarthritis

- Pregnancy complications (such as preeclampsia)

- Sexual dysfunction

- Sleep apnea

- Stroke

There are several different measures—besides the number on the scale—that can help gauge weight loss progress. My favorite is waist size; extra inches around the midsection are a good indication of excess fat in the abdomen, surrounding the organs, and this visceral fat is really bad for you. It increases the risk of both CVD and diabetes. I also like to use cholesterol, blood sugar, blood pressure, and heart rate to evaluate progress. Body mass index (BMI) is another popular measurement, but it has some drawbacks. It uses height and weight to calculate overweight and obesity, but it doesn't account for muscle mass, so if you lose 10 pounds of fat and gain 10 pounds of muscle, your BMI won't change although your health status (and heart health) will! Many professional athletes have very little body fat but still appear to be overweight on a BMI chart because of muscle mass. You can get body fat measured by a doctor or by a trainer at just about any gym. However, DEXA (dual-energy x-ray absorptiometry) is the gold standard for measuring body fat. It's actually used for osteoporosis screening, so the next time you go in for one of these, ask for your body fat percentage, too, if you're concerned about your weight.

The good news is that losing just 5 to 10 percent of your weight or several inches off your waist can lower the risk of heart problems by impacting the following:

- Reducing blood pressure by 10 points in those with hypertension

- Reducing blood sugar by 50 percent in people newly diagnosed with diabetes

- Reducing the chances of getting diabetes by 50 percent in those at risk for the disease

- Reducing total cholesterol by 10 percent, LDL (bad) cholesterol by 15 percent, and triglycerides by 30 percent and increasing HDL (good) cholesterol by 5 to 10 percent

- Reducing all-cause mortality by 20 percent, death from diabetes by 30 percent, and death from obesity by 40 percent

But here comes the bad news: Only one out of six people (17 percent) is able to lose 10 percent of their body weight and keep it off for a year. Dieting is tough. It's like playing the slots in Vegas; you only hear about the winners, not the millions of

METABOLISM BY THE NUMBERS

Your metabolism is basically an internal furnace; it's the energy your body expends doing everything you need and want it to, from sleeping to digesting to exercising. It's how you burn calories, and there are three primary aspects to it.

1. **Resting metabolism.** Your body devotes 60 to 75 percent of daily calorie output to just keeping your body functioning. It takes energy to filter urine, pump blood, and even think! Here's a sneaky way to increase your resting metabolism: Build muscle. It takes more energy to maintain a pound of muscle than it does to maintain a pound of fat. If you can preserve that muscle while you drop fat, you can avoid the decrease in metabolism that frequently occurs during weight loss.

2. **Digestion (a.k.a. the thermic effect of food).** About 10 percent of daily calorie output goes toward digesting the food you eat. Fun fact: It takes more energy to digest protein (versus carbs or fat), which gives credence to the theory that thinner people may not only move more but eat more protein.

3. **Physical activity.** Most people expend 15 to 30 percent of their daily calories on exercise. The more you work out (within reason), the more calories you burn. This is the aspect of metabolism that you have the most control over. That's why another goal of this section, beyond supplementation, is to get you to increase your overall metabolism through aerobic and resistance exercise as well as by increasing your protein intake.

losers (or "nonlosers," in the case of weight). We have all sorts of high-calorie foods and drinks at our disposal, and typical modern life is fairly sedentary, what with desk jobs, YouTube, and suburban sprawl, which makes it so you have to drive to get anywhere. Plus, your body doesn't like to lose weight. Once you finally wrestle the scale into submission, your metabolism slows down, which makes it easier to put pounds back on even when you don't increase the amount of food you're eating

(see "Metabolism by the Numbers" [above] for a way to avoid this conundrum). This is why it's so important to pay attention to the type of food you're eating and how you're exercising.

WHAT WORKS

1. (tie) Whey protein powder 50 to 60 grams a day in divided doses between meals, ideally in isolate form

Why protein powder? It's an easy way to increase protein intake; it helps suppress appetite while building and preserving muscle mass; it takes more energy to digest than carbs and fat; and it may lower blood pressure and improve cholesterol and blood sugar levels. Hundreds of human studies show it can do all of these things, and it's safe for most people in moderation. There is no other dietary supplement in the world that can come close to making all of these claims—except fiber, of course.

The Recommended Dietary Allowance for protein is 0.8 grams per kilogram of body weight (there are 2.2 pounds per kilogram), but I think this is too low, especially if you need to lose weight and increase muscle. I believe that for every 2 pounds you weigh, you should get 1 gram of protein daily. The average woman weighs 154 pounds, so that's 77 grams of protein a day. If you look at daily intakes based on this recommendation, most people have a deficiency of it. Multiple studies, including a recent USDA clinical trial, have found that 50 to 60 grams of whey protein daily (in addition to what is obtained through diet) has been associated with more significant weight loss compared to other protein powders, such as soy. In my opinion, when you're getting this much protein over a long period of time, you'll do well with any type of concentrated protein source (powders).

Protein powders can be either animal- (whey, casein, or egg whites) or plant-based (soy, brown rice, hemp, or pea).

Always look for products that are in isolate form, which usually contain no more than 100 to 125 calories per 20 to 25 grams of protein, no sugar and less than 5 grams of other carbs, no fat or cholesterol, very little sodium, and almost no lactose. There's simply no better way to pack so much protein into so little space than with a powder (no protein bar is able to do this).

Research has shown better weight loss and muscle building with animal-based protein powders versus plant protein sources, probably because the animal powders have higher amounts of the branched-chain amino acids (BCAAs), such as leucine. These BCAAs have the ability to stimulate muscle protein synthesis to a greater degree than other amino acids. And more muscle mass equals a higher metabolism. Or it could just be that plant proteins need more studies in larger amounts than were tested. Bottom line: Use a protein powder that you'll actually take on a daily basis (using a blend of powders or rotating them improves compliance for some dieters).

1. (tie) Soluble and insoluble fiber powder 10 to 15 grams of each a day

Fiber can help with appetite suppression, weight loss, blood sugar control, and cholesterol reduction. It also appears to temporarily increase metabolic signals in the

---

MOYAD TIP: Chase your protein drink with a glass of water. Protein is dehydrating and can increase the risk of constipation.

THE 411 ON PROTEIN POWDERS

When you go to the protein powder aisle at the store, you're usually confronted by a variety of different products with all sorts of odd words on them, like hydrolysate and micronized. Here, how to make sense of what you're seeing.

- Whey protein, which comes from milk, is digested and absorbed in less than an hour. It comes in three basic forms: concentrate (cheapest), isolate, and hydrolysate/micronized (most expensive). They are similar in many wheys (sorry, I couldn't resist), except the concentrate form has a greater chance of causing an allergy in people who are allergic or sensitive to dairy products. It's also only about 80 percent protein because it contains fat and carbs. My favorite is the isolate form—meaning it's all protein, no sugar (or other carbs), fat, cholesterol, or multivitamins. As a result, it's low in calories. It's also good for people with lactose intolerance. Hydrolysate/micronized powders contain amino acids that are already partially broken down, which theoretically makes them easier to absorb.

- Casein is another milk protein powder, but it takes longer (5 to 10 hours) to digest and absorb than whey does and it contains almost no lactose (0.1 percent or less). Since it takes longer to be absorbed, casein may help you feel

body so that metabolism increases for several hours. There have been at least 14 human studies done with a type of soluble fiber called glucomannan, which expands in the stomach, keeping you full. Subjects taking between 3,000 to 4,000 milligrams a day (in capsules) for 4 to 16 weeks lost up to 10 pounds or more. Still, it's expensive and we need more objective research.

Psyllium, another soluble fiber, has shown similar results in terms of heart health (not weight loss) at 10 to 15 grams per day. Psyllium and glucomannan (both are available in powder form), when combined with bran or other insoluble fiber products, such as bars or cereals, can also help you achieve that daily goal of 20 to 30 grams of fiber. (While soluble fiber comes in powder form, you'll usually find insoluble fiber in foods and bars, not supplements.) Its heart-healthy benefits and potential to aid weight loss combined with its flexibility (powders, bars, etc.) make fiber a must-do for anyone fuller longer. But it's not as tasty as whey protein, so some people have a hard time taking it daily. (Some prefer milk protein isolate products, which contain both whey and casein.)

- Egg white protein is a "medium absorbing" powder; it takes a few hours to be digested and is also lactose free.

- Vegetarian protein powders are lacking on the taste front. Soy protein powder isolate (again, look for the highest quantity of protein with the lowest calories) absorbs quickly like whey and has the highest quality and quantity of amino acids compared to any other plant protein. Soy protein is also allowed to advertise that it might lower cholesterol (at 25 grams per day). It's getting the most positive research I've seen in my lifetime in terms of heart disease and possibly cancer prevention, yet it has a bad rap because "experts" keep claiming it increases estrogen levels in men and women and ups the risk of thyroid and other diseases. But these claims are not founded on realistic research.

If you have any kidney disease or abnormal kidney function, you need to determine a safe protein intake with your doctor because, depending on your situation, it could be harmful.

who's trying to drop pounds. It also helps counteract the constipation that a high-protein diet can cause.

2. Alpha-lipoic acid (ALA) 800 to 1,800 milligrams a day in divided doses, ideally 30 minutes before each major meal

This compound may activate a metabolic master on-off switch—known as 5'-AMP-activated protein kinase, or AMPK—according to research, which means it may speed up metabolism. (The diabetes drug metformin, which can also cause weight loss, may do this as well.) In some small trials, it helped patients taking prescription medications that cause weight gain (such as antipsychotic drugs) lose weight; a study of more than 1,100 people taking 800 milligrams of an ALA supplement called Liponax daily for 4 months resulted in appetite suppression, weight loss (8 to 9 percent), and waist reduction (6 to 11 centimeters). It also led to blood pressure reductions of up to eight points systolic and six points diastolic.

One large clinical trial of ALA (the most impressive supplement weight loss study I have ever seen designed and published) included people with diabetes and without who were overweight or obese. The 360 subjects took either a placebo, 1,200 milligrams of ALA, or 1,800 milligrams of ALA (in three divided daily doses) for 5 months. After 20 weeks there was a 2 to 3 percent change in body weight on average in the high-dose ALA group and a 2- to 3-centimeter reduction in waist circumference. People taking the 1,200-milligram dose saw greater weight loss than a placebo, but there wasn't a statistical difference. More than 20 percent of the individuals in the 1,800-milligram group lost 5 percent or more of their weight compared to 10 percent of the people taking the placebo (which shows you how strong the placebo effect is in a good clinical trial). So, the impact of ALA on weight was excellent for a dietary supplement. It was equally impressive that approximately one-third of the participants had diabetes, another third had high cholesterol, and another third had hypertension. In other words, this trial included men and women who were having a tough time losing weight and needed to make it a priority. Studies like this one are never seen in the supplement world, only the drug world. Of the thousands of weight loss supplements out there, there has never been a study done this well—or with results that were better than the placebo—

with so many diverse individuals, which is why it was accepted into a major medical journal (the *American Journal of Medicine*).

Participants were also given 4 weeks prior to the start of the trial (this is called a run-in phase and is a critical part of any good study) to reduce total caloric intake by 600 calories per day (they ate a minimum of 1,200 calories daily so they couldn't cheat and lose weight by severely restricting calories). This close monitoring of dietary changes throughout a study needs to be seen more often in weight loss research, especially considering that after a month or two, people usually start cheating. Keeping close track of the dietary changes helps keep the study groups equal so the true effects of the supplement can be seen.

Overall, side effects were similar to a placebo except that more individuals in the ALA groups complained of an itching sensation (13 cases compared to three in the placebo group). The itching did not lead to dropouts and was not predictive of who would lose weight. ALA can also cause a harmless urine smell similar to what many people experience after eating asparagus, and it can lower blood sugar too much in very rare circumstances.

ALA is one of the most exciting supplements for weight loss because it is heart healthy, has a long track record of safety in other areas of medicine, and appears to help men and women get their metabolisms going, along with diet and exercise. In fact, this is arguably the only supplement I have ever endorsed for weight loss apart from fiber and protein. Companies usually avoid recruiting subjects for studies who have diabetes or who are taking medications that promote weight gain because it's very difficult to get good results!

HONORABLE MENTIONS

5-HTP is an intermediate metabolite in the conversion of L-tryptophan to serotonin, which basically means taking it leads to more serotonin production. Increasing serotonin levels may result in fewer cravings, especially for sugar. Drugs that increase serotonin or impact its receptors are well known to cause appetite suppression, as exemplified by the drug lorcaserin, which is FDA approved for weight loss.

There were three interesting studies of weight loss with 5-HTP. In one clinical trial, obese individuals who took 300 milligrams three times daily for 12 weeks saw significantly reduced calorie intake (more than with a placebo) and a 50 percent reduction in carbohydrate intake. I would take it with meals, but more is not better. Start low and don't exceed the dosage recommended above because too much can cause nightmares or vivid dreams, drowsiness, dizziness, nausea, and diarrhea (serotonin impacts the intestines and brain). Most important, 5-HTP should not be combined with any other medications that also impact serotonin levels, such as antidepressants, without talking with your doctor. Because it's a precursor to serotonin, I believe it can increase the risk of serotonin syndrome (a serious side

effect of excessive serotonin production that can lead to hospitalization) and can possibly deplete other neurotransmitters.

Kidney bean extract is touted as a carbohydrate blocker because it deactivates an enzyme in the gut (amylase) that digests carbohydrates, preventing their absorption, if you take it before starchy meals (bread, pasta, pizza). Studies have shown 5 to 10 pounds of weight loss with doses of 455 to 3,000 milligrams daily. The supplement forces people to be more aware of carb intake, but it can backfire by providing a false sense of security; some people who take it eat *more* carbs and gain weight (I've seen it happen, folks). I'm not aware of any safety issues, so give it a try for 3 months.

MCT oil (a mix of coconut and palm kernel oils, which are medium-chain triglycerides), in combination with a ketogenic (70 to 90 percent fat) diet, can cause significant weight loss in overweight and obese kids and adults. I'm a big fan of it, but compliance is a huge problem. (See the Epilepsy section, page 185.)

WHAT'S WORTHLESS

Note: Buckle up, folks! I'm about to take you on a very long and ugly ride past all the weight loss supplement roadkill—those products that just don't work. And remember: Any supplement that helps you lose weight by significantly increasing your heart rate or blood pressure is never worth the risk, even if losing weight helps you lower your cardiovascular disease risk in the long term.

Apple cider vinegar. Taking several teaspoons of this in a glass or two of water suppresses your appetite by upsetting your stomach (you just don't feel like eating afterward). But studies have shown little to no weight loss.

Bitter orange. You can find this in many ephedra-free weight loss supplements. Derived from the unripe dried fruit and fruit peel of *Citrus aurantium,* it usually contains a small percentage (1 to 6 percent) of the compound synephrine, which may increase heart rate and blood pressure, especially when taken with other stimulants. In other words, it's not worth the risk!

Caffeine pills. Caffeine boosts blood levels of epinephrine, a hormone that increases metabolic rate and helps burn fat. However, in clinical studies, caffeine pills have not worked better than a placebo, and they often increase heart rate and blood pressure. Other herbs with caffeine in them include coffee bean extract, kola nut, yerba mate, and guarana, and these aren't helpful for weight loss either.

Capsaicin. The active ingredient in chile peppers, capsaicin may slightly increase metabolism, but results with this supplement have translated to minimal or no weight loss. Eating real chile peppers makes more sense because it forces you to drink more water, which has the ability to make you feel slightly more full.

Chromium. This mineral can poten-tially help regulate insulin or increase insulin sensitivity, especially in people with diabetes. Studies have also looked at chromium's ability to increase metabolism, but so far they have shown only a minor benefit or none at all. I'm more excited about combining this supplement with other compounds, such as biotin, to improve the overall health of diabetics (see the Diabetes and Prediabetes section, page 173).

Conjugated linoleic acid. This is a big seller, but there has always been the question of whether this product raises cholesterol (it is partially a trans fat) or C-reactive protein (an inflammatory marker) or other markers of heart disease, which is not a good thing. It's naturally found in meat and milk (from cows, goats, and sheep) and may prevent fat formation. One yearlong study found an average weight loss of 4 pounds with 3 grams of conjugated linoleic acid (CLA) daily, but there have been just as many studies showing that CLA does not work any better than a placebo.

Exotic fruit–based products (acai, African mango, lychee). Some people think that exotic fruits work as weight loss aids because they're found in areas that have a low obesity rate. But, no surprise here, neither acai nor lychee has any credible studies. African mango contains high amounts of soluble fiber, and in one impressive study there was significant weight and waist loss with it, but the problem is that until another study can repeat these results (and without funding by investors in the product), I remain skeptical.

"Fat" appetite suppressant shots. The thinking here is that taking a small dose of fat (monounsaturated, polyunsaturated, or saturated) sends a signal to the brain that helps control appetite. These shots (like the kind you order in a bar), which are often a combination of oat and palm oil, may have some small benefit and most likely work in a somewhat similar way to fish oil or plant oil pills. But couldn't you just take a teaspoon or two of canola, olive, coconut, or safflower oil? Or how about peanut butter? Sorry to burst any bubbles, but during the time this book was being put together, one of the best studies of oat and palm oil was published, and it did not beat the placebo!

Fish oil. Small amounts (1,000 to 2,000 milligrams a day) of the active ingredients EPA and DHA have been touted for weight loss (they may increase satiety by a small amount), but recent human studies have not supported a consistent or impressive impact on pounds. Some studies suggest just eating fish (it's also high in protein) might be a better option.

Green tea pills. These contain EGCG, an antioxidant found in high amounts in a variety of teas, which increases metabolism and stimulates fat burning. However, many of the studies used an average of 520 milligrams of EGCG along with 100 milligrams or more of caffeine but saw only a minor (1 pound on average), if any, impact. Concentrated caffeine in this amount can increase anxiety, nervousness, stress, insomnia, and high blood pressure. An 8-ounce cup of brewed green tea contains 200 milligrams of EGCG and 45 milligrams of caffeine, and I would just stick with that!

Gymnema sylvestre. This compound, which is similar to glucose, is derived from a plant that grows wild in India and Africa. It goes to the same taste buds on the tongue that sugar does, and it's supposed to be able to reduce cravings for or the taste of sweets, as if you received a sugar fix. However, study results have been inconsistent, so it's not worth it at this time.

hCG (human chorionic gonadotropin). This is a popular liquid dietary supplement for appetite suppression that people usually take when they're on very low-calorie diets (500 calories or less). However, hCG has not really worked better than a placebo in clinical trials. Some patients end up paying thousands of dollars and lose weight long term simply due to caloric restriction. In other words, it's the extremely low-calorie diet that's leading to the weight loss, not the hCG.

Hoodia. Hunters used to eat this South African plant to suppress appetite on long trips in the Kalahari Desert. Despite considerable investment in the product, it has not lived up to expectations, and in clinical studies it caused side effects—such as headaches, dizziness, nausea, vomiting, fatigue, gas, and even blood pressure increases—and there was no weight loss. Pass!

Hydroxycitric acid (HCA). This compound is the active ingredient in many weight loss supplements (it's currently

457

being promoted on TV as the principal ingredient in *Garcinia cambogia,* a weight loss product). It supposedly blocks an enzyme that turns excess carbohydrates into fat and may also increase brain levels of serotonin. Yet, in well-done research studies it's been a dud, which has also been my experience with it. And recently there has been the potential for serious toxicity when combined with other serotonin-enhancing drugs, such as antidepressants.

Irvingia gabonensis. This is just a proprietary seed extract of the African mango, also known as IGOB131, which is supposed to suppress appetite and improve metabolism via multiple unproven pathways. It had great early research, but since then the methodology has been questioned, and I do not believe its ability to create weight loss is much better than a placebo. (I hope I'm wrong.)

Glutamine. This amino acid has been advertised as a replacement for glucose for brain fuel. Instead of giving in to your sugar craving, you take this. But these claims are based on animal studies, and human studies have not found it to be effective for weight loss. It's also touted on the Internet as a sugar substitute that can reduce cravings for it. In reality, when you cut out most of the sugar in your diet for a long period of time, sugar cravings are reduced anyway. In other words, the benefit is not caused by the supplement but by the behavior that takes place around the supplement.

DHEA and 7-Keto-DHEA. DHEA (dehydroepiandrosterone) can be converted into male and female hormones in the human body and potentially stimulate the metabolism. Currently, there's a lot of hype about 7-Keto-DHEA, which supposedly stimulates the metabolism without altering hormones, but good studies just aren't there. Plus, there is some hint that 7-Keto may increase thyroid function a bit, and if this is the case, it could raise heart rate and blood pressure in the short term and lead to thyroid abnormalities (increased or decreased thyroid hormone) in the long term. I would just love to see a really good study done with 7-Keto, but I've worked with both of these products for more than a decade and they just don't get me excited for weight loss. I hope someone proves me wrong!

Raspberry ketone. This is one of the major aromatic compounds in raspberries (it's a chemical that gives the fruit its scent), and it's commonly used as a fragrance in cosmetics and as a flavoring agent in food products. It has never really had a good published study, but since it resembles capsaicin in structure somewhat, researchers theorize it may crank up metabolism the way capsaicin does, although it hasn't been shown to be beneficial for weight loss either. I smell a rat—or a mouse—because only mouse studies have shown a potential benefit.

Resveratrol. This dietary supplement (resveratrol is a compound found in red wine) is supposed to have antiaging effects and help you lose weight, but in some of the better recent studies with men and women, subjects haven't seen weight loss or heart-healthy changes. Pharmaceutical companies have tried to make some magic out of this compound for a variety of conditions, but there has been no magic happening yet.

Sensa. This is a pricey blend of flavorless, scented starch crystals that you sprinkle on food. It's supposed to enhance the smell of food and trigger a feeling of fullness in the brain. The company-sponsored studies have not been published or peer reviewed at the time of my writing this, and a large number of subjects who started the study did not finish it. I don't think Sensa makes any sense, and you shouldn't spend your cents (get it) on it.

Vitamin D. When you lose weight, vitamin D levels in the blood increase naturally because it gets released from the fatty tissue that you're burning. But the vitamin itself doesn't help with weight loss.

WHAT ARE THE OPTIONS FOR KIDS?

If your child has a large amount of weight to lose, please talk to a medical professional. Just be careful; you don't want to create a sense of pill dependence (drug or supplement) at such a young age, unless it's really necessary.

LIFESTYLE CHANGES

Eat heart healthy. Low carb, low fat, vegan, paleo, Weight Watchers, Jenny Craig, gluten free—as long as it's heart healthy (lowers blood pressure, blood sugar, cholesterol, heart rate, weight, or waist size) and *mentally* healthy, then I support it. That's the Moyad rule on dieting.

Limit liquid calories. Alcohol, sugary sodas, fruit juices, and smoothies all contain calories, and there's evidence that your body doesn't recognize liquid calories in the same way it does solid calories. So you may not register the same sense of fullness even though you've downed a similar number of calories. Reducing or eliminating these drinks is one of the easiest ways to lose weight. That's why almost every diet program tells you to cut out alcohol, soda, and fruit juices first!

Exercise strategically. My favorite saying about exercise and weight loss comes from my daughter: "Abs are made in the kitchen, not on the treadmill." Research has clearly demonstrated that you do *not* need to exercise to lose weight or waist size! Diet trumps exercise. (I feel a *however* coming on . . .) However, the reason exercise—both cardio and strength training—makes sense for 99.9 percent of people who want to drop pounds is that it improves mood, heart health, and metabolism and prevents muscle loss. It can help you keep the weight off.

Have you ever heard of HIIT (high-intensity interval training)? The concept is simple. You alternate between doing harder, more intense exercise followed by easier "recovery" bouts (often it's 30 seconds to 2 minutes of hard work followed by an equal or longer amount of rest, repeated several times). And you can do it in as little as 20 to 30 minutes, versus

45 minutes of low- to moderate-intensity exercise. Research shows that it improves fitness levels as well as longer exercise bouts do, and it may even target fat better. A recent study also suggested that HIIT doesn't make you hungry the way moderate exercise might. You shouldn't do it every day (it's challenging), but a couple of times a week in addition to other workouts can make a difference in weight and body composition (the amount of fat and muscle that you have). Even beginners can do it because the harder intensities are relative to fitness level; you run or bike at a level that's tough for you, not your neighbor.

Make small changes. Try to cut back by 100 to 200 calories a day—that's one roll at dinner—so you don't feel like you're depriving yourself and you take weight off gradually, which is easier to maintain. I'm a firm believer that you need to pick a way of eating that works with your personality because you want to be able to stick with it long term.

Bulk up. Most people get half of the recommended 25 to 30 grams of fiber daily. Eating $\frac{1}{3}$ to $\frac{1}{2}$ cup of All-Bran, Fiber One, or other cereals (13 to 15 grams) and some flaxseed or chia seeds in the morning is an easy way to get your daily dose without having to run to the bathroom. Look for products with mostly insoluble fiber plus some soluble fiber, including fruits, veggies, beans, seeds, some cereals, oatmeal, and some bars. Most protein and fiber bars are worthless because they have either too few calories and fiber or too many calories and too much cheap soluble fiber, which can cause gas and bloating. Plus, they don't do much for weight loss.

Check your meds. Numerous prescription drugs can increase the risk of weight gain, including antidepressants, hormonal agents, beta-blockers, and steroids. I'm not saying to take yourself off them; just talk with a trusted doctor about your options.

APPENDIX

DR. MOYAD'S 70-POINT RESEARCH CHECKLIST

RESEARCH IS LIKE a courtroom, where the preponderance of the evidence *usually* leads to the right answer. But all studies are not equal; in fact, some are just downright worthless or even misleading. I mention a ton of studies in this book. Several were very well done and others left room for improvement (in these cases, I try to point out any shortcomings).

I've compiled this list of criteria that I look for in a research paper to determine whether it's low, moderate, or high quality—or in rare cases very high quality, such as a study that would be similar to what drugs go through to get FDA approval. (Unfortunately, this level of study is rare in the supplement world. I will certainly call your attention to it if it exists, though.) These criteria can overlap to a small or large degree. And yes, for all you skeptics and conspiracy theorists, I use the same criteria when analyzing drug studies!

The point of this Appendix is to show you what I look for in a study (because I love diving into the nitty-gritty details!) when evaluating a supplement—or any health intervention, for that matter. It will help you dig deeper, if you choose to, and understand how I came to the conclusions found in this book. It's a long list and some of you may enjoy how I parse the information. Ultimately, I hope this checklist helps you understand that when you read a story about a new study, there's *always* more to the story.

461

1. *Was there an abstract presented at a medical meeting that had similar results as the published research?*

I am an MD, which I like to say stands for medical detective (at least in my case). As part of my job, I attend a ton of meetings where researchers present their findings in a condensed form, called an abstract. It's during these presentations that I get an inside look at what went on during studies, and they are a forum for wider coverage and even criticism.

According to surveys, one-third to one-half of the research presented at many of these meetings never makes it into a medical journal, for multiple reasons—maybe it's negative results or the sheer time investment involved in publishing a paper or laziness or who knows what. Sometimes, if the research does get published, there are serious omissions or changes from what was presented at the meeting, often because the publication process is more rigorous and selective (I think a paper should always mention if the research was presented at a meeting prior to publication). For instance, one abstract presentation I attended concerning a diet and supplement study done with cancer patients omitted the fact that the participants with more aggressive forms of cancer failed to respond to the intervention when the research was formally published! Cancer patients who only read the article would think the intervention worked for everyone. This is misleading, and it's why I have this criterion on my radar.

Another advantage to following medical presentations at major meetings is that it helps to place other research papers on the same topic into better perspective. For example, when I saw at several meetings that ginger supplements were helping patients with nausea caused by a variety of factors, from pregnancy to cancer treatment, and then papers that aligned with the research started to get published, I believed it added credibility to the supplement's case. A lot of research never sees the light of day, but I take notice! The takeaway here is that sometimes you have to go beyond what is published in a paper. Hearing these abstracts is just one part of the whole puzzle. I'm always looking for the full story, and there's only so much room to tell that story in a medical journal. *Note:* You can often find these abstract presentations (as well as published research papers) online if you go to the conference organizer's Web site, such as the Academy of Nutrition and Dietetics.

2. *Are the active ingredient(s) standardized, and is the dosage identified?*

A study should tell me what was tested in terms of the active or principal ingredient and dosage. Did all of the participants receive the exact same standardized ingredient, and can this be proven? Standardization means that pill after pill and batch after batch there is good certainty that the product will contain the same amount of the intended active ingredient. Researchers should always reveal the company that provided the pill and the test used to determine its contents; this is a major shortcoming in supplement studies. For example, a good red yeast rice extract study for lowering cholesterol would report the exact amount or range of the active ingredient (monacolin K) found in each capsule, and a good valerian study for sleep would mention the percentage of valerenic acids in the total dosage of the pill. This is important information because it tells the consumer what to look for when shopping for a supplement. If you know a study of ginseng for memory used a 1,000-milligram dose with an 8 percent ginsenoside content, you can look for a similar product and be more confident that you might see a benefit. Standardization ensures better safety because it prevents people from getting too high or too low a dose, and it also helps researchers and health care professionals compare clinical trials. Many "experts" used to claim that saw palmetto only worked when a capsule contained a certain amount of fatty acids and sterols, but when the largest studies followed those guidelines, the pill did not work better than a placebo. Oops!

Unfortunately, many herbal dietary supplement products don't list the active ingredient or the researchers don't know what the active ingredient is, (arthritis products can have 5 to 10 ingredients for example) so consumers have to either purchase the exact product studied or just make a blind purchase and hope it works. I hear all the time that an herbal product works like an adaptogen (a compound that's supposed to keep your body in healthy balance), or that it has multiple ingredients that help many body functions. I call B.S.! Pills do not work by magic; specific ingredients do specific things to different parts of the body.

3. *Did researchers give participants adequate instructions for taking the pill(s) being tested (and other behaviors)?*

If the rules of the study are too loose, it's hard to trust the results or know how to copy them in the real world. Good research studies will clearly outline a series of rules for taking the pills and any other behaviors, and they will emphasize how important it is to follow these instructions. When studies aren't this detailed, participants may start following their own set of rules, which can skew results, and sometimes they just lose interest because there's not enough guidance. Researchers are supposed to make it clear that participants should report any major behavioral changes to the research team so they can be recorded. For example, if you're studying the effect of a weight loss pill, you're likely going to tell participants not to exercise so you can see the effect of just the pill. If one of the participants decides to work out daily for 2 weeks straight (and many do this, in my experience), you want to be aware of this information. Many past cholesterol-lowering supplement studies showed dramatic reductions in cholesterol, but some participants also decided to exercise and eat like they had a fitness TV show contract!

4. *Was allocation concealment adequate?*

It's not just important that the researchers and participants are unaware of which study group they're in; how the participants are assigned to those groups—called allocation concealment—is even more important. Were individuals assigned to placebo and intervention groups without influence from the researchers and was that concealment maintained throughout the study? Readers also need to know why the researchers believe no participant was influenced more or less in any group. Double-blind trials (see #22), where neither the researchers nor the participants know which group is which, help, but even in these situations a person working with the study might unconsciously place people with a better prognosis in the treatment group and those with a poorer prognosis in the placebo group.

Studies that do not use good allocation concealment tend to report results that are far better than what the pill actually can produce. Good allocation concealment eliminates as many confounding variables as possible, ensuring that the two groups are as equal as possible, except for the pills assigned. Many good studies (but not enough supplement studies) now use a centralized or independent service that performs all of the steps around randomization and allocation concealment, making it impossible for investigators to know beforehand who was allocated to what type of treatment.

5. *Were the size and duration of the study appropriate?*

Better researchers will work with a statistician to determine how large and long a study needs to be to show a benefit, if there is one. Otherwise, the process becomes a guessing game, and many researchers like to play this game, my friends. The larger and longer the study, the greater the cost, but the greater the accuracy as well (and the more likely the results will reflect what to expect in real life)!

Imagine if the recent vitamin E and Alzheimer's study (see the section on Alzheimer's disease, page 65) was only a 3-month trial. It would have shown nothing. And if the good saw palmetto studies would have lasted 3 to 6 months instead of 12 months, they would have reported a potential benefit where one did not exist. Some of the strongest placebo responses happen in the first few months of a trial; in order to get at the truth, a large, long study helps even the playing field.

6. *Did the study test an* a priori *hypothesis?*

This basically means, did the researchers know exactly what they were testing *before* the study began, or did they just throw something against the wall to see if it would stick? If the research protocol does not clearly define the hypothesis before the study begins, then it can create a huge bias in favor of the pill. This is a critical piece of information that many studies, including supplement studies, do not provide. Why? The chances that your study will fail to be impressive with an *a priori* hypothesis are much higher since you don't have any wiggle room to pull out favorable results. Basically, this is about transparency. If you want to see if your supplement lowers cholesterol and it doesn't, you might do 100 other tests on the pill to see what it can do. Then, lo and behold, it appears to raise vitamin D levels! This is deceptive, even if it *might* be true, because this was not the focus of the study.

7. Are the assessment points, or intervals, fixed in terms of number and time and well defined?

Researchers check for results at certain intervals, depending on the length of the study. It might be only at the end, or it may be after every few months. The number and timing of these assessments should be fixed, and there should be multiple intervals where all participants are evaluated. For example, a glucosamine study on osteoarthritis that evaluates participants' knee pain every 3 months over a period of 2 years and includes two imaging studies or x-rays at year one and two and four blood tests at 6, 12, 18, and 24 months allows for equitable comparisons between the groups. Some supplement studies will not have these rigorous features, which makes it difficult to understand the pill's true benefit.

8. Did the author honestly report any bias, and did she actually write the paper and control the data?

Conflicts of interest need to be spelled out in the paper to allow for objective analysis of the results. Conflicts don't negate the findings of a positive study, but revealing them does provide perspective for the reader now and in the future when making comparisons with other study results. For example, if you are an investigator studying cold and flu remedies and you are a speaker or consultant for the company or you get royalties from the sale of the supplement, then this should be clearly reported. The Federal Trade Commission has stepped up surveillance of this practice on television and the Internet, but it needs to be reported more in published papers. (Good medical journals will spot this bias and make sure it doesn't get introduced in the published study, but even medical journals can miss bias.)

One other thing I look for is whether the author actually wrote the paper and controlled the data. (You have to sign a document verifying that you're the one who wrote it.) Many companies will do the writing for the author and control the data, which is crazy. When this happens, it usually introduces some bias into the publication.

9. Is the statistical analysis between and/or within groups clearly defined?

The best studies compare supplements or drugs to a placebo or at least to another established or accepted treatment option (often referred to as a standard of care), which is considered a "between group" comparison. If the stats don't show that a pill works better than a placebo but the researchers or statisticians are still impressed with the results, they'll perform what's known as a within group analysis. They'll look at the group who took the pill and compare the beginning and end results.

Let's say you have a dietary supplement that you believe lowers cholesterol over 4 weeks compared to a placebo. But it turns out the supplement dropped bad cholesterol (LDL) by 15 points while the placebo group experienced a 10-point reduction, and when the statistician compared the results, they were not significant, meaning the difference isn't large enough to support the claim. However, since a 15-point reduction by a dietary supplement is nothing to sneeze at, you ask the statistician to ignore the placebo group and just compare the before and after cholesterol levels within the supplement group to see if the difference is statistically significant.

A within group analysis helps researchers determine if something has any effectiveness, but it can be used inappropriately to suggest an intervention works when it really doesn't (like with many testosterone-boosting supplements). The ideal scenario is for the between group analysis to show a benefit, but within group results can be interesting and relevant as well. Regardless, these comparisons should always be spelled out in the research paper. If a study does not mention it, I feel the researchers aren't being transparent, and it gets a lower grade on my list.

10. *How is this supplement clinically relevant and what is the market competition? What's novel about the findings?*

Researchers need to accurately and objectively assess how a new treatment is similar, worse, or better than what's currently available to the consumer. Is the study actually adding something to the health market other than a high price? I see osteoarthritis supplement companies do a small study and claim that the results are groundbreaking. They fail to mention, however, that there are tons of products in this same category that have claimed similar benefits. How is their product different or better than what is already out there? Unless the results are impressive and fulfill an unmet—or inadequately met—need for patients, I'm not going to give it a high grade.

11. *Was compliance predicted, measured, reported, and statistically compared?*

Compliance—meaning the study participants followed instructions—can be tracked in many ways. Researchers can count pills, but I like to see them using blood or urine tests to prove subjects took their pills, and if some subjects didn't, I want to know what percentage failed to do so, why they failed to do so, and how this affected the results. Heck, I can't remember to take my multivitamin more than a few days a week, so how can someone remember to take several pills a day, every day for months or even years? It may seem obvious, but compliance can completely change the outcome or interpretation of a study. Researchers should evaluate compliance and report why there was any lack of it and whether it made an impact on the results.

In one of the largest calcium and vitamin D supplement studies for the prevention of bone fractures that was ever completed (called the Women's Health Initiative, or WHI), the researchers were brilliant because they analyzed the group of women who took their supplements regularly as well as those who didn't. They found a potential significant reduction in certain types of fractures for those who took their supplements most days of the month compared to no impact in those who took them irregularly. If the researchers hadn't looked at compliance, the results would have suggested that the supplements are completely worthless! Now we know that compliance in this category is critical.

12. *Did the researchers calculate confidence intervals (95 percent)?*

One of the ways you can feel good about the results of a study is to look at the confidence interval, or CI. It tells you how large the variation in results was. A 95 percent CI, which is ideal, means that 95 percent of the results (e.g., cholesterol, prostate-specific antigen or PSA, or uric acid levels) fell within a particular range, and the researchers should note this.

For example, let's say a dietary supplement reduces blood cholesterol by -40 points and there's a 95 percent CI of -32 to -45. This means the average reduction was 40 points, but 95 percent of the participants experienced a 32- to 45-point drop. Higher-quality studies generally have a tight or smaller range. A larger variation (say, if the results above spanned -1 to -51) makes me less confident because the results were all over the map.

13. *Are the study conclusions justified by the data collected?*

There's no room for embellishment here. The conclusions should be objective and straightforward. When researchers conclude that a supplement "clearly" offers a benefit against a disease, when it was only tested in a preliminary study, then you know there's bias. I once peer reviewed and rejected multiple papers that suggested the supplement tested was profoundly better than anything else on the market despite being evaluated in just a small number of individuals.

Here's how it should be done: When a group of researchers at the Mayo Clinic made their conclusions about American ginseng and its impact on cancer fatigue (a very impressive study and findings), they wrote, "There appears to be some activity and tolerable toxicity at 1,000 to 1,200 mg/day doses of American ginseng with regard to cancer-related fatigue. Thus, further study of American ginseng is warranted." It's stoic, unbiased, and completely reflects the findings of this well-done clinical trial. I love to see studies like this!

14. *Were confounding variables corrected for? Were groups similar at the beginning of the study? Was multivariate analysis used or were only baseline characteristics compared?*

This basically means, did the researchers identify or try to remove any variables that might somehow cause misleading results? Making sure treatment groups are similar (e.g., in terms of age, gender, and body mass index) and treated equally throughout a study is one way to do this. However, if there were differences, you want to check to see if the researchers performed what's called a multivariate analysis, which accounts for these differences. The larger and better the study, the more confounding variables are accounted for so, in the end, there's little to no difference between the groups except for the pill being studied.

Vitamin D is a classic example of confounding variables. For years, researchers thought that high vitamin D blood levels might help reduce the risk of weight gain or obesity because in so many studies men and women with much higher blood levels of D were skinnier! But when further research looked into weight and waist size—confounding variables—and statisticians added this into their analyses, the weight loss claim fell apart. Why? Vitamin D likes to hang out in fat tissue. So as people gain weight, their blood levels of vitamin D go down because the D shifts to the fat. And as they lose weight, D is released

from the fat into the blood. In the studies, skinnier folks had higher vitamin D counts because they don't have fat for D to escape to. Vitamin D *wasn't* the trigger for weight loss after all.

Here is a short list (sarcasm alert #264) of things that can influence the results of dietary supplement studies and even nutrient levels.

- Age
- Alcohol
- Blood pressure/cholesterol
- Body mass index, weight, and waist size
- Diabetes and other diseases (a.k.a. comorbidities)
- Diet
- Education level
- Environment
- Gender
- Genetics/family history
- Infections and illnesses
- Medical procedures
- Medications (prescriptions, over-the-counter drugs, and dietary supplements)
- Menstrual cycle and other hormone fluctuations in men and women
- Occupation
- Physical activity/exercise
- Pregnancy/lactation

- Race/ethnicity
- Sleep
- Stress (physical and mental)
- Tobacco use (never used, ex-, current, and even secondhand)

15. Does the study provide a name and contact information for correspondence?

This is a minor point but still important. Good researchers are proud of their findings (negative, positive, or neutral) and are willing to defend or explain them, so most studies today list a contact person for correspondence. I'm always e-mailing some researcher in hopes of getting more information about the results of a study. But that doesn't mean the person will or can answer my questions, unfortunately, which always makes me nervous.

16. Is there an estimate of the cost of the treatment/intervention?

Many bone-headed "experts" do not want to consider cost when judging an intervention, but you can't tell me this isn't relevant to compliance! Look at all the Viagra, Cialis, Levitra, and other commercials. You think it's so simple: Just go get your prescription and then wait for your erection. But drug companies' own research suggests that 50 to 66 percent of men never refill their first prescription. And cost—at $10 to $25 per *pill*—is always at or near the top of the list of reasons they don't want more.

So if a dietary supplement is a lot cheaper than a prescription drug—even

though it might not work as well—I often rate it higher when analyzing a study (and vice versa).

17. Have the researchers clearly defined the medical condition they're testing?

While many conditions are fairly black and white in terms of how they're defined, the science of diagnosing isn't as exact as you would think. You always want to know exactly how the researchers view a condition and how they diagnosed participants (through a clinical exam, x-ray, questionnaire, blood test, or some combination of these).

18. Was the supplement delivery system easy to use, and who provided the supplements (a.k.a. pill practicality)?

When I think of delivery, I think of pizza! I love it, will continue to eat it several times a month forever, and can give you a list of all my favorite (and least favorite) places to get it in Ann Arbor. Pizza fans are passionate about their pies. Supplements and their delivery system can garner a lot of love and hate as well, not unlike pizza. Do you take a small pill once a day or 8 to 10? Do you have to measure out multiple scoops or liquid drops in water? The more complicated it is to take something, the less likely most folks are going to use it in the real world (and it can affect study compliance). Up to 50 percent of people report using lifesaving daily prescriptions irregularly within 1 to 2 years of starting it, even when they're tiny pills! So I do grade supplement delivery systems, and researchers should be sensitive to ease of use when testing participants.

I also like to know who provided the supplements for the clinical trial because it lets the consumer compare ingredients and buy what was used in the actual research. If a study used a Centrum Silver multivitamin, then you can compare it to products at Costco, Sam's Club, Walgreens, or wherever. Without this information, the study isn't really providing guidance. I think it also shows a lot of guts in some cases, especially in the really objective studies, because the product—and maybe the entire company—is on the line.

19. Is there dilution that leads to pollution and confusion?

I like to know how many ingredients the researchers tested. Was it just one (ideal) or a few? The more ingredients you add, the greater the potential to dilute the effects of that pill and to make it difficult to really know which ingredients are providing which benefits. It also introduces potential contaminants and interactions (a.k.a. pollution). There are a ton of osteoarthritis supplements that claim to be superior to the standard glucosamine or chondroitin products, but when you look at the ingredients, they're just another version of those standard supplements with some added herbs. But this doesn't justify the cost, in my book (and this *is* my book!). Companies would argue that every single ingredient is necessary, and I would argue that this makes no sense but does make cents for them. Also, the more ingredients you put

in a pill, the less room you have for the truly active ingredients, unless you want to be swallowing a quarter-size supplement every day!

20. Was the study diverse and does it reflect a real-world sample of participants (a.k.a. the whitewashing of clinical trials)?

Clinical trials have a major problem in general with lack of diversity. This is embarrassing and at times shameful. If a pill is truly effective, then it has been tested to some degree in diverse populations, both men and women and various races. If a study only looked at men, I want to know, because the results won't necessarily be the same in women. If a study only involved Caucasians, I want to know as well, because African Americans or Asians, for example, might respond differently. And it's not just men or Caucasians who watch commercials and buy supplements. As a medical detective, I want to know who was tested and what the differences were among groups so I can pass on the truth and increase consumer confidence.

21. Did researchers accurately and objectively assess the effects of different dosages (a.k.a. the dose response)?

A few years ago a company with an exotic supplement tested a high-dose and a low-dose version of its product in patients and saw the same slightly positive results. The researchers' conclusion seemed to be, okay, you can take either the high or low dose.

Good luck! If you test two dosages with no placebo group, I could (and will) easily argue that the reason they worked equally was that neither dose really works at all. You just don't know unless the different dosages are compared to something that's not the product, such as a placebo or the "standard of care," which is what large, well-done trials do.

22. *Was it truly a double-blind study, close to it, or not at all?*

The hot buzzwords in research are "randomized, placebo-controlled, double-blind trial." A study like this essentially tries to eliminate any potential bias or influence from both researchers and participants. So many experts demand this level of proof for dietary supplements and drugs, and while it sure sounds good, it does not necessarily mean a study is high quality. Do you know how many supplement company representatives, and even health care professionals, walk up to me every year and try to convince me their products work because they've been through "randomized, placebo-controlled, double-blind trials"? I simply roll my eyes and yawn. I wish that was all it took to prove a supplement's worth (don't get me wrong, it helps, but there's a lot more to look at). Time and time again, I have seen one well-done clinical study trump the findings of four or five previous weak or poorly done randomized trials.

Double-blinding is a strict method used in good studies to ensure that the researchers, participants, and any other health care workers involved in the trial have no idea who's getting the intervention (the real pill) or the placebo. If an investigator knows who's who, it's possible he might subconsciously provide more care and attention to the supplement group, which can skew results. Sometimes being too close to a product distorts your thinking even though you don't consciously want to interfere (and sometimes there are simply people who do want to skew results!).

Researchers should pay meticulous attention to making the placebo look, feel, smell, and weigh the same as the treatment pill because if participants know or think they know they're getting a placebo, it can influence results. This happened with some studies of saw palmetto for urinary health. The researchers didn't make the pills the same size, color, weight, and odor, so some people figured out what they were taking.

Just an FYI: A single-blind study means the researchers knew who was getting what, but the participants didn't. And there really are some studies out there where everyone knows who's getting what treatment!

23. *Did an objective, outside authority on the subject write an editorial on behalf of the study?*

Important, earth-shattering studies—positive, negative, or neutral—often get editorials. And these have one purpose: objective overview. I would much rather read an editorial on a study, which is often in the same issue of the journal as the study, than the study itself. It provides a complete overview of the subject, objectively explains the pros and cons of the findings, and analyzes the significance of the results. Some journals are beginning to provide quick editorial comments on the last page of the study, and this helps graders like me catch everything. (Sometimes you have to wait a few weeks or even months to get a really good editorial written by an objective authority on the subject.)

24. *Did the research team assess the participants' expectations of treatment, attitudes toward treatment assignment (the groups they were assigned to), or sense of treatment credibility?*

Knowing subjects' expectations and opinions of the treatment helps determine their mind-set and how this might translate to real-world findings. If you have some really skeptical people in the study and they report a benefit, then this bodes well for the product's effect in all kinds of personalities in the real world. All physicians have patients who think pills won't do anything, might do something, or will cure all their ills, so I think it's helpful to know if those same mind-sets were reflected in a study's subjects. I have seen supplement researchers do a nonplacebo study on one group where everyone who was recruited thought supplements were the cure to all of life's problems. Guess what the results were?

When researchers recruit participants,

they might not reveal the exact product, but they may tell them, for example, that the clinical trial is testing a new vitamin D pill or a protein powder for muscle strength. Just like in jury selection, researchers are trying to recruit an objective jury, not one that's biased for or against the treatment. It sounds simple enough, but not many studies reveal why they believe their participant pools are objective.

25. *Who funded the study?*

Follow the money. Knowing who funded the research and the role of each source helps determine how truly independent a study is. That's not to say research funded by a supplement company can't be trusted; it just needs to be included in the paper. Did the company only provide money or did it design the study, analyze the results, and write the paper? If it was the latter, this can be an indication of potential bias or commercial motivation. Transparency is critical in research. When investigators found ginger supplements helped reduce nausea from chemotherapy, the fact that the study was not funded by a commercial source only served to validate the findings even more.

26. *Did the researchers clearly describe and standardize inclusion and exclusion criteria for the study?*

I want to know the exact criteria that needed to be met by a subject to be eligible for the study and what criteria excluded someone. These rules for participating need to be strict in order to really determine if a pill works. Let's say you want to do a vitamin D study to determine if high doses can reduce the risk of an upper respiratory tract infection, and you want to include only healthy men and women 18 years or older. You would at the very minimum need to *exclude* individuals already taking high-dose vitamin D supplements; anyone on immunosuppressive drugs or drugs that could impact vitamin D metabolism; anyone with a history of abnormally high blood calcium, kidney stones, liver or kidney disease, or other diseases causing higher blood calcium; anyone who's pregnant or considering becoming pregnant; and so on. Unless you let the reader know how strict your standards for participation were, it's impossible to trust that the study was done adequately or to know who the pills will work for.

27. *Did participants give informed consent?*

All participants have the right to know exactly what they have signed up for in any clinical trial, including all the rules and potential risks. Participants also have the right to quit the study at any time, for any reason. Signing an informed consent form shows that subjects were not coerced or duped into the clinical trial. Many medical journals will not allow a paper to be published unless there was some type of informed consent given or researchers provided oversight in this area.

28. *Did the researchers use intention-to-treat (ITT) and per-protocol completer (PPC) methods?*

Results that are applicable to the real world require rules and analysis that apply to the real world. An ITT analysis means that all participants will be counted in the final analysis regardless of what happens to them during the study (whether they are noncompliant, skip check-ins, withdraw, or even die). This generally yields results that are very conservative but also closer to what happens in the real world, where people quit taking their meds, start a new diet, take up or quit exercising, and so on.

Researchers should also do what's called a PPC analysis, which looks at the subset of the ITT group who completed the study *without* any major protocol violations (i.e., they followed the rules). Many studies never report ITT; they only provide some version of PPC because they want to give you what I call the Las Vegas Effect. This happens when only the winners are advertised and the vast majority of losers are ignored. In the end, this results in a study that could be seriously biased because only the "perfect" people were looked at—not the real world at all.

More supplement studies need to provide ITT data. One very large trial on alpha lipoic acid for weight loss did include ITT and PPC analyses, and both showed a significant benefit over the placebo. This outstanding methodology is part of the reason it was one of the very few weight loss supplement studies to be published in a high-tier journal (the prestigious *American Journal of Medicine*).

29. *Were the investigators/assessors clearly described?*

Simply put, I want to know who did what, where, and how. When all the players are mentioned on paper, I want to know what positions they occupied in the game. There are groups called contract research organizations (CROs) that conduct safe (in general), independent clinical trials for anyone who has the money. Some of them are run well and professionally, others not so much. Regardless, if the study authors don't reveal this information, it's difficult to assess the credibility of the clinical trial site and the investigators involved. All of this transparency helps to further elevate the status of a study and the reliability of the results.

30. *Did an institutional review board (IRB) or another regulatory body approve the study?*

An IRB is usually made up of a diverse group of individuals (from lawyers to doctors to statisticians), and they help determine if a research study can or should be conducted and what the risks and benefits are. The board can also offer recommendations after reviewing a study. Although independent boards can be a real pain in the gluteus maximus, can cause delays, and can be costly, they are critically important to making sure a study is well designed, as safe and ethical as possible, and appropriate. If I see a study that has

not gone through any IRB approval, then I get nervous. Higher-quality trials usually have approval, and many of the top journals now require it for publication.

31. *What is the Jadad score, or was the study included in the* Cochrane Database of Systematic Reviews?

There are several quality-based scoring systems that are now applied to clinical trials and published studies. Although it does have some shortcomings, one of the most popular is the Jadad score, which was named after the doctor who developed it. The higher the score, the better the quality of the study and the more comfortable you can be with the results. You can find this score in an editorial or article on the study. I give each study I review a Moyad score (again, higher numbers are better), but I also like to see how it does with other systems, such as Jadad.

The *Cochrane Database of Systematic Reviews* journal does an outstanding job of evaluating studies, and I frequently look to see what its take is on a trial. The journal doesn't provide a numerical score, but it does make conclusions based on the quality and quantity of all the data.

32. *What is the quality of the journal publishing the study?*

Medical journals, like running shoes, come in all shapes, sizes, and levels of quality. There are low-tier journals that will publish almost anything (some supplement studies will steer toward these), and there are top-tier journals that are really tough to get into unless a study is super high quality. In general, the higher the tier, the more rigorous the process for being accepted (they commonly use the Moyad criteria I've outlined here).

Some higher-tier journals have been accused of only publishing supplement studies with negative results, and although this used to be the case for some journals, I think it happens rarely today. For example, the positive results on vitamin E and Alzheimer's disease that were published in the *Journal of the American Medical Association*—one of the best journals in the world—is a testament to this change in tide. I have reviewed studies for many journals over the years and, without a doubt, the journal matters. When I see a major study published in a top journal, I know 99 times out of 100, the methodology and study design were outstanding. When it comes to lower-level publications, they're generally not as stringent with their acceptance guidelines, so I never quite know exactly what I'm going to get (life is like a box of chocolates).

Another sensitive topic related to journals is advertising. Some critics argue that since high-tier publications accept tons of pharmaceutical advertising, they're more partial to those drugs. In general, I don't think this is the case, but the potential for bias is concerning in some instances. There's a new movement afoot to eliminate or reduce influential advertising, which I support, but then journals would have to look to taxpayers, authors, and private donors to foot the bill for publication.

33. *Were the study limitations identified and discussed?*

Any published paper that does not list the limitations of the research (usually in the discussion or conclusions sections) comes across as more of an advertisement than a study, and it should not be accepted for publication until this information is provided. Every study—no matter how good—has limitations (not enough minority participants, too small a number, too short, compliance problems, drop-outs, and so forth). Lack of a discussion on limitations is one of the biggest problems I see when reviewing a paper for a medical journal.

Here's an example of why addressing limitations is so important: In one study of omega-3 blood levels and brain size, the authors noted that a big limitation was taking only one blood sample for each participant over 8 years; more samples would have provided more accuracy. When I was reading the paper, I wasn't exactly sure how many samples they took until it was clearly spelled out for me. Authors should never fear the limitations of their study.

34. *Does the mechanism of action really make sense—or just cents?*

If the research seems to imply that a supplement works by magical means, with no specific mechanism of action, then I worry. Any good trial will rely on other comparable studies to identify why the product works (or not). For example, it makes sense that CoQ10 might help reduce the side effects of statins because previous research has shown that statins can reduce CoQ10 levels in some individuals to a large degree. The supplement is addressing a deficiency created by the drug. Good researchers will always try to explain how a product works because this means they have a solid grasp of the subject, which also partially reflects the credibility of the study.

35. What medications (other than the treatment and placebo) were allowed, and were they documented and mentioned?

Studies that record each and every medication taken in addition to the treatment or placebo improve the accuracy and limitations of the results. Most Americans take some kind of pill, and consumers want to know if a supplement will impact their current drug regimens. The only way to find out is to test the supplement, and the only way to fully evaluate the results is to know what other drugs were allowed. This documentation falls under the inclusion and exclusion criteria process, but it's even more methodical and exact. When the landmark AREDS trial (see the Cataracts section, page 127) allowed subjects to take a specific multivitamin (Centrum) along with the eye health supplement or placebo, the researchers later found that the multivitamin might have lowered the risk of cataracts. Documenting this information not only made the study more transparent (and better), but it also launched a series of studies that indeed found multivitamin users have a slightly to moderately lower risk of the most common type of cataract.

36. What has my personal history been with the product along with the sum of the research?

I have been working with supplements probably longer than just about anyone, so my experience with a product has to count for something. I have consulted with thousands, if not tens of thousands, of patients and health care professionals on supplements. When someone tells me L-theanine at 100 milligrams per day has many side effects, I'm less inclined to believe it because I have used the supplement for many years in my practice without problems and know the studies inside and out.

When a 1970s-era paper stated ginseng was dangerous, I knew there must have been other stimulants in the ginseng product the researchers tested. I had worked with ginseng for many years and had published articles on it as well. I'm not saying I toss out a study if it doesn't match what I've seen, but I include my experience in my overall evaluation. This brings me to one of the most important things I consider with any supplement: If it's not heart healthy or heart neutral then I don't generally recommend it for most medical conditions. Sometimes this information will be reported in a study, but often it just comes down to my experience with the supplement in the real world.

37. Is there a country/supplier bias?

There are many countries that rely on food and supplements for a substantial part of their gross national products. Some of the supplement studies coming out of those countries only report positive findings, and the companies involved in the production of the supplements often fund these trials. Ginseng from Korea and China, maca from Peru, policosanol from Cuba, and tongkat ali from Malaysia—they all have many positive studies to their credit, but unless other groups can replicate these findings, they're not as credible.

There's also a strong possibility of something I call US bias, which happens when a supplement company funds a study in a remote area of the world and then, after getting good results, claims that the product will work on people in the United States just as well. You can't say that a supplement that works well with indigenous people in the jungles of the Amazon will be beneficial for people in the United States, who have entirely different diets and lifestyles. Sometimes it does, but many times it does not.

38. Was the number needed to treat (NNT) versus the number needed to harm (NNH) reported/calculated?

These are powerful calculations that allow the reader (and health care worker) to truly identify the benefit-to-risk ratio. NNT is the number of people who would need to take the pill over a given time period to see a benefit in one individual. NNH is the number of people who would need to take the pill over a given time period to see it harm one individual. Good pills have a very small NNT and a very large NNH. For instance, melatonin for jet lag has an NNT

of about 2 (50 percent of people who take it see a benefit, in other words). Wow! And vitamin C for kidney stones has an NNH of more than 600 (out of every 600 people who take it for 1 year, only one person has a negative reaction). Unfortunately, these calculations are done in very few large studies.

39. Are there both objective and subjective clinical outcome measurements?

Studies that incorporate and report both subjective and objective measures when possible are rated higher and more likely to be effective. For example, a supplement that reduces pain (subjective) and improves healing in the joint (objective because joint space width changes can be determined by an imaging test) is powerful compared to one that just improves pain *or* joint healing. Some studies only have objective (lowered cholesterol, bone loss) or subjective (hot flashes, headaches) components, but research today is increasingly making it possible to look at both so the consumer knows exactly what to expect from the drug or supplement.

40. Is the research paper clear and easy to understand overall?

Confusing papers with an excess of medical vernacular and scientific terms do not usually arrive at tangible, realistic, or practical results (and often they are trying to hide something!). Every effective study has some simplicity that needs to be conveyed. Great studies do not have to try very hard to convince readers because they speak for themselves to a large degree.

41. Is the participant recruitment and compliance method (a.k.a. sampling procedure) identified?

If the researchers recruited subjects from a "supplements fix all the world's problems" convention or a "prescription drugs are the only answer" rally, then there's going to be a problem. Obviously, I embellished here to make a point, but some studies do recruit in wacky ways. Did they advertise on the radio and television or recruit in newspapers and clinics—all of which are helpful in reaching a diverse population—or did they simply cherry-pick to find perfect candidates so they could report a benefit?

Ideally, you want to recruit a diverse group of individuals—in terms of age, gender, and race—who have a neutral opinion on supplements (similar to picking an impartial jury). I know I can get bumped from jury duty if during questioning I claim, "I can spot a guilty person from a mile away!" However, some studies would not eliminate such a candidate!

In addition, it's always good to know how individuals were incentivized. Were they paid or given gifts or free products? A good study does not need to pay much or anything because the subjects are more than willing to help answer such an important research question (prostate cancer prevention or Alzheimer's treatment, for example). Regardless, disclosing incentives helps maintain transparency.

42. What clinical trial phase is it (Phase 1 to 4 or a preliminary clinical study)?

By law, dietary supplements cannot claim any druglike benefits. They can only make structure and function claims: "X product promotes, supports, or maintains healthy cholesterol or digestive health." This is insane because for the most part, supplements should be treated like drugs. I'm not saying they should be available only by prescription (no way), but when a supplement clearly impacts a disease, the FDA should consider allowing it to make some level of claim in its advertising, especially when the cost of the treatment is so much less than the standard of care or could be added to the standard of care quickly and easily.

This is why I rank all supplement studies similar to drug studies: A Phase 1 trial primarily looks at safety or effective dosage; a Phase 2 trial tests a specific dosage for treatment benefits; Phase 3 is the crème de la crème of phases because it's the one that can garner FDA approval for a drug (meaning it really, *really* works); and a Phase 4 trial is when researchers are trying to learn even more about an already FDA-approved drug, such as safety issues and efficacy in certain patient populations. Some dietary supplement studies, such as the recent trial showing vitamin E reduced functional decline in patients with mild to moderate Alzheimer's disease, are done so well that they're equivalent to a Phase 3 study. These are the ones to really pay attention to!

43. *Did researchers give participants post-clinical trial assessments or questionnaires?*

Ahhh, more truth serum. Good studies, in many cases, regardless of the results, ask participants what they thought of the intervention or pill after taking it and whether they would continue using it. Few supplement studies include these post-trial questionnaires because many times they reveal that people enjoyed taking the placebo also or would not want to continue taking the pill being studied because the small benefit they received was not dramatic enough. Regardless, including these comments improves my confidence in the overall results because it speaks to the real-world impact.

44. *Did the researchers do a post hoc analysis to determine the true efficacy of the product?*

Post hoc (Latin for "after this") analysis is not a new study but just a further analysis of the groups after the study has been completed (researchers might contact the participants to get an update on their health or to find out if they're still taking the supplement or drug, for example). This type of analysis can help determine who really responded (or failed to respond) and whether the results are holding up. For example, in the FLEX and FIT osteoporosis trials, researchers learned that even after some people stopped their osteoporosis medication, years later it was still helping them because their number of fractures

had not really increased despite having slightly more bone loss. If former participants are still seeing results after the study, it provides further confidence in the findings.

In the famous trial of vitamin E and selenium (called SELECT), the researchers would have had no idea of the extent to which these supplements could increase the risk of prostate cancer had they not followed up with the men after the study was officially concluded. Even after the subjects stopped taking their pills, they had a significantly increased risk years later. Often these post hoc results help to garner more funding for further research.

45. *Was a power calculation for sample size and type I and II errors adjusted for?*

Good clinical studies mention the power calculation in the statistics section of the paper. This demonstrates how the researchers arrived at the number of participants and how they were able to minimize the chances of a type I error (saying something happened with a pill when it was just chance or luck) or a type II error (saying nothing happened with a pill when in reality it did something). Good researchers will perform these calculations before the study to justify their approach, and they will publish this statistical analysis in the paper.

A power calculation can involve some pretty hairy statistical terms, but this is what it looks like in a paper: In the largest multivitamin study of healthy individuals ever conducted (Physicians' Health Study II, or PHS II), the authors reported in their statistical analysis section, "The PHS II was estimated to have 80 percent power to detect a 10 percent reduction of the multivitamin . . . with an average compliance of 75 percent during the entire treatment period, and no interaction with other randomized components." That's just a jargony way of saying the study was so large and well done that we can feel confident that the results really do apply to real life!

46. Did researchers allow people who had previously taken medication for the same condition to participate in the trial, or did they have to stop taking it well in advance?

Some drugs remain in the body for days and others are still effective for years after the drug was stopped (like osteoporosis medication), so a good study will report exactly what previous treatments could have affected the objectivity of the clinical trial. This is precisely where some supplement trials have screwed up. Participants were not stopped from taking medications that could have impacted the trial results. Medication is, of course, part of the inclusion and exclusion criteria (see #26), but I think of it as a criterion all to itself because there are so many medications and pills that can impact clinical studies. It's a constantly moving target. Researchers should be clear about which drugs, supplements, and even food products (such as cholesterol-lowering margarines) were

not allowed, either before (potential subjects who took them could not participate) or during the study.

47. Were primary (always), secondary, and other endpoints identified before the study started?

Any high-quality study—even one as small as 10 individuals or as large as 30,000—has to ask itself one basic question *before it starts*: "What are we primarily trying to determine in this study?" It is almost impossible to clearly answer more than one question because of the time, cost, and energy involved in creating the appropriate study design. In the Women's Health Initiative study, researchers were trying to determine whether calcium and vitamin D supplements could reduce the risk of hip and possibly other fractures. While the *a priori* hypothesis (see #6) is more general (calcium affects bone mineral density, so does it positively impact bones and fractures?), the primary endpoint is more specific and clinical (will calcium and vitamin D reduce the risk of hip fractures?).

Now, the researchers might have also wanted to know if calcium and vitamin D could reduce tooth loss or colon cancer risk (secondary endpoints), but they did not have the time or resources to answer these questions. However, let's just say that in this study it appeared there was a lower rate of breast cancer after taking these supplements, and the researchers then came out and said they believed calcium and vitamin D reduce breast cancer risk (more like a tertiary endpoint). There would be anarchy! Okay, maybe not anarchy, but most folks would say that this is speculation and inappropriate because the study was not designed to answer this.

Some supplement trials are really bad at defining endpoints. Many years ago, a study found a tremendous reduction in the risk of most major cancers with 200 micrograms of selenium daily, but this is not what the study was originally designed to test. The primary endpoint was a reduction in skin cancer risk only in individuals with low blood levels of selenium. After taking selenium there was no overall reduction in skin cancer, but there was an *increase* in one type of skin cancer. However, researchers and consumers became obsessed with the finding that it might reduce the risk of other major cancers, such as colon and prostate. This was part of the evidence used to generate a clinical trial that cost well over 100 million taxpayer dollars. In the end, the study did not work—surprise! When researchers become obsessed with secondary endpoints from a study and ignore the primary endpoint, the chance for chance (random) findings increases.

48. *What kind of study are you doing (prospective, parallel, crossover, cross-sectional, retrospective, case series, and so on)?*

Studies come in all shapes and sizes, and each one has benefits and limitations. Researchers need to be clear what type of study they did. In general, supplement trials that are prospective, which means looking forward in time, are usually more accurate than retrospective designs, which involve looking back at data, or a case series. But all of these are important. A parallel study is when one group gets a placebo or competitive product and the other gets the supplement; a crossover is when the groups start parallel but then switch at some point during the study, so the placebo/competitive product group takes the supplement and vice versa. Both are prospective studies. A good retrospective study can beat a below-average prospective study, and a well-done case series, where many patients were followed meticulously, might be as good as any retrospective study. A cross-sectional study is essentially a snapshot in time to determine the prevalence of a condition or habit, and it's usually done via survey. For example, how many people in a given population you're surveying (maybe patients in a doctor's office) took vitamin D supplements between January and July.

One of my favorite supplement studies ever done involved just five people! They took cranberry supplements and researchers monitored their oxalate levels, which can increase the risk of kidney stones when high. Sure enough, oxalate rose dramatically. This spurred some supplement companies to reduce or at least test the amount of oxalate in their cranberry products. So this tiny yet well-done study had as much impact as a major study! This is an example of why all types of studies matter to some extent. Sometimes you can find great quality in a small study, but you have to really keep your eye out for these rare examples.

49. *How was the study randomized, and was it done appropriately?*

It is one thing to have a randomized study and quite another to have a *real* randomized study. So you may be wondering, *What in the heck does that mean, Dr. Moyad?* You can randomize patients—assign them to treatment or placebo groups in a way that minimizes any potential bias—using very objective methods or more subjective methods. The latter, while still being considered random, can create bias in favor of a pill or group without the researcher realizing it.

Let me give you an example: If a computer collects the names of all the participants, assigns each one a number, and then randomly assigns each number to a group—as if you were flipping a coin—then we can be confident in the randomization process (this is known as a computer-generated sequence). However, if a human being looks at a list of participants and their characteristics and personally places them in the different groups—even if this person is using a "random" process—bias could be introduced (i.e., the researcher might place participants who may be more likely to respond to the pill in the intervention group). You can tell if a study is randomized correctly because the groups will be even in every way, except for the pill being

taken, of course. The subjects will have similar weights, medication use, smoking status, ages, and so on.

50. *Is there raw, anonymous data available for future use and evaluation?*

Even though a researcher may have only been interested in data regarding one aspect of a trial, she should still provide other information that was collected during it. This allows statisticians and other researchers to solidify the original findings and possibly even make future conclusions based on the data.

If I was testing a multivitamin to determine if it could lower the risk of cataracts overall, I may only look at the total number of cataracts that occurred in my groups, but I should also provide data on the type of cataract each person acquired, even if I don't do anything with it. That information could be important down the line for determining whether my supplement, or other supplements like it, might help or harm cataracts (or have no impact). Making extra data available only serves to improve transparency and confidence in the results. Remember, "raw" means "naked" and good researchers do not mind having other folks see them naked! (I see a T-shirt opportunity: GOOD RESEARCHERS DO IT IN THE RAW!)

51. *Were the study participants representative of an average population, or were they from areas with rare deficiencies?*

Some supplement studies take place in Third World countries, where nutrient deficiencies run rampant, and then the researchers try to say that the benefits seen also apply to people in the industrialized world, where vitamin and mineral deficiencies are scarce. This just doesn't make sense. For example, one of the largest reductions ever seen with a supplement in terms of total mortality and cancer risk, especially stomach cancer, was from a famous Chinese study that was published in the *Journal of the National Cancer Institute*. Investigators found that supplementation with beta-carotene, selenium, and vitamin E appeared to reduce the risk of cancer after just 1 or 2 years. However, the population involved had some potentially significant nutrient deficiencies, and the study could not be replicated in other areas of the world, especially in the United States, where people have normal nutrient intakes. In fact, the nutrients tested in that Chinese study can cause real harm in otherwise healthy individuals, depending on the situation. Bottom line: You can't cure a bunch of scurvy patients with vitamin C and then announce that everyone in the United States needs vitamin C.

52. *Are the references supplied in the paper adequate or misleading?*

Good papers reference other studies that help explain why the study was done and that provide background and apples-to-apples comparisons. Bad studies put in ridiculous references to make it look like the researchers did their homework, when they really did not. I read many supplement studies that refer to a rat, mouse, or test-tube trial and then suggest that the pill clearly works in humans, too. Yikes! I see this often in weight loss, arthritis, and sexual health studies. Test-tube and animal trials are preliminary, not definitive, and should be described as such.

53. *Did the researchers register their trial at clinicaltrials.gov or another reputable site before starting so there is no last-second sleight of hand?*

Objective researchers will usually insist that their clinical trial gets registered on a public domain site like clinicaltrials.gov before the trial begins. By doing this, they document for everyone to see the exact questions they're trying to answer (remember the *a priori* hypothesis in criterion #6 and the primary and secondary endpoints in criterion #47?). It prevents them from pulling a fast one after the results are in and suggesting a product is really good for something that they weren't even testing (happens all the time).

54. *Is regression to the mean (average) resolved?*

In many cases, a pill can work really well the first 4 weeks you take it because it's new to your body and there's probably some placebo effect. Over time, though, most participants regress to a point that reflects the real results of a pill, which is known as regression to the mean. This is more reflective of the average response that a typical user can expect. (It's like falling in love. In the beginning it's all puppies and roses and you're floating on clouds, but

483

after a while you settle into a warm, fuzzy, comfortable partnership without those ecstatic highs.)

Drugs and supplements for weight loss, pain, sexual dysfunction, and even cholesterol or blood pressure all have to address this issue of better reflecting real results seen over time. Some pills take a short time to regress to the mean, like cholesterol (usually less than 6 months), and others can take a year or longer (like vitamin D and osteoarthritis supplements). I'd rather see one randomized study with more than 300 individuals done over at least 3 to 4 months than three 20-person randomized studies done over 1 month. The larger the number of individuals in a study and the longer the time, the greater the statistical accuracy of the results will be since they will more accurately demonstrate what happens in the real world.

55. *Have the results been replicated by other sources or independent researchers?*

This one is simple: The results of a study are more believable when researchers around the world have tested the same product and arrived at a similar result. When researchers in Europe, the United States, and Asia all showed benefits for alpha-lipoic acid and peripheral neuropathy, it was more believable than just seeing one study from one place. As a medical detective, I'm always on the lookout for other studies that have been done (and this is where those abstracts presented at medical meetings—criterion #1—can be espe-

cially helpful). Sometimes you have to wait for years, and other times there will be a bunch of similar studies published at the same time.

56. *Is there reverse causation?*

Smokers (whether current or former) and sick people can really mess up a study and its statistics by potentially contributing to false or misleading results, often known as reverse causation. This can be confusing, so here's an example: Some studies over the years have found that people who are overweight have a greater chance of living longer than people who are a normal weight or underweight. But if the lower/normal weight group contains smokers or sick people, who are more likely to be thinner than the nonsmokers and healthy people and also more likely to die, the results are skewed. On the surface, the results imply that being thin makes you more likely to die early, but in fact it's the underlying smoking or sickness factor that makes you thin and more likely to die.

57. *Did the researchers incorporate a run-in phase with or without the pill before the official study began?*

This is essentially like doing a dry run to see which participants are more likely to be compliant. For several weeks before the official clinical trial starts, subjects may be told to take a pill (placebo) daily. The more compliant participants are more likely to continue into the official trial. In the large STEP study of saw palmetto that was published in the *New England Journal of Medi-*

cine, researchers noted, "All potentially eligible participants were assigned to a one-month, single-blind, placebo run-in period and were excluded if their rate of adherence was less than 75 percent, as measured by a capsule count." During the run-in phase, results showed that there was an enormous placebo pill response (improved urinary flow) for men with non-cancerous prostate enlargement, so researchers gleaned quite a bit of information before the study ever started! Many trials are so darn expensive and time-consuming, and some participants take the study seriously while others do not. So, it's in the researchers' and public's best interest to ensure they have compliant subjects.

58. Is the pill safe for kids, during pregnancy, and for heart and mental health?

This is the essence of first do no harm (remember that groovy dude Hippocrates and his famous oath?). Cardiovascular disease has been the number one cause of death in the United States for more than a century, and we don't need any supplements that will only add to this ongoing epidemic. Supplements should have to meet the same safety criteria that drugs do (if it's not safe, then why would you take it?). Ideally, a supplement should also be safe for kids and during pregnancy, but that's not always going to happen, and this is usually not tested for. My research team is submitting a proposal to treat early stage prostate cancer with a pill you would take for 6 months, but I insisted that we also look at the impact it has on cardiovascular parameters.

59. Were side effects/adverse events (objective and subjective) monitored and clearly and statistically reported at different time intervals?

Patient self-reported side effects are subjective (headache, nausea, reduced libido); objective side effects include abnormal blood tests or increases in blood pressure, for example. Researchers should monitor *any* potential side effect, list them all, and statistically calculate which ones were more common than the placebo. Ideally, side effects seen in supplement studies should be graded the same way they are in drug trials, where grade 1 and 2 effects are more minor and 3 and 4 are more serious. I also want to know if the side effects resulted in hospitalization or dropout or if they were minor and had no impact on the study. Even good supplements will cause side effects in some people, and researchers should not shy away from this fact.

60. Was the study site(s) identified? (Two or more are better than one.)

Larger, well-done studies are usually performed at multiple sites, which encourages objective findings because it allows for a checks-and-balances system as opposed to one site doing all the work and controlling the results. Multisite studies usually also involve a greater number of—and more diverse—participants. Good studies will be transparent and list all of the locations used as well as contact information for the principal investigator (the person in charge) at each site.

61. *Is the statistical analysis appropriate and accurate, and was it also completed and checked by an independent statistician?*

Statistics is a specialty for good reason. Deciding which statistical tests to run on data is about as easy as deciding which of your children is your favorite! It's really, really tough and should be handled by a competent statistician. Good researchers will typically consult with one or two usually independent statisticians to make sure that they are getting it right.

What everyone looks for among all the stats is something called a P value, which essentially tells us the probability or chances the results achieved were accurate. The smaller the P value (e.g., P = 0.001 vs. P = 0.05), the more likely it is that the results are correct (you want a very small chance that you got it wrong). A minimum cut-off value for statistical significance is usually P = 0.05 (there's a 5 percent chance that the results are not what they appear to be or, to say it another way, a 95 percent chance the results are accurate), but researchers are gunning for P = 0.01 or lower (there's a 1 percent chance that the results are not what they appear to be or a 99 percent chance the results are accurate). This is why I often say that medical studies and pills are just probabilities with no guarantees, so pick one with the highest probability that it will work in someone like you!

62. *Are the treatment results statistically significant, clinically significant, both, or neither?*

Statistically significant means the P value (see #61) was 0.05 or less. Clinically significant means the results might actually change the clinical practice of medicine or patient care when your doctor hears about or reads them. When researchers compared red yeast rice to a generic low-dose statin drug for reducing cholesterol, there was no statistical difference between them; they both worked similarly well. However, many folks cannot tolerate statin drugs, but they can tolerate red yeast rice. This is a clinically significant finding because so many people need a different option— besides simply not taking anything—when they become statin intolerant. I like to see both statistical and clinical significance with a dietary supplement—at the very least clinical significance—but if there's neither, that's a bad sign.

63. *Did researchers do an appropriate subgroup statistical analysis?*

Subgroup analysis tries to identify groups of patients who are more or less likely to respond to current or future treatment. For example, when researchers gave the probiotic *Lactobacillus casei* Shirota to bladder cancer patients, those with a greater or larger tumor burden did not respond as well as those with a single or smaller tumor.

Analyzing subgroups can help to individualize or personalize treatment, but it can also greatly mislead doctors and patients into thinking there is something there that isn't. So researchers use other factors to help determine the accuracy of subgroup analysis, including asking things like, was the subgroup hypothesis determined before the study, could chance or luck explain the results, have other studies observed this effect, was this looked at within-group or between-group or even between other studies, what was the impact overall on the entire group, and does it make sense from a scientific or mechanistic standpoint? Regardless, these subgroup analyses have to be identified and scrutinized in research papers. They provide additional insight right after the study concludes but do not have more importance than the primary endpoint findings.

64. Did the researchers provide supplementary data/information at the time of publication?

Most good, large studies make additional data available that isn't presented in the main published paper due to a lack of room or information overload, usually through the publishing journal's Web site. This supplementary information can really add to the credibility of the research or help to raise and answer other questions related to the study. It demonstrates how meticulous some researchers are in terms of not only gathering data but also analyzing every aspect of it in order to make sure the right answer is arrived at.

65. Are the tables and figures provided in the study clear and easy to understand?

Why the heck does this matter? Well, the tables and figures in some studies are just downright confusing, and they should be able to stand alone, which means they should give you a clear picture of the information on their own so you don't have to refer to the paper to figure out what's going on. A figure or table that is so twisted and difficult to read just serves to hurt the research.

66. Did the researchers use validated outcome measures, such as questionnaires, or did they simply make something up?

For most medical conditions today there are validated questionnaires and tests that have been evaluated in many studies to make sure they accurately measure the disease in question (and any improvements). There are validated instruments for measuring fatigue, sexual health, osteoarthritis, hot flashes, pain, quality of life, and many other things. These pre-tested tools—many of which are very simple and straightforward—make the results far more believable than DIY options, however well intentioned and researched. Many osteoarthritis studies use the validated Western Ontario and McMaster Universities Arthritis Index (WOMAC). It's a disease-specific, self-administered questionnaire for patients with osteoarthritis of the knee or hip. It has three separate dimensions with 24 individual scenarios, which measure pain (five scenarios), stiffness (two scenarios), and physical function (17 scenarios). Here's a secret: Testosterone supplements are notorious for using non-validated questionnaires in an effort to prove they actually work!

67. Was there a washout period before the study began?

The washout period also happens at the beginning, but it's the period (often several weeks) before the official clinical trial begins when participants are told to stop using any pills, such as prescription medicines or supplements, or performing any activities that could somehow impact the results of the study. In the published results, the study authors should mention the washout period and what it was trying to accomplish.

68. What was the withdrawal/dropout rate, and why did people leave the study?

As in real life, sometimes subjects in clinical studies just stop taking the pill. It may be due to side effects, boredom, lack of any effect, bad memory, and so on. If there's a large dropout rate, the results can be less reliable, but the study authors should always report this and clarify why people left the study.

Let's say 50 men started a hair loss study that involved taking a supplement, and 40 dropped out, mainly because they were experiencing erectile dysfunction (ED). The remaining 10 ended up growing some hair and had mild or no ED. If the researchers failed to report the withdrawal/dropout rate, the reader could be convinced that this was a miracle pill for

hair loss with minimal toxicity. This might sound like a crazy example, but this happens all the time in studies where large numbers drop out for many reasons.

69. and 70. Miscellaneous items

I was so close to an impressive number like 70 that I'm taking up two slots for miscellaneous items. Every study brings up at least one or two unique questions that I have to add to my list. For example, the Physicians Health Study II for cancer prevention stopped after an average of 11.2 years, but it looked as if the results were getting better with time, so why didn't the researchers let the trial go for a few more years? Did they run out of money, or did the statistician suggest the results would not get better or worse over time when looking at the numbers? The authors didn't answer this in the paper because it was already one of the longest and largest supplement clinical trials ever conducted in medical history. Still, for me, this information is critical and could affect the level of certainty about taking a multivitamin long term.

In the red yeast rice clinical trials for cholesterol reduction, many failed to report whether grapefruit juice was allowed or if the supplement worked better with or without food. The reason these factors were important is because the active ingredient in the supplement is similar to the drug lovastatin, which should not be consumed with grapefruit and is absorbed better with food. When questions like these go unanswered, you get an incomplete picture of the pill. These are details that can make a great study even better.

DR. MOYAD'S RESEARCH CRITERIA

You can use this checklist to do your own study evaluation and check a piece of research against my ideal criteria. Here, you can note how the research stacks up—or falls short—in each area. By the time you've gone through the list, you should have a good idea as to whether or not you're working with quality research, or if it leaves something to be desired.

Note: Some items on the checklist carry more weight than others, and this is partially based on the type of study. Also, some of these criteria could overlap to a small or large degree. Refer to the detailed breakdowns of each criterion in this chapter for a complete explanation.

_____ 1. Abstract presentation at a medical meeting with similar or different results?

_____ 2. Active ingredient(s) standardized and dosage identified?

_____ 3. Adequate instructions given to all participants?

_____ 4. Allocation concealment adequate?

_____ 5. Appropriate size and duration?

_____ 6. A priori hypothesis?

_____ 7. Assessment points/intervals fixed in terms of number and time and well defined?

_____ 8. Author honesty/reports bias or conflict of interest?

_____ 9. Between group or within group statistical analysis defined?

_____ 10. Clinical relevance/competition and novel findings?

_____ 11. Compliance predicted, measured, reported, and statistically compared?

_____ 12. Confidence intervals (95% CI)?

_____ 13. Conclusions of the study justified by the data collected?

_____ 14. Confounding variables corrected for, groups similar at the beginning of the study, and multivariate analysis used?

_____ 15. Contact info?

_____ 16. Cost estimate of the treatment?

_____ 17. Definition of the medical condition being tested clear?

_____ 18. Delivery system easy to use and supplier of supplements identified?

_____ 19. Dilution that leads to pollution and confusion?

_____ 20. Diversity/real-world sample of participants?

_____ 21. Dose-response assessed?

_____ 22. Double-blind? Was anyone blind?

_____ 23. Editorial written by a true expert in the field that supports or negates the study's findings?

_____ 24. Expectations of treatment, attitudes toward treatment assignment, or sense of treatment credibility assessed for the participants?

_____ 25. Funding source(s)/independence explained?

_____ 26. Inclusion/exclusion criteria for the study described clearly?

_____ 27. Informed consent?

_____ 28. Intention-to-treat and per-protocol completer methods used?

_____ 29. Investigators/assessors described clearly? Contract research organization or similar used?

_____ 30. Institutional review board (or another regulatory body) approval?

_____ 31. Jadad or another scoring system used?

_____ 32. Journal quality?

_____ 33. Limitations of the study were identified and discussed?

_____ 34. Mechanism of action clearly explained?

_____ 35. Medications (other than treatment and placebo) documented?

_____ 36. Moyad personal history and experience with this category/product? (only I can assess this one)

_____ 37. Nation/supplier bias?

_____ 38. Number needed to treat vs. number needed to harm reported/calculated?

_____ 39. Objective and subjective outcome measurements?

_____ 40. Paper clear and easy to understand?

_____ 41. Participant recruitment and compliance method described?

_____ 42. Phase of trial or preliminary clinical study?

_____ 43. Post–clinical trial assessments or questionnaires given to participants?

_____ 44. Post hoc analysis?

_____ 45. Power calculation for sample size and type I and II errors adjusted for?

_____ 46. Previous treatments for the same condition allowed or at least stopped well in advance of clinical trial?

_____ 47. Primary endpoint and others (secondary) identified before the study began?

_____ 48. Prospective vs. parallel vs. crossover trials vs. retrospective vs. cross-sectional vs. case series study?

_____ 49. Randomized appropriately?

_____ 50. Raw, anonymous data available for future use and scrutiny?

_____ 51. Real-world participants/situation?

_____ 52. References used in paper adequate?

_____ 53. Registered at clinicaltrials.gov or a similar site before starting?

_____ 54. Regression to the mean (average) resolved?

_____ 55. Results replicated by other sources or independent researchers?

_____ 56. Reverse causation corrected for?

_____ 57. Run-in phase to test for compliance and other potential issues?

_____ 58. Safe for kids, during pregnancy, and for heart and mental health?

_____ 59. Side effects/adverse events (objective and subjective) monitored and clearly reported at different time intervals?

_____ 60. Site(s) of the study identified?

_____ 61. Statistical analysis appropriate?

_____ 62. Statistically significant but not clinically significant or vice versa or both or neither?

_____ 63. Sub-group analysis appropriate?

_____ 64. Supplementary data/information available at the time of publication?

_____ 65. Tables and figures stand alone?

_____ 66. Validated outcome measures used (questionnaires and tests)?

_____ 67. Washout period before the official study began?

_____ 68. Withdrawal/dropout rate and reasons for leaving the study reported?

_____ 69. and 70. What more could have been done? Or what was actually done (good or bad) that is unique to this study?

INDEX

Underscored page references indicate boxed text.

ACKNOWLEDGMENTS

First, I want to thank my wonderful teammate and new friend Janet Lee who helped not only bring my life's work to the page but helped me create a book that I wished I would have had when I was starting my career. (At least the current and future health care professionals and patients have ample objectivity in this discipline now.) I also want to thank Jess Fromm at Rodale for her kindness, guidance, leadership, and dedication to this book. I would be honored to work again with Janet and Jess (another understatement).

Thank you also to: Marilyn Hauptly, Elizabeth Neal, Carol Angstadt, Kristen Downey, and Wendy Hess Gable at Rodale for their hard work on this project; Trisha Calvo for championing this book from the start; and Heather Hurlock for introducing me to the Rodale team.